D1593999

ALLERGY & IMMUNOLOGY

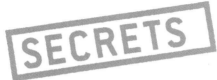

ALLERGY & IMMUNOLOGY

SECRETS

Second Edition

M. Eric Gershwin, M.D.
Division of Rheumatology, Allergy, and Clinical Immunology
University of California, Davis, School of Medicine
Davis, California

Stanley M. Naguwa, M.D.
Division of Rheumatology, Allergy, and Clinical Immunology
University of California, Davis, School of Medicine
Davis, California

ELSEVIER
MOSBY

ELSEVIER
MOSBY
An Affiliate of Elsevier

The Curtis Center
170 S Independence Mall W 300E
Philadelphia, Pennsylvania 19106

ALLERGY AND IMMUNOLOGY SECRETS   ISBN: 1-56053-619-5
Second Edition

NOTICE

Medicine is an ever-changing field. Standard safety precautions must be followed, but as new research and clinical experience broaden our knowledge, changes in treatment and drug therapy may become necessary or appropriate. Readers are advised to check the most current product information provided by the manufacturer of each drug to be administered to verify the recommended dose, the method and duration of administration, and contraindications. It is the responsibility of the licensed prescriber, relying on experience and knowledge of the patient, to determine dosages and the best treatment for each individual patient. Neither the publisher nor the author assumes any liability for any injury and/or damage to persons or property arising from this publication.

Previous edition copyrighted 2001.

International Standard Book Number   **1-56053-619-5**

Acquisitions Editor: Linda Belfus
Developmental Editor: Stan Ward
Publishing Services Manager: Joan Sinclair
Project Manager: Cecelia Bayruns

Printed in the United States of America.

Last digit is the print number: 9   8   7   6   5   4   3   2   1

CONTENTS

CONTRIBUTORS

Rahmat Afrasiabi, M.D.
Associate Clinical Professor, Division of Rheumatology/Allergy and Clinical Immunology, Department of Internal Medicine, University of California, Davis, School of Medicine, Davis, California; Enloe Hospital, Chico, California

Pearl Barzaga, M.D.
Staff Physician, Allergy Department, Kaiser-Permanente Medical Group, Hayward, California

Andrea Borchers, Ph.D.
Visiting Scholar, Division of Rheumatology/Allergy and Clinical Immunology, Department of Internal Medicine, University of California, Davis, School of Medicine, Davis, California

Christopher Chang, M.D., Ph.D.
Associate Professor, Division of Rheumatology/Allergy and Clinical Immunology, Department of Internal Medicine, University of California, Davis, School of Medicine, Davis, California

Gurtej S. Cheema, M.D.
Assistant Professor, Division of Rheumatology/Allergy and Clinical Immunology, Department of Internal Medicine, University of California, Davis, School of Medicine, Davis, California

Gordon Garcia, M.D.
Assistant Clinical Professor, Department of Pediatrics, University of California, Davis, School of Medicine, Davis, California; Kaiser Foundation Hospital, Sacramento, California

M. Eric Gershwin, M.D.
Division of Rheumatology, Allergy, and Clinical Immunology, University of California, Davis, School of Medicine, Davis, California

Rosemary Hallett, M.D.
Assistant Clinical Professor, Division of Rheumatology/Allergy and Clinical Immunology, Department of Internal Medicine, University of California, Davis, School of Medicine, Davis, California

Maurice E. Hamilton, M.D.
Clinical Professor, Division of Rheumatology/Allergy and Clinical Immunology, Department of Internal Medicine, University of California, Davis, School of Medicine, Davis, California

Russell J. Hopp, D.O.
Professor, Department of Pediatrics, Creighton University School of Medicine; St. Joseph Hospital, Omaha, Nebraska

Nicholas J. Kenyon, M.D.
Assistant Professor, Division of Pulmonary and Critical Care Medicine, Department of Internal Medicine, University of California, Davis, School of Medicine, Davis, California

Fu-Tong Liu, M.D.
Professor and Chair, Department of Dermatology, University of California, Davis, School of Medicine, Davis, California

Samuel Louie, M.D.
Professor, Division of Pulmonary and Critical Care Medicine, Department of Internal Medicine, University of California, Davis, School of Medicine, Davis, California

Stanley M. Naguwa, M.D.
Division of Rheumatology, Allergy, and Clinical Immunology, University of California, Davis, School of Medicine, Davis, California

Cristina Porch-Curren, M.D.
Clinical Fellow, Division of Rheumatology/Allergy and Clinical Immunology, Department of Internal Medicine, University of California, Davis, School of Medicine, Davis, California

Bruce T. Ryhal, M.D.
Clinical Professor, Division of Rheumatology/Allergy and Clinical Immunology, Department of Internal Medicine, University of California, Davis, School of Medicine, Davis, California; Senior Physician, Department of Allergy, Kaiser-Permanente Medical Center, Roseville, California

Arif M. Seyal, M.D.
Clinical Professor, Division of Rheumatology/Allergy and Clinical Immunology, Department of Internal Medicine, University of California, Davis, School of Medicine, Davis, California; Chief, Department of Allergy and Clinical Immunology, Kaiser-Permanente Medical Center, Roseville, California

Calvin So, M.D.
Clinical Fellow, Division of Rheumatology/Allergy and Clinical Immunology, Department of Internal Medicine, University of California, Davis, School of Medicine, Davis, California

E. Bradley Strong, M.D.
Assistant Professor, Department of Otolaryngology-Head and Neck Surgery, University of California, Davis, School of Medicine, Davis, California

Suzanne S. Teuber, M.D.
Associate Professor, Division of Rheumatology/Allergy and Clinical Immunology, Department of Internal Medicine, University of California, Davis, School of Medicine, Davis, California

Robert D. Watson, M.D., Ph.D.
Allergy Department, MedClinic, CHW Medical Foundation; Mercy General Hospital, Sacramento, California

Mark Zlotlow, M.D.
Assistant Clinical Professor, Department of Pediatrics, University of California, Davis, School of Medicine, Davis, California; Assistant Chief, Allegy Department, North Valley CSA, Permanente Medical Group, Roseville, California

PREFACE

The incidence of allergic disease has become almost epidemic. Indeed, allergies are among the most common chronic problems of childhood and the most frequent complaints of adults. Several national studies have demonstrated that up to 20% of people in the United States suffer from allergic rhinitis and up to 10% suffer from asthma. More than 90% of patients with allergies require some form of intermittent drug therapy. These overwhelming statistics, as well as the chronic and sometimes restrictive nature of allergies, result in significant stress for patients and families. However, despite the widespread nature of asthma and allergies and the fact that they have been well characterized throughout reported medical history, the basic disease process is only now being defined. Indeed, there are large numbers of etiologies that interact in the common pathways of allergic disease.

Because of the ubiquitous nature of allergies, physicians in many disciplines are called upon to treat allergic patients. Although the majority of research on allergy occurs at large university medical centers, the bulk of medical care is delivered throughout the community by primary care physicians. At the University of California, we have emphasized the need for continued and intensive education of our housestaff in order to improve the care of people who suffer from allergic disease. The specialization of allergy and immunology, one of the most exciting disciplines in medicine, attracts students from both pediatrics and internal medicine. In addition, with the growing numbers of adult-onset allergy, even gerontologists need to be kept abreast of advances in the management of immunologic problems. In this volume, our goal has been to bring together important issues for housestaff and for primary care physicians of all backgrounds. We have provided readers with useful materials to help them in their broad examinations and perhaps even stimulate a career in allergy and immunology. Most importantly, we hope it improves the care of patients.

The editors appreciate the valuable contributions of our authors. We particularly thank Nikki Phipps for her hard work in putting this manuscript together.

M. Eric Gershwin, M.D.
Stanley M. Naguwa, M.D.

TOP 100 SECRETS

These secrets are 100 of the top board alerts. They summarize the concepts, principles, and most salient details of allergy and immunology.

1. Although the prevalence rate for atopic dermatitis is 10–12%, less than 15% have disease after puberty.

2. There has been a 75% increase in self-reported asthma from 1980 to 1994.

3. The probability of asthma at 3 years of age is 55% based on family risk factors, IgE levels, frequent illness, and excessive psychosocial factors.

4. The hygiene hypothesis appears to explain the increased incidence of allergies and asthma based on vigorous use of Th1 T cells.

5. Cysteinyl-leukotrienes are up to 1,000-fold more potent than histamine and 100-fold more potent than prostaglandins in inducing bronchoconstriction.

6. VLA-4/VCAM-1 promotes adherence of eosinophils, along with interleukin-5.

7. The major enzyme in the cytoplasmic granules of mast cells is tryptase.

8. Mast cells are derived from CD34+ hematopoietic progenitor cells.

9. Glucocorticoid therapy decreases the proportion of bronchoalveolar lavage fluid cells expressing IL-4 and IL-5 and promotes a shift towards Th1 responsiveness.

10. Most litigation cases involving mold toxicity are based on bad science.

11. Allergens that are airborne present the greatest hazard to human health because of their ability to penetrate the respiratory tract.

12. Most common aeroallergens are carried on particles between 2 and 60 μm in diameter.

13. To treat allergy effectively, it is important to know to what the patient is allergic and also to what the patient is exposed.

14. Most common aeroallergens are proteins or glycoproteins between 10 and 100 kd in size.

15. The best test for evaluation of suspected food allergy is the double-blinded food challenge, not skin tests or allergen-specific IgE tests.

16. A tryptase level can be obtained as evidence of recent anaphylaxis.

17. Allergen-specific IgE tests are considered less sensitive, take more time, and are more costly than skin tests.

18. Beta blockers may increase skin sensitivity to skin tests.

19. Intradermal skin testing is the preferred diagnostic method for evaluation of venom and drug allergies.

20. Allergy is responsible for only about 50% of the cases of chronic rhinitis.

21. The finding of nasal polyps in children should lead to a work-up for cystic fibrosis.

22. First-generation antihistamines may cause psychomotor impairment even when the patient does not feel sedated.

23. Eighty percent of cases of allergic rhinitis begin before the age of 20 years.

24. Asthma is a syndrome of related inflammatory airway disorders characterized by airway hyper-responsiveness, reversible airflow obstruction, and episodic symptoms of wheezing and dyspnea.

25. The severity of asthma, from mild intermittent to severe persistent, should be determined in each patient based on the updated 2002 guidelines of the National Asthma Education and Prevention Program, which are available at *http://www.nhlbi.nih.gov/guidelines/asthma/asthgdln.html.*

26. Allergic rhinosinusitis and gastroesophageal reflux disease are two concomitant conditions that require treatment in up to 70% of asthmatics.

27. Most asthmatics have moderate to severe persistent disease and require aggressive anti-inflammatory, controller therapy.

28. Combination therapy with long-acting beta agonists and moderate-dose inhaled corticosteroids can provide better disease control than high-dose inhaled corticosteroids alone.

29. The sphenoid sinus drains into the spheno-ethmoidal recess located on the sphenoid rostrum, lateral to the septum and medial to the superior turbinate.

30. The physical examination can be unremarkable even in the presence of an active infection of the sinuses.

31. Hyposmia/anosmia is most commonly seen with nasal polyposis.

32. Headache can be found with rhinosinusitis but is uncommon in the absence of other symptoms of rhinosinusitis.

33. The predominant immunoglobulin of nasal secretions is IgA.

34. Unilateral maxillary rhinosinusitis is of concern because it may reflect an obstructing malignant lesion.

35. When urticarial lesions have a purpuric component, are painful, and last for longer than 24 hours, one should suspect urticarial vasculitis and perform a skin biopsy.

36. There is significant association between thyroid autoimmunity and chronic urticaria. The patient may be clinically and biochemically euthyroid.

37. Autoantibodies to the IgE receptor FcεRI may be an important cause of chronic urticaria.

38. Atopic dermatitis is termed "the itch that rashes." No primary lesion is present, but the severe pruritus leads to scratching and excoriation.

39. Atopic dermatitis usually presents in childhood; has a chronic, relapsing course and a characteristic distribution (adults: flexor surfaces and hands; infants: face and extensor surfaces); and is associated with pruritus.

40. Adult-onset atopic dermatitis is less common without a history of childhood atopic dermatitis. Other diagnoses should be considered.

41. Infectious agents can complicate atopic dermatitis, most commonly *Staphylococcus aureus*. *S. aureus* colonizes 90% of atopic dermatitis skin versus 5% of healthy patients.

42. Food allergies are associated with 20–30% of children with atopic dermatitis, most commonly egg, milk, peanut, soy, and wheat.

43. Food is not a common trigger for adults with atopic dermatitis.

44. Increased ocular pressure has been seen with both systemic and topical corticosteroids.

45. The safety of ketorolac (Acular) has not been established in aspirin-sensitive people.

46. Oral decongestants can precipitate an attack of acute closed-angle glaucoma.

47. Tumor necrosis factor alpha is the primary agent for upregulation of adhesion molecules.

48. Interleukin-5 is the principal cytokine for promoting eosinophils.

49. Generalized urticaria, pruritus, flushing, and angioedema are the most common manifestations of anaphylactic reaction.

50. Patients taking oral or ophthalmic beta-adrenergic antagonists may be more likely to experience severe and protracted anaphylaxis.

51. The combination of H_1 antihistamines (e.g., diphenhydramine, 1 mg/kg up to 75 mg) and H_2 antihistamines (e.g., cimetidine, 300 mg) is more effective than either administered alone.

52. Epinephrine injected intramuscularly into the anterolateral thigh produces high and more rapid peak plasma levels and should be considered as a preferred route and site of administration during moderate and severe anaphylaxis.

53. A low level of autoimmunity is crucial to normal immune function.

54. Autoimmune diseases can be divided into organ-specific autoimmune diseases and systemic autoimmune diseases.

55. Diseases mediated by immune complexes include systemic lupus, polyarteritis nodosum, and poststreptococcal glomerulonephritis.

56. Environmental risk factors are critical to the induction of autoimmune disease because the concordance of autoimmunity among monozygotic twins is less than 50%.

57. The term *food allergy* refers to an adverse reaction to food mediated by the immune system. Most adverse reactions to food are not immune-mediated.

58. The presence of IgE to a food does *not* equate to clinical reactivity to a food!

59. Food allergy is confirmed in about 2% of the adult population and 5–8% of the pediatric population.

60. The big eight foods associated with food allergy in the U.S. are cow's milk, egg, peanut, soy, wheat, tree nuts, crustaceans, and fish. Sesame is gaining importance.

61. Patients who have had only mild systemic allergic reactions to foods may have life-threatening anaphylaxis the next time they accidentally ingest the food and should thus be referred to an allergist to design an anaphylaxis action plan.

62. Risk factors for death from food-induced anaphylaxis include delayed or no use of self-injectable epinephrine; a history of asthma; allergy to peanut, tree nut, or seafood; and age (adolescents and young adults).

63. This website should not be a secret: *www.foodallergy.org*.

64. A positive RAST test will become negative if one follows RAST-positive patients over several years.

65. Venom-specific IgE may be detected by RAST even in the absence of positive skin tests and vice versa.

66. An estimated 40–50 people die each year from insect sting allergy, but this number may be artificially low, because many cases may go unrecognized and misdiagnosed as myocardial infarction or cerebrovascular accidents.

67. Provision of Epi-Pens is the standard of care in patients with stinging insect hypersensitivity.

68. Clinical presentations of delayed reactions following Hymenoptera stings have included Guillain-Barré syndromes as well as serum sickness-like reactions.

69. Most adverse drug reactions do not involve immune mechanisms.

70. Skin testing for drug allergy is most accurate when the drug is penicillin or a protein and the suspected reaction is a type I, or IgE-mediated, mechanism.

71. Drug-induced anaphylaxis involves IgE, or allergic, antibodies, and mast cells.

72. Drug-associated excipients, preservatives, or contaminants may cause an allergic reaction in some people.

73. Consider ABPA in steroid-dependent asthma patients and particularly in patients with cystic fibrosis.

74. Initial testing for allergic bronchopulmonary aspergillosis (ABPA) may include skin testing for *Aspergillus* sp., total IgE, and a chest x-ray.

75. A high index of suspicion is needed for the diagnosis of hypersensitivity pneumonitis (HP).

76. Early diagnosis of HP allows a good prognosis and should prevent progression to end-stage disease.

77. The acute and chronic forms of HP differ in presentation and prognosis; both require a detailed exposure history to identify causative triggers.

78. Hypersensitivity serologies (specific IgG) are helpful, but not diagnostic of HP per se.

79. Systemic corticosteroids (and avoidance measures) are the main treatments for ABPA and HP.

80. Common features of immunodeficiency include frequent, prolonged, or severe infection; poor response to therapy; infection with unusual organism or organism of low virulence; failure to thrive; diarrhea or malabsorption; dermatitis; autoimmune disease; malignancy; inflammatory disease; hematologic disorder; infection from live vaccines; and family history of immunodeficiency or consanguinity.

81. Primary immunodeficiencies that may present in adulthood include IgA deficiency, common variable immunodeficiency (CVID), IgG subclass immunodeficiency, complement deficiency, and specific antibody deficiency of normal immunoglobulins.

82. Primary immunodeficiencies that may be asymptomatic include IgA deficiency, CVID, and complement deficiency.

83. Common features of antibody or B-cell immunodeficiency disorders include recurrent sinopulmonary infections, sepsis, aseptic meningitis, autoimmune diseases, hematologic disorders, and increased incidence of malignancy.

84. Common features of T-cell immunodeficiency disorders include failure to thrive, opportunistic infections, viral infections, disseminated infections, chronic diarrhea, dermatitis, and increased incidence of malignancy.

85. Common features of phagocytic disorders include lymphadenitis, skin and visceral abscesses, cellulitis, and gingivitis.

86. Common features of complement deficiency include pyogenic bacterial infections, neisserial meningitis, and autoimmune disease.

87. Immunotherapy typically takes 3–5 years to achieve a sustained clinical improvement.

88. Immunotherapy causes antibody changes, cytokine changes, or cellular changes.

89. Beta-blocker therapy is a contraindication for immunotherapy.

90. Prompt administration of epinephrine is the treatment of choice for a systemic reaction.

91. Immunotherapy may inhibit the progression of allergic rhinitis to allergic asthma.

92. Twenty-nine percent of adults in the U.S. use complementary and alternative medical therapy.

93. The majority of botanical supplements have not been studied for safety.

94. Drug interactions with dietary supplements remain a major clinical concern.

95. The overall improvement of upper respiratory infections with certain echinacea preparations is very small.

96. To make an accurate diagnosis of mastocytosis, the patient must meet one major and one minor criterion or three minor criteria.

97. The primary mast cell growth factor is the c-kit ligand, or stem cell factor.

98. The most common skin presentation of systemic mastocytosis is urticaria pigmentosa.

99. There is no consistently observed genetic pattern to systemic mastocytosis.

100. There is no known cure for systemic mastocytosis. Treatment of symptoms is the mainstay of therapy.

CHAPTER 1

EPIDEMIOLOGY AND GENETICS OF ALLERGIC DISEASE

Russell J. Hopp, D.O.

EPIDEMIOLOGY OF ALLERGIC DISEASES IN THE UNITED STATES

1. **What is the current prevalence of atopic dermatitis in the U.S.?**
   The International Study of Asthma and Allergies in Childhood (ISAAC) evaluated the current prevalence of atopic eczema with the question, "Ever had an itchy rash which was coming and going for at least 6 months?" In the sole U.S. site, Seattle, the 12-month prevalence was 9.4% for adolescents aged 13–14 years. There was a lifetime prevalence of 19.4%. Lifetime prevalence rates of up to 20% have been recently reported.

2. **What is the prevalence of allergic rhinoconjuntivitis in the U.S., according to the ISAAC study?**
   The ISAAC study evaluated the current prevalence of allergic rhinoconjuntivitis with two questions:
   1. In the past 12 months have you had a problem with sneezing or a runny or blocked nose when you did *not* have a cold? Or the flu?
   2. If yes, has this nose problem been accompanied by itchy-watery eyes?
   Two sites in Chicago and one site in Seattle asked these questions of over 7000 children 13–14 years of age. The 12-month prevalence ranged from 12% to 22%.
   Strachan D, Sibbald B, Weiland S, et al: Worldwide variations in prevalence of symptoms of allergic rhinoconjunctivitis in children: The International Study of Asthma and Allergies in Childhood (ISAAC). Pediatr Allergy Immunol 8:161–176, 1997.

3. **What were the results of the Third National Health and Nutrition Examination Survey (NHANES III) in regards to the prevalence of allergic rhinitis?**
   In 1988–1994, NHANES III collected data about seasonal and perennial allergic rhinoconjuntivitis. Based on survey data, the prevalence of allergic rhinitis is 19.9% for ages 6–11 years, 26.8% for ages 12–17 years, and 29.6% for ages 18 years and older. Of the 71 million people with allergic rhinitis, based on the current U.S. population, 13.6 million have continuous symptoms.
   Ma X, Fick RB, Kaplowitz HJ: Prevalence of allergic rhinoconjunctivitis in the United States: Data from the Third National Health and Nutrition Examination Survey, 1998–94 (NHANES III). Am J Respir Crit Care Med 161:A325, 2000.

4. **What percentage of the U.S. population has positive allergy skin tests?**
   The NHANES II survey of allergy skin test reactivity in the U.S. from 1976 to 1980 reported that the rates of skin test response to one or more common allergens were highest in adolescents and young adults. More males than females and more blacks than whites were positive. In the 6- to 11-year age-group, 18% of whites and 28% of blacks were positive. In the 12- to 17-year age-group, 23% of whites and 36% of blacks were positive, with similar rates for subjects aged 18–24 years. Rates were lower in subjects older than 25 years for both racial groups.
   Gergen PJ, Turkeltaub PC, Kovar MG: The prevalence of allergic skin test reactivity to eight common aeroallergens in the U.S. population: Results from the Second National Health and Nutrition Examination Survey. J Allergy Clin Immunol 80:669–679, 1987.

5. **What is the current prevalence of asthma in children in the United States?**
    The Centers for Disease Control and Prevention (CDC) released a comprehensive report in 1998 that documented a 75% increase in self-reported asthma from 1980 to 1994. This increase crossed all races, both genders, and all age groups. Children demonstrated remarkable increases: 160% in children 0–4 years and 74% in children aged 5–14 years.

    NHANES III determined prevalence of asthma by a physician diagnosis at any time, with symptoms in the past year. The prevalence was 6.6% in ages 6–11 years and 9.6% in ages 12–17 years.

    Centers for Disease Control and Prevention: Forecasted state-specific estimates of self-reported asthma prevalence United States, 1998. MMWR 47:102–125, 1998.

6. **How is asthma defined for mortality and prevalence analysis?**
    Since 1979 the Ninth International Classification of Diseases (ICD-9) has been the basis for defining asthma for mortality analysis, using codes 493-493.X. The CDC uses data from the National Health Interview Survey (NHIS). In 1997 the NHIS changed the asthma current prevalence question to the following two questions:
    1. Has a doctor or other health care professional ever told you that your child has asthma?
    2. During the past 12 months has your child had an episode of asthma or an asthma attack?
    This rate has been termed asthma attack prevalence. The rates (per 1000) since the change in the questions are summarized in Table 1-1.

    Akinbami LJ, Schoendorf KC, Parker J: US childhood asthma prevalence estimates: The impact of the 1997 National Health Interview Survey redesign. Am J Epidemiol 158:99–104, 2003.

TABLE 1-1. RATES PER 1000 SINCE REVISION OF QUESTIONS	1997	1998	1999	2000
Overall prevalence	54.4	53.1	52.7	55.3
White/non-Hispanic	52.2	52.1	49.9	53.4
Black/non-Hispanic	67.5	68.1	74.1	76.8
Hispanic	51.3	47.4	44.5	42.1
0–4 years	41.2	46.5	42.1	43.5
5–10 years	58.5	53.0	57.2	57.5
11–17 years	60.4	68.0	56.2	61.5

7. **What is the prevalence of adult-onset asthma according to the NHIS?**
    Adult-onset asthma has not gained a national or international sense of urgency as has pediatric-onset asthma. The data from the NHIS (1980–1999), however, suggest increasing trends. Per 1000 people, rates were given for ages 15–34, 35–64, and ≥ 65 years. Until 1996 the question related to self-reported asthma. Since 1997 the data are reported as asthma attack prevalence (see question 6). The results are presented in Table 1-2.

TABLE 1-2. ASTHMA ATTACK PREVALENCE (RATES PER 1000)								
Age	1980	1985	1990	1995	1996	1997	1998	1999
15–34	30.0	36.1	37.3	57.8	67.2	44.2	37.5	42.2
35–64	29.9	30.8	38.4	50.1	46.2	37.0	35.7	33.4
≥ 65	31.9	38.6	36.3	39.4	45.5	27.3	28.7	22.5

8. **Summarize the results of NHANES III in regard to adult-onset asthma.**
NHANES III (1988–1994) based current prevalence on a physician diagnosis at any time, with symptoms in the past year. In ages 20 or older the prevalence was 4.5%, and by race the highest prevalence was among non-Hispanic blacks at 5.1%. The prevalence of work-related asthma was 3.7%.

9. **What were the results of the Behavioral Risk Factor Surveillance System (BRFSS) in regards to asthma prevalence?**
The BRFSS surveyed asthma prevalence in adults ≥ 18 years in 2001. Random phone surveys were based on two questions: (1) Have you ever been told by a doctor, nurse, or other health professional that you have asthma? and (2) Do you still have it? The overall current asthma rate was 7.2%, with ranges in the 50 states and the District of Columbia from 5.3% to 9.5%.

EPIDEMIOLOGY OF ALLERGIC DISEASES OUTSIDE THE U.S.

10. **What is the current prevalence of atopic dermatitis worldwide?**
The ISAAC study found that the 12-month prevalence results for children aged 13–14 ranged from virtually nonexistent in China and Albania to between 15% and 20% in Nigeria, United Kingdom, Finland, and Sweden.

  The worldwide literature on atopic dermatitis as of 2002 was reviewed by Schultz-Larsen, who found that the prevalence rates for atopic dermatitis were 10–12% and that less than 15% of patients maintain their disease after puberty.

  Schultz-Larsen F, Hanafin JM: Epidemiology of atopic dermatitis. Immunol Allergy Clin North Am 22:1–24, 2002.

KEY POINTS: EPIDEMIOLOGY

1. The prevalence of atopic disease continues to increase.

2. Major relative risk factors for the development of asthma include *Alternaria* and house dust allergy as well as use of antibiotics before 1 year of age.

3. Respiratory syncytial virus appears to play a key role in the development of asthma in some children.

4. The prevalence of asthma in children 6–7 years of age ranges from 10.2% to 26.8%.

11. **What other studies have addressed the prevalence of atopic dermatitis outside the U.S.?**
- In a German study based on doctor diagnosis, the prevalence of atopic eczema in children 6 years old was 15.7% in East Germany and 12.9% in West Germany.
- In Germany, a recent time-trend evaluation of eczema or eczema symptoms in 1994/1995 and 1999/2000 in children aged 6–7 and 13–14 years using the ISAAC written and video questionnaires showed some increase in prevalence and symptoms.
- In Danish children aged 5–16 years, the prevalence was 7%, based on symptoms and doctor diagnosis.
- A lifetime rate of 24%, based on questionnaires, was found in Norwegian children aged 7–12 years.
- In children 3–11 years in the United Kingdom, the current prevalence is 11.5%, with a lifetime rate of 20%, based on clinic chart data.
  von Mutius E, Martinez FD, Fritzsch C, et al: Prevalence of asthma and atopy in two areas of West and East Germany. Am J Respir Crit Care Med 149:358–364, 1994.

12. **What is the prevalence of allergic rhinoconjunctivitis?**
    In the ISAAC study (see question 2 for survey format), the 12-month prevalence data ranged from less than 5% in several former Soviet bloc nations to well over 25% in Nigeria, Paraguay, and Hong Kong and near 25% in Argentina, Canada, and Australia. The United Kingdom was similar to the U.S. at 12–22%, depending on the site. In Germany, a recent time-trend evaluation of rhinitis symptoms in 1994/95 and 1999/2000 in children 6–7 and 13–14 years using the ISAAC written and video questionnaires showed an increase, especially in girls.

13. **What is the current prevalence of asthma in children?**
    The ISAAC study found a global prevalence of 10.2% in children aged 6–7 years, with the Oceanic area of New Zealand and Australia having a regional prevalence of 26.8% at the high end and the Eastern and Northern European region having the lowest prevalence at 3.2%. Rates in children aged 13–14 years ranged from 26% in the Oceanic region to 4.4% for the Eastern and Northern European region. Rates in the United Kingdom were the highest for all Western European regional countries: over 19% for the UK versus 13.0% for all Western European countries, inclusive of the UK. In Germany, a recent time-trend evaluation of asthma and asthma-like symptoms in 1994/95 and 1999/2000 in children 6–7 and 13–14 years using the ISAAC written and video questionnaires showed a substantial increase, especially in girls.

    Strachan D, Sibbald B, Weiland S, et al: Worldwide variations in prevalence of symptoms of allergic rhinoconjunctivitis in children: The International Study of Asthma and Allergies in Childhood (ISAAC). Pediatr Allergy Immunol 8:161–176, 1997.

14. **What is the prevalence of adult-onset asthma in Europe?**
    The European Commission Respiratory Health Study I (ECRHS I), a multicenter survey of the prevalence and determinants of asthma in adults 20–44 years of age, is probably the most recent comprehensive study of disease symptoms in young adults. In the 45 centers reporting data, the median 12-month prevalence of asthma attacks was 3.1%; of treatment for asthma, 3.5%. The maximum prevalence in any center was 9.7% for attacks and 9.8% for treatment. In 12 industrialized European countries the risk for asthma symptoms among different occupations was highest in farmers, followed by painters, plastic workers, cleaners, spray painters, and agricultural workers.

    Variations in the prevalence of respiratory symptoms, self-reported asthma attacks, and use of asthma medication in the European Community Respiratory Health Survey (ECRHS). Eur Respir J 9:687–695, 1996.

15. **What is the prevalence of adult-onset asthma in Canada?**
    At six sites in Canada reported in 2001, the ECRHS survey reported that 4–6% of men and 4.9–9.7% of women were using asthma medication. The prevalence rates for wheezing were as high as 30% for men and 35% for women in the previous year.

INTERRELATIONSHIP OF THE ATOPIC DISEASES

16. **What are the known relationships between the common allergic diseases?**
    Atopic dermatitis, the most usual early presenting atopic disease, is a herald for the development of allergic rhinitis and/or asthma. Nearly 50% of children with atopic dermatitis later develop either rhinitis or asthma.

17. **Summarize the results of NHANES III in regard to interrelationships among atopic diseases.**
    In NHANES III (1988–1994) data, prevalence was determined by a physician diagnosis at any time and with symptoms in the past year. The prevalence of asthma was 6.6% in children aged 6–11 years, 9.6% in children aged 12–17 years, and 5.9% in adults 18 years of age or older.

Further analysis, based on reports of allergic symptoms and/or atopy (as determined by positive skin tests), revealed that 80% of the 6- to 11-year-old group, 86% of the 12- to 17-year-old group, and 93% of adults 18 years or older with asthma also had concomitant atopic or allergic manifestations.

18. **What were the results of the ISAAC study?**
The ISAAC study evaluated the prevalence of asthma and asthma symptoms, allergic conjunctivitis, and atopic dermatitis in children aged 6–7 years and children aged 13–14 years throughout the world in the mid 1990s. The symptoms of asthma (A), allergic rhinoconjunctivitis (AR), and atopic eczema (AE) for the previous 12 months were compared by regression analysis (Table 1-3).

TABLE 1-3.   REGRESSION ANALYSIS OF SYMPTOMS

Comparison	Regression Coefficient	Significance
A versus AR	0.75	$p < 0.0001$
A versus AE	0.74	$p < 0.0001$
AR versus AE	0.71	$p < 0.0001$

A = asthma, AR = allergic rhinoconjunctivitis, AE = atopic eczema.

FACTORS INFLUENCING THE DEVELOPMENT OF ATOPIC DISEASES

19. **Are there differences in the risk factors for the various atopic diseases?**
Despite the close relationship between the atopic diseases, there are distinct differences in the risk factors for the development of these diseases. The development of asthma, in particular, has been causally associated with both allergic and nonallergic factors. In contrast, allergic rhinitis, by definition, is due totally to atopy, and the major risk factor, beyond a genetic predisposition, is allergen exposure. Atopic dermatitis is probably more similar to asthma, but the biggest risk factor is atopy. In addition, certain factors may reduce the development of an allergic disease. Breast-feeding may be the most classic example.

20. **What is an odds ratio?**
Epidemiologic data are commonly expressed as a relative risk or odds ratio. A relative risk is used with cohort studies and an odds ratio with case-control studies. A ratio of 1.0 indicates no effect, a ratio > 1.0 indicates some effect, and a ratio < 1 indicates that the studied "risk" factor is actually of benefit.

21. **How are atopy, allergy, and allergic rhinitis defined in epidemiologic studies?**
Being atopic or allergic is defined as having evidence for specific IgE, regardless of the clinical diagnosis. Evidence for specific IgE is defined, in various reports, as a positive immediate skin test with a typical wheal and flare, a positive RAST, or an IgE level greater than two standard deviations above the mean. The last criterion is generally less useful. In most epidemiologic studies, allergic rhinitis, a clinical diagnosis, is either self- or parent-reported, or the condition may be termed "allergic rhinitis" if compatible symptoms are reported. It is uncommon to see both atopy and self-reported allergic rhinitis used together to define allergic rhinitis.

22. **What are the risk factors for atopy?**
The most common reason for being atopic is parental atopy. The risk for being atopic is 1.4 if only one parent is atopic. If both parents are atopic, the odds ratio (risk) is 2.8. Other studies have shown that 90% of atopic children have at least 1 atopic parent, that 66% of children are atopic when one parent is atopic, and that 75% of children are atopic if both parents are atopic. That fact that children with two atopic parents can be found to be nonatopic (at the time of testing, of course) suggests that environmental factors necessary for sensitization must also exist.

23. **What risk factors have been shown to be conducive to the development of asthma? With what level of risk?**
See Table 1-4.

TABLE 1-4. CAUSATIVE FACTORS AND RELATIVE RISK	
Causative Factor	**Relative Risk or Odds Ratio (Single Report Unless Noted)**
Specific allergen positive skin tests	*Alternaria*: 5.0
	Housedust: 2.9
Passive smoke exposure	Pooled analysis of 60 studies: 1.21
Prematurity	Birth weight < 1500 gm: 1.61
	Respiratory distress syndrome: 2.95
	Prematurity: 1.34
Familial factors: adoption	Adoptive mother atopic: 3.2
	Adoptive father atopic: 1.9
Weight	Highest quintile for weight: 2.3 for boys, 1.5 for girls
Antibiotics	Use of antibiotics: 2.74
	Use before 1 year: 4.05

24. **What other factors have been shown to influence the development of asthma but with less quantifiable risk?**
See Table 1-5.

25. **If a parent has asthma, what risk factors may enhance the development of asthma in the offspring?**
In a study from the National Jewish Center for Immunology and Respiratory Medicine, 150 mothers with asthma were recruited at the time of pregnancy. Twenty-eight fathers were also asthmatic. At age 3 years, the child's asthma status was identified, and the risk factors for the development of asthma were assessed (Table 1-6).
At age 6–8 years, the prevalence of asthma in the same children was reassessed. Significant associations with current asthma were found: 6-month IgE levels, parenting difficulties, bilateral asthma (both parents), higher number of respiratory infections in the first year of life, IgE level at age 6, positive skin tests at age 6, child's behavior at age 6 (fearfulness, depression), and child's psychological risk (adjustment problems). There were multiple significant interactions.

26. **What advice can a physician provide for the possible effect of pets on asthma or allergy development?**
In large part, patients (and parents) are looking for any conceivable excuse to keep their pets. In practical terms, if a child is already allergic to pet and nonpet allergens, there is no benefit

TABLE 1-5.   OTHER CAUSATIVE FACTORS WITH LESS QUANTIFIABLE RISK

Causative Factor*	Subjective Risk (Author's Opinion)
Gender: boys before age 10, girls after puberty	Well documented
Bronchial hyperresponsiveness	Rarely measured before development of asthma, but its presence in an atopic person is a moderate risk
Atopic dermatitis in infancy or early childhood	Moderate risk
Atopy	Moderate risk
Maternal age at conception	Advancing age decreases incidence
Family history of asthma in a first-degree relative (especially mother)	Increases risk
Preterm birth	Possibly increases risk
Having older siblings	Possibly reduces risk
Low birth weight	Possibly increases risk
Racial/ethnic group	In U.S., it is closely associated with socioeconomic factors. African-Americans and Puerto Ricans have higher risks
Socioeconomic factors	Higher in lower income families
Air pollution	Small risk if any
Attendance at day care	Small risk
Cockroach exposure	Moderate risk
High endotoxin exposure	Possibly reduces risk
Alum-containing vaccinations	? (Theoretically increases TH2 responses)
Respiratory syncytial virus (RSV) infection	With a serious RSV infection, the risk is probably higher

*These factors may interact.

in keeping the pets. If a child is allergic to nonpet allergens but not pets, there is no help in acquiring a pet, but it is not necessary to eliminate an existing pet. If a child has asthma and is pet-allergic, the pet should be removed from the home. If a newborn is joining a household with a pet(s), then and only then will dog or multiple pet exposures provide potential benefit. If a child develops pet allergies or nonpet allergies before age 7, the above recommendations prevail.

27. **Does breast-feeding reduce the risk for development of asthma?**
The pooled odds ratio for the effect of breast-feeding for more than 3 months on the develop-ment of asthma was calculated to be 0.80. Breast-feeding has numerous beneficial effects for

TABLE 1-6. ASTHMA STATUS AND RISK AT AGE 3 YEARS	
Factors	Probability of Asthma at Age 3 Years (%)
No risk factors	2
Psychosocial stressors	6
IgE > 10 IU at age 6 months	7
Frequent illness (> 8)	7
Frequent illness and IgE > 10 IU	22
Frequent illnesses, IgE > 10 IU at age 6 months, and excessive psychosocial factors	55

infants and should remain the choice for nutrition for newborns. Its benefit as an asthma prophylaxis appears conservative, but it may be significant if breast-feeding can be increased.

Gdalevich, M, Mimouni D, Mimouni M: Breast-feeding and the risk of bronchial asthma in childhood: A systematic review with meta-analysis of prospective studies. J Pediatr 139:261–266, 2001.

28. **What other factors may reduce the risk for development of asthma?**
    - An increased ingestion of omega-3 fatty acids, common in a diet rich in fish, may have a modest effect in reducing asthma prevalence.
    - Day care may decrease asthma risk at age 6 if the mother does not have asthma.
    - Rural living seems to be protective against the development of asthma, although the nation of residence may have some influence.
    - A recent report showed that asthma is reduced in children with allergic rhinitis who underwent immunotherapy (IT) versus those with allergic rhinitis receiving placebo. This study points out the importance of aggressively treating an allergic disease, which may influence the development of a second allergic disease.

29. **What risk factors have been shown to be conducive to the development of allergic rhinitis? With what level of risk? What factors may reduce the development of allergic rhinitis?**
    See Table 1-7.

30. **What risk factors have been shown to be conducive to the development of atopic dermatitis? With what level of risk? What factors may reduce the development of atopic dermatitis?**
    See Table 1-8.

31. **How may the "hygiene hypothesis" explain the increased incidence of asthma and allergy?**
    It has been proposed that living in a highly developed country may be a detrimental risk factor for development of asthma or atopy. This hypothesis is supported, in part, by studies showing that family size and indoor pets offer a protective effect against the development of atopic diseases. Results from such studies focus on the concept of TH1 and TH2 CD4+ T cells. TH1 cells are responsible for thwarting serious infectious agents, whereas TH2 cells are seemingly involved with atopic responses. If children use their TH1 T cells more vigorously, less stimulation of TH2 occurs. If the hygiene hypothesis has merit, it probably has more validity in highly developed nations but may also play a role in rural versus urban differences in developing nations.

TABLE 1-7.   RISK FACTORS FOR ALLERGIC RHINITIS AND LEVEL OF RISK

Risk Factors for Allergic Rhinitis*	Risk (Qualitative or Quantitative) for Allergic Rhinitis Diagnosis or Symptoms
Month of birth	May be a factor for regions with high seasonal pollens counts
Western life style	Increased
Parental allergy	Increased
Parental atopy	Increased
Lower birth order	Increased
Multiple gestation	Increased
Younger birth mother	Increased
Food allergy (atopy)	Increased
Traffic related air pollution	Increased
Not breast-feeding	Increased
Atopy (+ allergy skin tests)	Increased
Childhood farm environment	Decreased
Breast-feeding	Decreased

*These factors may interact.

TABLE 1-8.   RISK FACTORS FOR ATOPIC DERMATITIS AND LEVEL OF RISK

Risk Factors for Atopic Dermatitis*	Risk (Qualitative or Quantitative) for Atopic Dermatitis
Parental atopic dermatitis	Increased
Parental allergy	Increased
No siblings	Increased
Animal exposure in bedroom	Increased
Heavy traffic exposure	Increased
Higher socioeconomic advantages	Increased
High newborn eosinophilia	Increased
Low breast milk IgA	Increased
Maternal lactobacilli GG ingestion during pregnancy and during breast-feeding	May reduce
Strict maternal dietary restrictions and breast-feeding	May reduce or postpone
Domestic hard water	Increases

*These factors may interact.

32. **What is the role of air pollution in the development of an allergic disease?**
Because air pollution, increased diesel particulates, and ozone are common urban air problems, it has been suggested that the increase in asthma incidence may be associated with these pollutants. The most convincing argument against this theory, however, is the data from surveys of asthma and allergy in reunified Germany. The incidence of childhood asthma was no greater in East Germany, the more industrialized and polluted country, and atopy was more common in West Germany. The direct role of ozone, NO_2, and diesel particulates in the increased incidence of asthma in industrialized nations has not been adequately examined; evaluation should continue.

   Nicolai T, von Mutius E: Pollution and the development of allergy: The East and West Germany story. Arch Toxicol Suppl 19:201–206, 1997.

33. **What is primary prevention of asthma?**
Primary prevention implies that a clinical interaction stops the development of asthma in a person who otherwise has a high probability of developing it. The only studies that have shown primary prevention of asthma are those using immunotherapy versus placebo in patients with allergic rhinitis.

34. **Explain secondary and tertiary prevention of asthma.**
Secondary prevention reduces the severity of asthma (day-to-day clinical situation), whereas tertiary prevention reduces asthma-related morbidity and irreversible lung changes. These terms can apply to individual or population-based protocols.

GENETIC FACTORS IN ATOPIC DISEASE

35. **What is the current theory about the genetics of allergic diseases?**
From a genetic perspective allergy is multifactorial, which means that the susceptibility to the disease is determined by interactions between multiple genes and involves important nongenetic factors, such as the environment, for expression.

KEY POINTS: GENETICS

1. From a genetic perspective allergy is multifactorial.

2. The susceptibility to the disease is determined by interactions between multiple genes and involves important nongenetic factors, such as the environment, for expression.

3. The concordance of asthma in identical twins is very high.

4. To date, the major studies of serum IgE levels using segregation analysis have generally supported an inheritable model, but with varying genetic models, including major gene, either recessive or codominant.

---

36. **What is an asthmatic phenotype?**
When an investigator undertakes a protocol to determine a genetic basis for asthma, the enrolled subjects have to meet specific criteria accepted as "characteristic of a typical asthmatic" (Table 1-9). In many instances, these genetic studies are performed in collaborative fashion, often internationally. All investigators must enroll asthmatics that have uniform characteristics to provide a basis for studying a proposed candidate gene. It is important to note

TABLE 1-9.   POTENTIAL REPRESENTATIVE ATOPIC AND ASTHMATIC PHENOTYPES

Atopic	Asthmatic
Serum IgE at a specific "elevated" level + Skin test(s) to standardized allergens + RAST test(s)	+ Methacholine challenge (or) + histamine + Skin test to standardized allergen(s) Clinical diagnosis of asthma Reversibility to a beta agonist

that a particular component of the asthma phenotype, such as elevated IgE levels, can also be used as a trait for genetic association.

37.   **Define allergic versus nonallergic atopic diseases.**
Although somewhat contradictory at first glance, these concepts are well recognized in clinical medicine. Asthma and rhinitis are commonly classified as allergic (extrinsic) or nonallergic (intrinsic). Nonallergic asthma or rhinitis has no known allergic orientation; all known allergy skin tests are negative. However, the total IgE level may be slightly higher than in the normal population. Atopic dermatitis is also defined as allergic or nonallergic. Evidence suggests that nonallergic atopic dermatitis may be due to high levels of IgE to microbial components only. Such components are not available for standard allergy skin tests. These distinctions are important in defining a specific "atopic" phenotype and affect the results of genetic studies.

38.   **What types of subject populations are used in genetic studies of asthma?**
Various subject populations have been used, including sibling pairs (both with asthma), twin pairs, nuclear families (an index asthmatic with one or both parents), large nuclear families (an index asthmatic and three generations), founder populations (isolated communities), and population-wide or ethnic-limited genome searches (with a clinical diagnosis of asthma).

39.   **What is a segregation analysis?**
This method of analysis suggests the pattern of inheritance of a disorder or phenotype by observing how it is distributed within families. The absence or presence of asthma, atopy, or a serum IgE level can be used as the variable of interest. The analysis compares the affected phenotype in the families with the expected phenotype using various statistical models. The analysis can provide a suggestion for the mode of inheritance and determine whether a single or multiple genes are responsible.

40.   **What are candidate gene studies?**
A candidate gene study is an a priori approach. In essence, the search for the "asthma" gene is preselected, based on known biologic information. This method of genetic analysis attempts to determine whether the "asthmatic" proband, or surrogate, has a statistical association with specific polymorphisms (DNA sequence variations) occurring with the candidate gene or regions of chromosomes. If there is a significant association between the surrogate (e.g., a positive methacholine challenge) and a known marker on a specific chromosome, by inference the "gene" for the asthma condition or the surrogate marker for the asthma condition may be on that chromosome and near that repeat sequence loci. By using other loci on the same chromosome, the closeness or distance from known candidate genes can be determined. Association studies compare "affected" subjects versus controls, looking for statistical differences for the distribution of a given marker in a candidate gene.

41. What is a traditional logarithm of the odds (LOD) score?
In a linkage study the statistical association between a phenotype (e.g., asthma) and a candidate gene or a marker (e.g., Il-4 loci) is expressed as a logarithm ($\log_{10}$) of the odds score. It is a method of expressing the odds of linkage in conditions known to follow a mendelian mode of inheritance. LOD scores of 3 (1000:1 odds in favor of linkage) or higher are usually of more importance, although in complex disease values less than 3 may prove important.

42. What is a genetic polymorphism?
When used in genetic research, polymorphism refers to the variation in the sequence of nucleotides in the DNA on a particular chromosome.

43. What are microsatellites?
Microsatellites are identifiable repeats of nucleotides (polymorphisms) in the genome.

44. What is an SNP?
SNP refers to a single nucleotide substitution within a gene locus. The protein expression of the nucleotide substitution may or may not affect outcome. The best example in medicine is sickle cell disease. In asthma, the different amino acid substitutions (due to variations in the polymorphism of the beta-receptor gene) in the beta receptor may affect treatment outcome. Genetic studies may identify linkage between a candidate gene (for asthma) and known microsatellite(s) or potentially an SNP on a specific chromosome.

45. What constitutes a genome search for the genes for asthma or allergy?
The genome search approach takes an unbiased approach, relative to asthma biology, and may allow identification of unsuspected genes. The Collaborative Study on the Genetics of Asthma (CSGA) and others have detected a number of potential candidate gene areas for further research. Using the entire genome, linkages to specific marker areas are sought. Further evaluations using other markers on these "new" candidate genes can then be used to establish potential linkage, and unique reasons for the biology of "asthma." The genome search uses markers spaced at relatively even intervals throughout the genome.

Blumenthal MN, Rich SS, King R, Weber J: Approaches and issues in defining asthma and associated phenotypes map to chromosome susceptibility areas in large Minnesota families. The Collaborative Study for the Genetics of Asthma (CSGA). Clin Exp Allergy 28(Suppl 1):515, 1998.

46. To date, what genes have shown important linkage to asthma or allergic conditions?
See Table 1-10.

47. Define pharmacogenetics.
Pharmacogenetics is the study of a specific genetic alternation and its effect on treatment of a disease. A well-recognized example is the difference in the beta$_2$-adrenergic receptor (B2AR) polymorphisms at amino acid positions 16 (Arg16Gly) and 27 (Gln27Glu), and the effect of these polymorphisms on the use and response to beta$_2$ agonists. Polymorphisms for the 5-lipoxygenase *(5-LO)* gene and the leukotriene c(4) *(LTC4)* synthase gene may also affect the response to asthma therapy.

48. Have genetic studies been done in occupational asthma?
In large part genetic studies have focused on the allergic asthma phenotype, which generally means younger subjects with positive skin tests. Studies of occupational asthma would have a similar commonality—a specific allergen or chemical that induces an asthmatic response. Unfortunately, these subjects are infrequently seen, and sufficient numbers for a protocol are not readily available. Preliminary reports suggest an association with HLA-DR3 and low-molecular-weight respiratory sensitizers. Genetic associations have been shown for TDI-asthma

TABLE 1–10.	GENES WITH IMPORTANT LINKS TO ASTHMA OR ALLERGIC CONDITIONS
Chromosome	Allergy/Asthma Phenotypes or Candidate Genes Controlling Biologic Responses Potentially Critical in Asthma or Allergy
13	IgA levels(mucosal antigen regulation)
	Linkage to HDM allergy
	Linkage to atopic dermatitis
	Linkage to asthma in founder population
12	Linkage to asthma
	Linkage to total serum IgE levels
11	Beta-chain of high-affinity IgE receptor
	Polymorphisms of high-affinity IgE receptor
	Atopy (with strong maternal effect)
6	MHC region to asthma phenotypes
5	Linkage to total serum IgE levels
	Linkage to eosinophil levels
	Linkage to cytokines IL-4, IL-13, IL-5, and GMCSF
	Polymorphisms of IL-13 (and IL-4) and IgE
2	Linkage to total IgE
20	Linkage to a gene for a membrane-anchored zinc-dependent metalloproteinase (ADAM 33)

and polymorphisms to a glutathione-S-transferase locus, and with HLA DQA1*0104 and DQB1*0503.

49. **Have genetic studies been done in intrinsic (nonallergic) asthma?**
Adult nonallergic asthmatics are probably part of the "asthma" component of genome screen studies and may dilute results when included with allergic asthmatics, but in themselves they have not been the object of specific phenotype-directed protocols. The Epidemiological Study on the Genetics and Environment of Asthma (EGEA) has considered nonallergic asthma (intrinsic) as a separate phenotype in its ongoing studies.

50. **How can studies of structural gene variations assist in the genetics of asthma?**
If a candidate gene is a cause of asthma, a reasonable approach to elucidating the etiology of asthma is to study the various forms (polymorphisms) of a specific gene. To date, differences in the IL-4 alpha subunit, the beta chain of the high-affinity receptor for IgE, and the beta-adrenergic receptor have been found. The full question to be answered is whether these structural differences account for the disease itself or for different phenotypes or severity of the disease.

51. **What critical issue has been uncovered by genetic studies of serum IgE levels?**
Segregation analysis has been the predominant method in the attempt to determine the inheritance of IgE levels. A critical issue has been uncovered: the basal IgE level may be controlled by a gene(s) separate from the gene(s) responsible for the IgE response to specific allergens. This principle is evidenced by the fact that IgE is detectable in almost all humans, but specific IgE is *not* detected in all humans.

52. Summarize other results of genetic studies of serum IgE levels.

To date, the major studies of serum IgE levels using segregation analysis have generally supported an inheritable model, but with varying genetic models, including major gene, either recessive or codominant. Other authors have shown polygenic, genetic heterogeneity, and no genetic effect.

A suggestion has been made that a recessive gene may be responsible for basal IgE levels, as supported by the analysis of random families. A dominant gene may be involved in high IgE levels, as ascertained through asthmatic families.

53. Give a brief overview of the HLA system.

Human leukocyte antigen (HLA) is the major histocompatability complex in humans. The genetic control for the HLA system is located on chromosome 6. These genes encode proteins of three different types: class I, class II, and class III.

54. Describe class I molecules.

There are three class I loci: HLA-A, HLA-B, and HLA-C, each having multiple allelles. The class I allelles specific to the individual code for HL antigens that reside on nucleated cells. These antigens can be tissue-typed.

55. Describe class II molecules.

Class II molecules are encoded by the DR, DP, and DQ regions of the HLA complex. The class II molecules mostly are limited to cells responsible for immunity. There are different loci for each of the three class II regions, and these alleles code for the specific class II molecules that reside on T and B lymphocytes. Since class I and class I molecules are encoded by genes, they can be used as markers for determining the likelihood of inheriting other genetic traits, such as highly specific IgE responses (see below).

56. What are class III molecules?

Class III molecules are complement proteins.

57. What are allergenic epitopes?

The antigenic location on a large allergen that the human IgE antibody recognizes is the allergenic epitope. Each allergen has one or more major epitopes. These epitopes can be identified by a positive allergic skin test reaction. Peanut, for example, expresses 3 major epitopes, Ara h 1-3. Since these proteins are available for skin testing, it is possible to "fingerprint" each atopic patient to their exact epitope profile. The results can then be compared with their specific HLA characteristics, and statistical associations made between HLA type and specific epitope antigen-IgE response. Examples are shown in Table 1-11.

TABLE 1-11. ALLERGENIC EPITOPES		
Allergen	**HLA**	**Ethnic Group**
Der p 1 (house dust mite)	HLA-DPB1	
Bet v I (birch)	HLA-DR3	Caucasian
Amb a V (ragweed)	HLA-DR2	Caucasian
Lol p I-III (rye grass)	HLA-DR3	Caucasian

ACKNOWLEDGMENT

The author acknowledges the assistance of Mark L. Johnson, Ph.D., Creighton University Medical Center, Osteoporosis Research Center.

WEBSITES

1. ATS CME symposium: The RSV Asthma Link: The Emerging Story. Available at http://www.thoracic.org/mepframe.html.

2. The Collaborative Study on the Genetics of Asthma (CSGA): A genome-wide search for asthma susceptibility loci in ethnically diverse populations. Available at http://cooke.gsf.de.

BIBLIOGRAPHY

1. Akinbami LJ, Schoendorf KC, Parker J: US childhood asthma prevalence estimates: The impact of the 1997 National Health Interview Survey redesign. Am J Epidemiol 158:99–104, 2003.

2. Arif AA, Delclos GL, Lee ES, et al: Prevalence and risk factors of asthma and wheezing among US adults: An analysis of the NHANES III data. Eur Respir J 21:827–833, 2003.

3. Asher MI, Keil U, Anderson HR, et al: International Study of Asthma and Allergies in Childhood (ISAAC): Rationale and methods. Eur Respir J 8:483–491, 1995.

4. Barnes KC, Freidhoff LR, Nickel ER, et al: Dense mapping of chromosome 12q13.12q23.3 and linkage to asthma and atopy. J Allergy Clin Immunol 104:485–491, 1999.

5. Barnes KC, Neely JD, Duffy DL, et al: Linkage of asthma and total serum IgE concentration to markers on chromosome 12q: Evidence from Afro-Caribbean and Caucasian populations. Genomics 37:41–50, 1996.

6. Blumenthal MN, Rich SS, King R, Weber J: Approaches and issues in defining asthma and associated phenotypes map to chromosome susceptibility areas in large Minnesota families. The Collaborative Study for the Genetics of Asthma (CSGA). Clin Exp Allergy 28(Suppl 1):51–55, 1998.

7. Bodner C, Godden D, Seaton A: Family size, childhood infections and atopic diseases. The Aberdeen WHEASE Group. Thorax 53:28–32, 1998.

8. Borish L: Genetics of allergy and asthma. Ann Allergy A thma Immunol 82:413–424, 1999.

9. Bracken MB, Belanger K, Cookson WO, et al: Genetic and perinatal risk factors for asthma onset and severity: A review and theoretical analysis. Epidemiol Rev 24:176–189, 2002.

10. Centers for Disease Control and Prevention: Asthma mortality and hospitalization among children and young adults-United States, 1980-1993. MMWR 45:350–353, 1996.

11. Centers for Disease Control and Prevention: Asthma United States, 1980-1990. MMWR 41:733–735, 1992.

12. Centers for Disease Control and Prevention: Forecasted state-specific estimates of self-reported asthma prevalence United States, 1998. MMWR 47:102–125, 1998.

13. Center for Disease Control and Prevention: Self-reported asthma prevalence and control among adults—United States 2001. MMWR 52:381–384, 2003.

14. Cookson WO: Asthma genetics. Chest 121(3 Suppl):7S–13S, 2002.

15. Cookson WO: Genetics and genomics of asthma and allergic diseases. Immunol Rev 190:195–206, 2002.

16. Cookson WO, Moffatt MF: The genetics of atopic dermatitis. Curr Opin Allergy Clin Immunol 2:383–387, 2002.

17. Gdalevich, M, Mimouni D, Mimouni M: Breast-feeding and the risk of bronchial asthma in childhood: A systematic review with meta-analysis of prospective studies. J Pediatr 139:261–266, 2001.

18. Gergen PJ, Turkeltaub PC, Kovar MG: The prevalence of allergic skin test reactivity to eight common aeroallergens in the U.S. population: Results from the Second National Health and Nutrition Examination Survey. J Allergy Clin Immunol 80:669–679, 1987.

19. Hall CB: Respiratory syncytial virus: A continuing culprit and conundrum. J Pediatr 135(Suppl):S2–S7, 1999.

20. Host A, Halken S: Can we apply clinical studies to real life? Evidence-based recommendations from studies on development of allergic diseases and allergy prevention. Allergy 57:389–397, 2002.

21. Howard TD, Meyers DA, Bleecker ER: Mapping susceptibility genes for allergic diseases. Chest 123 (3 Suppl):363S–368S, 2003.

22. Immervoll T, Wjst M: Current status of the Asthma and Allergy Database. Nucleic Acids Res 27:213–214, 1999.

23. Klinnert MD, Nelson HS, Price MR, et al: Onset and persistence of childhood asthma: Predictors from infancy. Pediatrics 108:E69, 2001.

24. Ma X, Fick RB, Kaplowitz HJ: Prevalence of allergic rhinoconjunctivitis in the United States: Data from the Third National Health and Nutrition Examination Survey, 1998–94 (NHANES III). Am J Respir Crit Care Med 161:A325, 2000.

25. Manfreda J, Becklake MR, Sears MR, et al: Prevalence of asthma symptoms among adults aged 20–44 years in Canada. Can Med Assoc J 164:995–1001, 2001.

26. Mannino DM, Homa DM, Pertowski CA, et al: Surveillance for asthma—United States, 1960–1995. MMWR 47:1–27, 1998.

27. Mansur AH, Bishop DT, Markham AF, et al: Suggestive evidence for genetic linkage between IgE phenotypes and chromosome 14q markers. Am J Respir Crit Care Med 159:1796–1802, 1999.

28. Maziak W, Behrens T, Brasky TM, et al: Are asthma and allergies in children and adolescents increasing? Results from ISAAC phase I and phase III surveys in Munster, Germany. Allergy 58:572–579, 2003.

29. Moller C, Dreborg S, Ferdousi HA, et al: Pollen immunotherapy reduces the development of asthma in children with seasonal rhinoconjunctivitis (the PAT-study). J Allergy Clin Immunol 109:251–256, 2002.

30. Nelson DA, Johnson CC, Divine GW, et al: Ethnic differences in the prevalence of asthma in middle class children. Ann Allergy Asthma Immunol 78: 16, 1997.

31. Nickel RG, Saitta FP, Freidhoff LR, et al: Positional candidate gene approach and functional genomics strategy in atopy gene discovery. Int Arch Allergy Immunol 118:282–284, 1999.

32. Nicolai T, von MutiusE: Pollution and the development of allergy: The East and West Germany story. Arch Toxicol Suppl 19:201–206, 1997.

33. Novak N, Bieber T: Allergic and nonallergic forms of atopic diseases. J Allergy Clin Immunol 112:252–262, 2003.

34. Nsouli TM: Inner-city disadvantaged populations and asthma prevalance, morbidity, and mortality. Ann Allergy Asthma Immunol 82:24, 1999.

35. Ober C, Cox NJ, Abney M, et al: Genome-wide search for asthma susceptibility loci in a founder population. The Collaborative Study on the Genetics of Asthma. Hum Mol Genet 7:1393–1398, 1998.

36. Oddy WH, Holt PG, Sly PD, et al:. Risk factors for asthma and atopic disease in six-year-old children: Exclusive breastfeeding is protective. Am J Respir Crit Care Med 159 (Part 2 of 2):A43, 1999.

37. Palmer LJ, Cookson WO: Using single nucleotide polymorphisms as a means to understanding the pathophysiology of asthma. Respir Res 2:102–112, 2001.

38. Peat JK, Li J. Reversing the trend: Reducing the prevalence of asthma. J Allergy Clin Immunol 103:110, 1999.

39. Persky VW, Slezak J, Contreras A, et al: Relationships of race and socioeconomic status with prevalence, severity, and symptoms of asthma in Chicago school children. Ann Allergy Asthma Immunol 81:266–271, 1998.

40. Schultz-Larsen F, Hanafin JM: Epidemiology of atopic dermatitis. Immunol Allergy Clin North Am 22:1–24, 2002.

41. Strachan D, Sibbald B, Weiland S, et al: Worldwide variations in prevalence of symptoms of allergic rhinoconjunctivitis in children: The International Study of Asthma and Allergies in Childhood (ISAAC). Pediatr Allergy Immunol 8:161–176, 1997.

42. Thomas NS, Holgate ST: Genes for asthma on chromosome 11: An update Clin Exp Allergy 28:387–391, 1998.

43. Troisi RJ, Speizer FE, Willett WC, et al: Menopause, postmenopausal estrogen preparations, and the risk of adult-onset asthma. A prospective cohort study. Am J Respir Crit Care Med 152:118–138, 1995.

44. Variations in the prevalence of respiratory symptoms, self-reported asthma attacks, and use of asthma medication in the European Community Respiratory Health Survey (ECRHS). Eur Respir J 9:687–695,1996.

45. von Mutius E, Martinez FD, Fritzsch C, et al: Prevalence of asthma and atopy in two areas of West and East Germany. Am J Respir Crit Care Med 149:358–364, 1994.

46. Wickens K, Pearce N, Crane J, Beasley R: Antibiotic use in early childhood and the development of asthma. Clin Exp Allergy 29:766–771, 1999.

47. Wilkinson J, Thomas NS, Morton N, Holgate ST: Candidate gene and mutational analysis in asthma and atopy. Int Arch Allergy Immunol 118:265–267, 1999.

48. Williams H, Robertson C, Stewart A, et al: Worldwide variations in the prevalence of symptoms of atopic eczema in the International Study of Asthma and Allergies in Childhood. J Allergy Clin Immunol 103:125–138, 1999.

49. Wjst M, Fischer G, Immervoll T, et al: A genomewide search for linkage to asthma. German Asthma Genetics Group. Genomics 58:18, 1999.

50. Worldwide variations in the prevalence of asthma symptoms: The International Study of Asthma and Allergies in Childhood (ISAAC). Eur Respir J 12:315–335, 1998.

CHAPTER 2

IMMUNOLOGY AND PATHOPHYSIOLOGY OF ALLERGIC DISEASE

Maurice E. Hamilton, M.D.

1. **What are immunoglobulins?**

   Immunoglobulins are a heterogeneous group of glycoproteins that constitute about 20% of total serum proteins and migrate with gamma—and, to a lesser extent, beta—globulins during protein electrophoresis.

2. **Describe the physical properties of immunoglobulins.**

   All immunoglobulins are composed of two identical heavy (H) chains and two identical light (L) chains covalently linked by disulfide bonds between cysteine residues. Each chain contains an amino-terminal sequence characterized by significant diversity in the amino acid residues, the variable (V) region, and a carboxy-terminal sequence with less variability, the constant (C) region.

   Within each chain are globular regions known as domains: the domains in the light chains are termed V_L and C_L, whereas those in the heavy chains are named V_H, C_H1, C_H2, C_H3, and C_H4 (Fig. 2-1). The segment of heavy chains between the first two constant domains, C_H1 and C_H2, forms the hinge region.

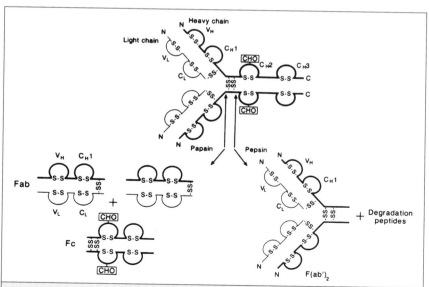

Figure 2-1. Basic structure of the antibody molecule and fragments. CHO = carbohydrate, thick lines = heavy chains, thin lines = light chains. (From Li JT: Immunoglobulin structure and function. In Adkinson NF Jr, Yunginger JW, Busse WW, et al (eds): Middleton's Allergy: Principles and Practice, vol. 1, 6th ed. St. Louis, Mosby, 2003, Fig. 5-1, p 54, with permission.)

3. **What is the structural basis for the classification of immunoglobulins?**
   Immunoglobulins are classified on the basis of structural differences in the constant regions of the heavy chains into five classes or isotypes—IgG, IgA, IgM, IgD, and IgE, corresponding to the heavy chains γ (gamma), α (alpha), μ (mu), δ (delta), and ε (epsilon), respectively. IgG and IgA may be further categorized into subclasses on the basis of antigenic differences in the structure of the C_H regions (IgG1–IgG4, IgA1, and IgA2).

4. **Describe the structural differences between the immunoglobulin classes.**
   Mu and epsilon chains consist of five domains (V_H, C_H1, C_H2, C_H3, and C_H4), whereas gamma and alpha chains are composed of four domains (V_H, C_H1, C_H2, and C_H3). IgG, IgE, and IgD exist only as the basic immunoglobulin unit consisting of two heavy chains and two light chains, whereas IgA and IgM also exist as polymers. In the circulation, IgA exits in both monomeric and dimeric forms. IgA in secretions exists as a dimer and includes a J chain and a secretory piece synthesized by epithelial cells. IgM is secreted as a pentamer composed of five immunoglobulin units joined by disulfide bonds and a J chain. Although the J chain is present in all polymeric immunoglobulin molecules with more than two basic units, the secretory component is uniquely associated with IgA.

5. **How are light chains classified?**
   Light chains are subdivided on the basis of antigenic differences in the constant regions into κ (kappa) and λ (lambda) types. In humans, the proportion of kappa to lambda chains is about 2:1.

6. **What are the products of enzymatic digestion of immunoglobulins by papain and pepsin?**
   Digestion of immunoglobulins by **papain** splits the molecule on the amino-terminal side of the disulfide bonds joining the heavy chains and yields two antigen-binding fragments (Fab), each containing an entire light chain and the V_H and C_H1 domains of a heavy chain, and a crystallizable fragment (Fc), composed of the carboxy-terminal halves of the heavy chains.
   Pepsin cleaves the heavy chains on the carboxy-terminal side of the disulfide bonds linking these chains to produce a divalent antigen-binding fragment, F(ab')$_2$, composed of two Fab regions and the hinge region with intact disulfide bonds, in addition to small peptides.

7. **Characterize the antigen-binding site and its relationship to antibody function.**
   Amino acids within the variable regions of the heavy and light chains form the antigen-binding site, which is closely associated with three segments on light and heavy chains that display significant diversity, the hypervariable regions.
   Binding of antigen to immunoglobulin induces conformational changes in the constant regions of the heavy chains. These changes permit the carboxy-terminal portion to bind to Fc receptors on the surface of lymphocytes and macrophages and to the first component of complement, C1q.

8. **Which genes encode immunoglobulins?**
   The κ light chain is encoded by genes on chromosome 2, whereas the λ light chain is encoded by genes on chromosome 22. Genes located on chromosome 14 encode the heavy chain.
   The light chain loci are composed of V (variable) gene elements, J (joining) segments, and C (constant region) exons. In addition to these elements, heavy chain loci contain D (diversity) segments between the V and J regions. The amino terminal region of each light chain is created by somatic linking of genes encoding variable (V_L) and joining (J_L) light chain elements. Similarly, the amino terminal region of each heavy chain is formed by linking of genes encoding a variable (V_H), diversity (D_H), and joining (J_H) region. The genes encoding the constant region of light chains contain a single exon, whereas the genes encoding the constant region of heavy chains contain exons corresponding to each of the heavy chain isotypes (IgM, IgD, IgG1, IgG2, IgG3, IgG4, IgA1, IgA2, and IgE).

9. **List the mechanisms responsible for immunoglobulin gene diversity.**

VJ/VDJ recombination, class switch recombination, somatic hypermutation, and gene conversion generate antibodies with diverse specificities. Somatic hypermutation refers to error-prone DNA polymerase repair of breaks in DNA strands introduced during class switch recombination. In humans, gene conversion does not appear to be a significant contributor to gene diversification.

Class switch recombination, somatic hypermutation, and gene conversion are dependent upon activation-induced cytidine deaminase (AID), an enzyme that catalyzes deamination of deoxycytidine (dC) to deoxyuridine (dU) on single-stranded DNA. AID is present only in activated B cells, and the AID master gene appears to regulate all B cell-specific modifications of vertebrate immunoglobulin genes.

KEY POINTS: GENERATION OF ANTIBODIES

1. VJ/VDJ recombination, class switch recombination, somatic hypermutation, and gene conversion generate antibodies with diverse specificities.

2. Interleukin-4 (IL-4) and IL-13 are the only cytokines capable of inducing IgE synthesis.

10. **How do immunoglobulin allotypes differ from idiotypes?**

Allotypes represent minor polymorphic or allelic variations in the amino acid sequences (usually a single amino acid substitution) in the constant regions of heavy and light chains that segregate according to Mendelian genetics. They usually do not alter function. Gm allotypes are associated with γ chains, Am allotypes with α chains, and Inv allotypes with γ light chains.

Idiotypes refer to antigenic determinants within the variable regions of heavy and light chains that may encompass the antigen-binding sites, particularly the hypervariable regions. Shared idiotypes on structurally different immunoglobulins are termed public- or cross-reactive idiotypes, whereas idiotypes expressed on only a limited number of closely related antibodies are called individual or private idiotypes.

11. **Discuss the relationship between anti-idiotypic antibodies and antigens.**

Some anti-idiotypic antibodies are believed to resemble the structure of the original antigen that induced antibody formation. Thus, if the antigen-binding site represents a negative image or "cast" of the antigen, then an anti-idiotypic antibody directed against the antigen-binding site may resemble a negative image of the antigen-binding site, or the original antigen itself. Anti-idiotypic antibodies form immune complexes that may modulate immune function and are potentially pathogenic.

12. **Characterize the function of IgG.**

IgG represents the predominant antibody in the secondary immune response and is the only immunoglobulin capable of crossing the placenta. IgG activates complement via the classical pathway. The ability of the IgG subclasses to bind complement varies, being greatest for IgG3 and IgG1. IgG2 is a poor activator of complement and IgG4 is unable to bind complement. The C1q binding site on IgG appears to be located in the C_H2 domain.

IgG Fc receptors (FcγR) on cells such as macrophages bind IgG1 and IgG3 via the C_H3 domain of the Fc region, mediating phagocytosis and antibody-dependent cell-mediated cytotoxicity (ADCC). Fcγ receptors have also been identified on B cells, neutrophils, basophils, eosinophils, and platelets.

13. **Characterize the function of IgM and IgA.**

IgM is the predominant antibody in the early immune response, the initial immunoglobulin expressed on the surface of B cells, and the most efficient complement-fixing antibody (requiring binding of antigen to only one antibody molecule).

IgA is the primary immunoglobulin class in secretions, including tears, saliva, and mucus, providing the primary defense against local pathogens.

14. Characterize the function of IgD and IgE.

IgD, like IgM, functions as a membrane-bound antigen receptor on the surface of B lymphocytes. Some data indicate that binding of antigen to surface IgD may stimulate B cell maturation. In addition, surface IgD may inhibit the induction of B cell tolerance.

IgE, a monomeric antibody with MW 190,000 daltons, binds to effector cells via its Fc portion and plays a key role in mediating allergic reactions and cytotoxicity to parasites following binding of specific antigen. Unlike other immunoglobulins, IgE does not activate complement via the classical pathway.

15. What is the proportion of each immunoglobulin class in the circulation?

In normal humans, IgG comprises about 75% of total serum immunoglobulins; IgA, 15%; IgM, 10%; IgD, 0.2%; and IgE, 0.004%.

16. Describe the location and kinetics of IgE production.

IgE-producing plasma cells are distributed primarily in lymphoid tissue adjacent to the respiratory and gastrointestinal tracts. The highest concentrations are found in the tonsils and adenoids. The half-life of IgE is only 1–5 days in the circulation versus about 14 days in human skin.

17. How do serum IgE levels vary with age?

IgE-bearing B lymphocytes are detectable by the eleventh week of gestation, but IgE synthesis is negligible in utero. Serum IgE levels increase after birth, attain median adult levels at age 3 years, peak between ages 7 and 14 years, and decrease rapidly after age 15. IgE levels are less than 80 IU/ml in most nonallergic adults.

18. What diseases are associated with elevated serum IgE?

Levels of IgE are elevated in patients with atopic diseases, including allergic rhinitis, allergic asthma, and atopic dermatitis. The quantity of IgE correlates with the severity of symptoms in patients with allergic rhinitis and atopic dermatitis. Total IgE levels are markedly elevated in allergic bronchopulmonary aspergillosis.

Increased levels of IgE are characteristic of Wiskott-Aldrich syndrome, hyperimmunoglobulinemia E syndrome, IgE myeloma, Hodgkin's disease, and acute graft-versus-host disease. IgE levels may also be increased with Epstein-Barr virus mononucleosis, Di George syndrome (thymic hypoplasia), Nezelof syndrome (cellular immunodeficiency with immunoglobulins), cystic fibrosis, and Kawasaki disease.

19. Are parasitic infections associated with elevated serum IgE?

Infections with metazoan helminthic parasites (e.g., *Ascaris, Schistosoma*, and *Trichinella* species) are frequently associated with elevated levels of serum IgE, whereas IgE levels are usually normal with protozoan infections (e.g., *Entamoeba, Giardia*, and *Toxoplasma* species). An exception is malaria, caused by plasmodial protozoans, in which serum IgE is typically increased. Most of the elevated IgE in parasitic infections is not specific for parasites.

20. To which receptors does IgE bind?

IgE binds by its Fc portion to high-affinity IgE receptors (FcεRI), present on the surface of mast cells, basophils, monocytes, eosinophils, non-B/non-T cells, and antigen-presenting cells, and to low-affinity receptors (FcεRII or CD23), present on B cells, some T cells, eosinophils, monocytes, macrophages, follicular dendritic cells, Langerhans cells, and platelets.

21. Characterize the high-affinity IgE receptor.

FcεRI on mast cells and basophils is a tetramer formed by an α-chain, a β-chain, and two γ-chains. The α-chain binds IgE, whereas the β- and γ-chains induce transmembrane signals that mediate cellular activation. The FcεRI β-chain contains two immunoreceptor tyrosine-based activation motifs (ITAMs) that amplify the signaling from this receptor and are associated with the Src-type protein-tyrosine kinase Lyn. Each of the γ-chains also contains two ITAMs. Following aggregation of receptor-bound IgE, these ITAMs are phosphorylated, which activates the protein-tyrosine kinase Syk and initiates a phosphorylation cascade that results in activation of the cell.

On antigen-presenting cells, including Langerhans cells, monocytes, and peripheral blood dendritic cells, FcεRI is a trimer composed of one α-chain and two γ-chains. In contrast, FcεRII is a single transmembrane chain.

Boyce JA: Mast cells: Beyond IgE. J Allergy Clin Immunol 111:24–32, 2003.

22. **Which cytokines regulate IgE synthesis?**
Interleukin-4 (IL-4) and IL-13 are the only cytokines capable of inducing IgE synthesis. IL-4 induces isotype switching from IgM to IgG4 and IgE, perhaps sequentially. IL-13 also promotes isotype switching to IgE production. IL-5, IL-6, IL-9, and tumor necrosis factor-α (TNF-α) stimulate IL-4-mediated IgE synthesis, whereas interferon-α (IFN-α), IFN-γ, transforming growth factor-β (TGF-β), IL-2, IL-8, IL-10, and IL-12 inhibit IgE synthesis.

23. **Describe the interactions between B and T cells required for IgE synthesis.**
In addition to IL-4 and IL-13, direct contact between B lymphocytes and activated T cells is required for switching to IgE production. B cells present processed antigen bound to major histocompatibility complex (MHC) class II molecules to T cell receptors. Other cell surface interactions are also necessary. These may occur between the B cell surface glycoprotein CD40 and its ligand CD40L on T cells and between CD23 on B cells and CD21 on T cells. The CD40-CD40L interaction induces B cells to express B7.1 (CD80), which binds to CD28 on T cells, thereby upregulating IL-4 production. Nuclear factor κB and B-cell-specific activator protein elements are also required for IgE synthesis.

24. **What is the function of membrane-bound immunoglobulin on B lymphocytes?**
B cells utilize membrane-bound immunoglobulin molecules as receptors for soluble antigens. Naïve B cells display both IgM and IgD surface receptors. B cell receptors (BCRs) also contain invariant transmembrane accessory molecules known as Igα and Igβ that contain cytoplasmic ITAM domains.

25. **Describe the events initiated by binding of antigen to the B cell receptor.**
After binding of antigen to the BCR, the Src-type kinases Blk, Fyn, and Lyn phosphorylate BCR ITAMs, which bind and activate Syk tyrosine kinase, thereby initiating a cascade that activates protein kinase C, the G proteins Ras and Rac, and mitogen-associated protein kinases (MAPKs). This action is facilitated by the costimulatory complex CD19-CD81-CD21 (complement receptor 2), which is activated by binding to complement component C3d.

Subsequent gene transcription leads to B-cell proliferation and differentiation into immunoglobulin-secreting cells with the capacity to express various immunoglobulin isotypes sharing the same antigenic specificity. The principal antibody produced in response to a primary antigenic challenge is IgM, followed by IgG, IgA, and IgE. During the secondary, or memory, response, IgG, IgA, and IgE account for most antibody synthesis.

26. **Characterize CD4+ and CD8+ T lymphocytes.**
CD4+ T cells, which comprise approximately 60% of circulating T cells, function as helper cells for B cell differentiation and mediate delayed-type hypersensitivity (DTH) reactions. CD8+ T cells participate in the host response against intracellular microorganisms and mediate cytotoxic and suppressor activities. Although CD4+ T cells have been categorized as helper-inducer cells and CD8+ T cells as cytotoxic-suppressor cells, both CD4+ and CD8+ lymphocytes can act as helper-inducer and cytotoxic-suppressor cells and produce similar cytokines.

Kalish RS, Askenase PW: Molecular mechanisms of CD8+ T cell-mediated delayed hypersensitivity: Implications for allergies, asthma, and autoimmunity. J Allergy Clin Immunol 103: 192–199, 1999.

27. **What is the primary difference between CD4+ and CD8+ T cells?**
    CD4+ T cells recognize antigens presented by class II MHC molecules (HLA-DR, -DP, and -DQ in humans). CD8+ T cells recognize antigens presented by class I MHC molecules (HLA-A, -B, and -C).

28. **Describe the structure and function of the major histocompatibility complex class I molecules.**
    Human major histocompatibility complex (MCH), or HLA, molecules are cell-surface glycoproteins that bind peptide fragments. Class I HLA molecules are heterodimers consisting of a transmembrane α chain (class I heavy chain) associated with β2-microglobulin. Class I HLA type is determined by three highly polymorphic genes on chromosome 6 that encode HLA-A, -B, and -C α chains. The α chain is composed of three extracellular domains (α1, α2, and α3), a transmembrane domain, and a short intracellular domain. The α1 and α2 domains combine to form the MHC peptide-binding groove. The α3 domain of the heavy chain interacts with CD8 molecules on T cells, restricting antigen presentation to CD8+ T cells.

29. **Describe the structure and function of the major histocompatibility complex class II molecules.**
    The major class II proteins are classified as HLA-DR, -DQ, and -DP. Class II HLA molecules consist of two transmembrane polypeptide chains designated α and β. Genes in the HLA-DR subregion encode the α chain, which is minimally polymorphic (with one common and two rare alleles), and two polymorphic β chains (DRB1 and DRB3). Each of these chains contains a shorts cytoplasmic anchor, a transmembrane domain, and two extracellular domains: α1 and α2 for the α chain and β1 and β2 for the β chain. Pairing of α1 and β1 chains creates the MHC peptide-binding groove. In addition to providing support, the β2 chain interacts with CD4 molecules, restricting antigen presentation to CD4+ T cells.

30. **What are the primary subsets into which CD4+ T cells differentiate?**
    Resting naïve CD4+ T cells (Th cells) release minimal cytokine, but after antigenic stimulation by antigen-presenting cells (APCs), Th cells synthesize IL-2 and are known as Th0 cells. Activated Th0 cells differentiate into Th1 or Th2 cells, depending upon the cytokine milieu.

31. **Characterize the subsets of CD4+ T cells.**
    See Table 2-1.

32. **Describe factors that promote development of Th1 versus Th2 cells.**
    Infection of monocytes by bacteria or viruses induces secretion of IFN-α and IL-12, which promote the formation of Th1 cells, and IFN-γ, which inhibits differentiation into Th2 cells. In contrast, IL-4 from mast cells or Th2 promotes the formation of Th2 cells and antagonizes differentiation into Th1 cells. Moreover, different subsets of dendritic cells (DC) preferentially stimulate different Th cells: DC1 produce large amounts of IL-12, favoring Th1 development, whereas DC2 produce little IL-12, favoring Th2 development. The DC2 cytokine profile appears to be mediated at least in part by surface histamine receptors H_1 and H_2, which decrease IL-12 secretion and stimulate IL-10 production.

33. **How do signal transducers and activators of transcription (STATs) interact with transcription factors to influence Th development?**
    For Th1 development, IL-12 signaling via STAT4 is required. IL-27 signaling via STAT-1 is also important. Signaling via these pathways activates T-box transcription factor expressed in T cells (T-bet), a factor selectively expressed in Th1 cells that induces production of IFN-γ and is nec-

TABLE 2-1.   SUBSETS OF CD4+ T CELLS

Characteristic	T Helper 1 (Th1) Cells	T Helper 2 (Th2) Cells
Type of response	Cell-mediated	Humoral-mediated
Activators	Microbes	Allergens, parasites
Functions	Cytotoxicity, DTH, monocyte activation	B cell helper, IgE synthesis, monocyte inhibition, eosinophil activation
Cytokines produced*	IFN-γ, TNF-β	IL-4, IL-5, IL-9, IL-25
Cytokine inducers	IFN-γ, IL-12, IL-18, IL-23, IL-27	IL-4, IL-5, IL-13
Cytokine inhibitors	IL-4, IL-10	IFN-γ, IL-12

*Both types of T helper cells secrete IL-2, IL-3, IL-10, IL-13, TNF-α, and GM-CSF. CD4+ cells may also produce CC chemokines such as eotaxin, MCP-3, MIP-1α, and RANTES.

essary for Th1 differentiation. In contrast, STAT6 upregulates IL-4 dependent genes and is activated by other Th2 cytokines. Signaling via STAT6 induces the transcription factor GATA-3, which enhances synthesis of Th2 cytokines and blocks Th1 differentiation. GATA-3 is expressed in Th2 cells and regulates the transcription of IL-4 and IL-5, mediating Th2 differentiation in the absence of STAT6.

Escoubet-Lozach L, Glass CK, Wasserman SI: The role of transcription factors in allergic inflammation. J Allergy Clin Immunol 110:553–564, 2002.

34. **How are Janus kinases (JAKs) related to STATs?**
JAKs and STATs represent two groups of protein-tyrosine kinases that are activated following binding of cytokines to their receptors. Most cytokine receptors signal using one of the four related cytoplasmic protein-tyrosine kinases known as Janus kinases (JAKs): JAK1, JAK2, JAK3, and TYK2. Different JAKs associate with the cytoplasmic domains of different cytokine receptors. JAK3 is the major signal transducer for the common γ chain shared by multiple cytokine receptors. Binding of cytokine to its receptor triggers tyrosine phosphorylation of both

KEY POINTS: T CELLS

1. CD4+ T cells recognize antigens presented by class II MHC molecules, whereas CD8+ T cells recognize antigens presented by class I MHC molecules.

2. CD4+ T cell subsets include Th1 cells, which mediate cytotoxicity, and Th2 cells, which function as B helper cells, stimulate synthesis of IgE, and activate eosinophils, thereby enhancing atopic responses.

3. αβ T cell receptors are members of the immunoglobulin supergene family and recognize peptide fragments that have been processed by antigen-presenting cells (APCs).

4. Activation of αβ T cells requires antigen recognition by TCRs and stimulation by IL-1 in addition to a costimulatory signal provided by binding of the T cell ligand CD28 to B7.1 (CD80) or B7.2 (CD86) on the surface of APCs.

the receptor and receptor-associated JAKs. This phosphorylated complex in turn phosphory-lates its respective signal transducer and activator of transcription (STAT), causing it to dimer-ize and migrate to the nucleus, where it binds to specific regulatory sequences in the promoters of cytokine-responsive genes.

35. Give an example of how JAKs are related to STATs.

As an example, binding of IL-4 to IL-4 receptor (IL-4R, a heterodimer composed of an α and a γ chain) activates JAK1, which is attached to the IL-4R α chain, and Janus kinase 3 (JAK3), attached to the IL-4R γ chain. This induces tyrosine phosphorylation of signal transducer and activator of transcription 6 (STAT6). Tyrosine-phosphorylated STAT6 translocates to the nucleus, where it initiates transcription of IL-4 responsive elements, including genes for ε heavy chain, VCAM-1, MHC class II, CD23, and cytokines for Th2 differentiation. Similarly, binding of IL-12 to IL-12R, which is associated with JAK2 and TYK2, leads to phosphorylation of STAT4, which translocates to the nucleus and mediates the biological effects characteristic of IL-12, including induction of IFN-γ and differentiation of Th0 cells into Th1 cells.

36. What is the effect of immunostimulatory deoxynucleotides on T-cell differentiation?

Immunostimulatory sequence oligodeoxynucleotides (ISS-ODNs) containing CpG motifs (char-acteristic of many bacterial genomes) promote Th1 and inhibit Th2 differentiation. ISS-ODNs also function as an effective Th1 adjuvant, producing immune responses to co-administered protein antigens similar to those following gene vaccination. Application of these techniques to ragweed-sensitive patients has demonstrated rapid improvement in allergic rhinitis symptoms following vaccination with Amb a 1 (the major ragweed allergen)-ISS-ODN conjugate.

Santeliz JV, Van Nest G, Traquina P, et al: Amb a 1-linked CpG oligodeoxynucleotides reverse established airway hyperresponsiveness in a murine model of asthma. J Allergy Clin Immunol 109:455–462, 2002.

37. How do toll-like receptors modulate the immune response?

Toll-like receptors (TLRs) represent a group of receptors that activate innate immune responses by recognition of pathogen-associated molecular patterns (PAMPs) used by pathogens, but not mammalian cells. Stimulation of these receptors leads to activation of the transcription factor nuclear factor κB (NF-κB), gene transcription, production of IL-12, and a Th1 immune response.

TLRs are especially prevalent on macrophages and dendritic cells but are also present on other cells types, including eosinophils, neutrophils, and epithelial cells. Endotoxin is recog-nized by TLR2 and TLR4, whereas bacterial-containing CpG motifs are recognized by TLR9.

38. Explain the "hygiene hypothesis."

The hygiene hypothesis proposes that improvements in public hygiene lower serious infections but increase the incidence of allergy and asthma. This hypothesis has been reinforced by reports of decreased prevalence of asthma among persons infected by hepatitis A, herpes sim-plex type I, measles, *Toxoplasma gondii*, or *Mycobacterium tuberculosis.*

Effects of infectious agents on Th1/Th2 cell populations have been invoked to explain these observations. Microbial stimulation, including stimulation by endotoxin, induces production of IL-10, which may decrease airway inflammation. Endotoxin is a potent inducer of IL-12 and IFN-γ, key regulators of Th1-type immune development. Endotoxin prevents most manifesta-tions of allergic asthma, including IgE synthesis, production of Th2 cytokines, and airway eosinophilia, but not airway hyperresponsiveness.

39. Which CD4+ T cells suppress autoreactive lymphocytes?

A novel population of CD4+ CD25+ suppressor T cells, known as regulatory T cells, produces large quantities of transforming growth factor-β and IL-10, thereby blocking proliferation of autoreactive lymphocytes in peripheral tissues. CD4+ CD25+ T cells induce tolerance to allo-geneic skin grafts and ameliorate graft-versus-host disease in murine models. However, in humans, co-expression of CD4 and CD25 may not be sufficient to identify regulatory T cells. In fact, increased numbers of CD25+ T cells have been reported in donor grafts of stem cell trans-plant patients who develop GVHD.

McHugh RS, Shevach EM: The role of suppressor T cells in regulation of immune responses. J Allergy Clin Immunol 110:693–702, 2002.

40. How do CD8+ T-cell subsets differ from CD4+ subsets?
CD8+ T cells are also divided into subsets based upon their cytokine profiles. CD8+ T cells that produce cytokines similar to CD4+ Th1 cells are designated T cytotoxic 1 (Tc1) cells, whereas those that produce cytokines similar to CD4+ Th2 cells are called T cytotoxic 2 (Tc2) cells.

41. Explain the mechanisms by which CD8+ cells mediate cytotoxity.
CD8+ T cells exhibit two distinct mechanisms for inducing cytotoxicity: Fas ligand and perforin. Fas ligand on CD8+ cells engages Fas on the target cell, thereby initiating apoptotic pathways that lead to activation of caspase 8 (exogenous pathway) and caspase 9 (endogenous pathway). Both caspase pathways activate caspase 3, which induces apoptosis.

Alternatively, cytotoxic cells may interact with perforin, a membrane pore-forming molecule, to create pores in the target cell. Cytotoxic enzymes such as granzyme B and granulysin are transferred from the cytotoxic cell into the cytosol of the target cell, leading to cell death. In addition, granzyme B induces apoptosis by activating caspase 8, caspase 9, and caspase-activated DNAse (CAD), an endonuclease that cleaves DNA.

42. Which T-cell subset is associated with oral tolerance?
Another type of Th cell, known as Th3, is preferentially induced by chronic oral administration of low doses of antigens. These cells synthesize large amounts of transforming growth factor-β, produce IL-10, and induce oral tolerance.

43. Describe the structure of T-cell receptors.
T-cell receptors (TCRs) are composed of two polypeptide chains (α and β or γ and δ) that are associated with the CD3 complex. TCR α and β polypeptide chains are somatically assembled from variable, diversity, and joining gene peptides to produce mature VαJα and VβDβJβ chains. Each T cell expresses a single type of TCR, either $\alpha\beta$ (> 90%) or $\gamma\delta$. In normal subjects, cells bearing $\gamma\delta$ TCR rarely express either CD4 or CD8.

44. Describe the function of T-cell receptors.
$\alpha\beta$ T-cell receptors are members of the immunoglobulin supergene family and recognize peptide fragments that have been processed by antigen-presenting cells (APCs). The antigenic response to polysaccharide and lipid antigens was previously believed to be restricted to T-cell indepen-dent activation of B cells. However, some CD4-CD8-T cells—mostly $\gamma\delta$ T cells—recognize anti-gens in an MHC-independent manner by interacting with lipids bound to HLA-like CD1 molecules. (The CD1 molecule is composed of an α chain and a β chain; α1 and α2 domains form a binding groove for glycolipid antigens.) In addition, a subset of CD4-CD8-$\gamma\delta$ T cells rec-ognizes proteins encoded by MHC class I–related chains (MIC).

45. Why are T-cell receptors important for T-cell survival?
Signaling through the TCR is necessary for T-cell survival and proliferation. In the cortex of the thymus, most developing $\alpha\beta$ T cells are initially negative for both CD4 and CD8 (double nega-tive) and subsequently express both CD4 and CD8 (double positive). CD4+CD8+ cells are then tested by positive selection: those with TCRs that react with class I MHC molecules develop into CD8+ T cells, whereas those that react with class II MHC molecules develop into CD4+ T cells. Selection of CD4+ and CD8+ T cells is also dependent upon the tyrosine kinases Lck and

zeta-associated protein 70 (ZAP-70), respectively. These cells then move to the medulla prior to transport to the peripheral tissues. T cells that are unable to recognize self-MHC do not survive (death by neglect). Similarly, autoreactive T cells that display very high avidity for self-peptides are eliminated (negative selection). Some γδ T cells also differentiate in the thymus, but many are produced outside the thymus and reside in the GI tract.

46. **How do antigens presented to TCRs on CD4+ cells differ from those presented to CD8+ cells?**
Antigens presented to **CD4+** T cells originate extracellularly and include allergens such as pollens, molds, and house dust mites in addition to extracellular bacteria, bacterial toxins, fungi, and vaccines. These exogenous proteins are endocytosed by antigen-presenting cells, degraded into peptides by lysosomal enzymes, bound to MHC class II molecules in late endosomes, and transported to the cell surface, where the peptide-MHC class II molecule combination is recognized by specific αβ T cell receptors on the surface of CD4+ T cells.

In contrast, antigens presented to **CD8+** T cells usually originate in the cytoplasm. These endogenous antigens may include intracellular infectious agents, tumor-associated antigens, and transplantation antigens. Endogenous antigens are degraded by proteasome into peptide fragments that are transported into endoplasmic reticulum by the transporter-associated protein (TAP). Interaction with β2 microglobulin stabilizes this complex, which is then transported by the Golgi apparatus into exocytic vesicles for transport to the cell surface, where the combination is recognized by specific αβ TCRs on CD8+ T cells.

47. **What are the requirements for activation of T cells?**
In addition to antigen recognition by TCRs, activation of αβ T cells requires stimulation by IL-1 (produced by macrophages and other APCs) and a second or costimulatory signal provided by binding of the T cell ligand CD28 to B7.1 (CD80) or B7.2 (CD86) on the surface of APCs. Once fully differentiated, neither CD4+ nor CD8+ T cells require costimulatory signals to respond to antigen.

In the presence of a costimulatory signal, binding of the TCR to antigen-MHC complexes induces phosphorylation by receptor-associated kinases Lck and Fyn of immunoreceptor tyrosine-based activation motifs (ITAMs) in the cytoplasmic portions of each chain of the CD3 complex, which consists of a large intracytoplasmic homodimer containing two CD3ζ chains, single transmembrane CD3γ and CD3δ chains, and two transmembrane CD3ε chains. This triggers an intracellular signaling cascade involving the proteins LAT, SLP-76, and ZAP-70. These proteins activate protein kinase C, phospholipase C, the G proteins Ras and Rac, and MAPKs, leading to transcription of genes that regulate T cell differentiation and proliferation. This process can be downregulated by the protein-tyrosine phosphatase CD45, which dephosphorylates protein-tyrosine residues on Src-family protein-tyrosine kinases.

T-cell activation also promotes the synthesis of IL-2 and expression of high-affinity IL-2R, both of which are required for T-cell proliferation, thereby limiting the response to T cells specific for the stimulating antigen. Another costimulatory molecule, CD152 or CTLA-4, is expressed on the surface of T cells about 48 hours after activation. CD152 also binds to B7.1 or B7.2 on APCs but, in contrast to CD28, inhibits the immune response.

48. **Summarize the molecular basis of immune tolerance.**
Anergy results from presentation of antigen to T cells in the absence of costimulatory signals. Without IL-1, the immune response is impaired or tolerance develops. Tolerance may also be induced in stimulated T cells via soluble mediators from T cells (immune deviation) or direct cell-cell contact (suppression). Deletion of T cells via apoptosis occurs when activated T cells, which express Fas, bind to Fas ligand on APCs or other cells.

Rotrosen D, Matthews JB, Bluestone JA: The immune tolerance network: A new paradigm for developing tolerance-inducing therapies. J Allergy Clin Immunol 110:17–23, 2002.

49. **Define and provide an example of a superantigen.**

Superantigens are bacterial products that activate T cells by binding to APCs via the β1 chain of class II MHC molecules outside the antigen-binding groove and to TCRs via Vβ chains outside the antigen-binding site. Since superantigens bind to all Vβ chains of a particular subclass, they activate all members of that TCR Vβ family, which may comprise up to 20% or more of T cells. For example, Staphylococcus exotoxins can activate all T cells bearing Vβ2 and Vβ5.1 TCR chains, causing the release of large quantities of cytokines and producing toxic shock syndrome.

50. **How does glucocorticoid treatment modify T cells in patients with allergic asthma?**

Treatment of allergic asthma patients with corticosteroids markedly decreases pulmonary γδ T cells, probably due to steroid-induced apoptosis. Glucocorticoid therapy also decreases the proportion of bronchoalveolar lavage fluid cells expressing IL-4 and IL-5, and increases the cells expressing IFN-γ, suggesting a shift toward a Th1 response.

51. **Describe the appearance and function of NK cells.**

Natural killer (NK) cells, which represent CD56+ cytotoxic lymphocytes, mature in the bone marrow under the influence of IL-2 and IL-15. When activated, NK cells appear as large granular lymphocytes. NK cells lack antigen-specific receptors. They kill cells via antibody-dependent cell-mediated cytotoxicity in addition to Fas and perforin mechanisms. Surface receptors on NK cells inhibit cytotoxic activity against class I MHC bearing cells.

52. **What is the origin of mast cells?**

Mast cells are derived from CD34+ hematopoietic progenitor cells. Mast cell–committed progenitors expressing c-kit (the receptor for stem cell factor) migrate from the bone marrow to mucosal or connective tissue sites, where they expand and differentiate into mature mast cells under the influence of stem cell factor (SCF) produced by endothelial cells, fibroblasts, and other stromal cells. IL-5 enhances proliferation of mast cells induced by SCF.

53. **List the mediators produced by mast cells.**

See Table 2-2.

54. **Define proteoglycans and identify the classes present in mast cells.**

Proteoglycans are macromolecules composed of glycosaminoglycan (GAG) chains covalently linked to a protein core. The presence of acidic GAGs explains the affinity of mast cell and basophil granules for basic dyes such as toluidine blue, which leads to the metachromasia that characterizes these cells. Proteoglycans bind histamine, neutral proteases, and carboxypeptidases and may facilitate the packaging of these molecules within the secretory granules.

Mast cell granules contain two classes of proteoglycans, heparin and chondroitin sulfates. Within mature human pulmonary mast cells, the ratio of heparin to chondroitin is 2:1.

55. **Identify the major enzyme present in mast cell cytoplasmic granules.**

The major enzyme in the cytoplasmic granules is tryptase, a neutral protease stored in active form in association with heparin. Tryptase digests peptide and ester bonds on basic amino acids and accounts for the IgE-mediated kininogenase activity described in mast cells. Tryptase also functions as a growth factor for airway smooth muscle cells, epithelial cells, and fibroblasts. Tryptase has previously been considered to be present in human mast cells but not other cell types. Recent studies have also identified tryptase in basophils, with some cells containing levels similar to mast cells.

56. **Characterize serum tryptase isoenzyme levels in mastocytosis and allergic diseases.**

Two forms of tryptase have been identified in humans: α-tryptase and β-tryptase. α-Tryptase is released constitutively from mast cells and represents a measure of mast cell mass or hyperplasia.

TABLE 2-2. MEDIATORS PRODUCED BY MAST CELLS

Preformed Mediators	Newly Synthesized Mediators
Biogenic amines	Cyclooxygenase products
Histamine*	Prostaglandin D_2
Neutral proteases	Thromboxane A_2
Tryptase	Lipoxygenase products
Chymase	Leukotriene B_4
Carboxypeptidase A	Leukotrienes C_4, D_4, E_4
Cathepsin G	Platelet-activating factor
Hydrolases	Cytokines
Arylsulfatase	
β-Galactosidase	
β-Glucuronidase	
β-Hexosaminidase	
Proteoglycans	
Heparin	
Chondroitin sulfate	
Chemotactic factors†	
Neutrophil chemotactic factors	
Eosinophilic chemotactic factor of anaphylaxis	
Cytokines	
IL-4	
TNF-α	

*Histamine is responsible for many of the phenomena associated with the early-phase reaction.
†Mast cell chemotactic factors initiate the late-phase reaction associated with allergic inflammation.

In contrast, β-tryptase is stored in mast cell secretory granules and provides an indicator of mast cell activation. Accordingly, systemic mastocytosis and anaphylaxis may be associated with elevated levels of α-tryptase and β-tryptase, respectively. Peripheral blood tryptase levels are usually normal in patients with asthma and other allergic disorders.

57. **Explain the characteristics of MC_T and MC_{TC} mast cells.**
Mast cells have been subdivided into MC_T and MC_{TC} cells based on their neutral protease content. MC_T cells contain tryptase but not chymase, whereas MC_{TC} cells contain both tryptase and chymase. In addition, MC_{TC} cells contain carboxypeptidase and cathepsin G.

    MC_T cells appear to play a major role in host defenses and constitute >90% of the mast cells present in the alveoli, airway epithelium, and airway lumen. MC_{TC} mast cells are located in the submucosa of the respiratory tract and appear to be primarily involved with angiogenesis and tissue remodeling. MC_{TC} cells are also the predominant mast cells in skin, synovium, and gastrointestinal submucosa.

58. **Describe the stimuli that activate mast cells.**
Activation of mast cells is triggered by linking of adjacent FcεRI receptor-bound IgE molecules by bivalent or multivalent antigens or by antibodies directed against either IgE or its receptor,

resulting in the rapid release of preformed mediators and the synthesis of newly generated mediators.

Mast cells may also be activated by various biologic, chemical, and physical stimuli. For MC_{TC} cells, these stimuli include complement fragments C3a and C5a (anaphylatoxins), basic polypeptides (polyarginine and polylysine), peptide hormones, substance P, radiocontrast media, calcium ionophores, drugs (opiates and muscle relaxants), melittin in bee venom, and cold. Among these nonimmunologic stimuli, only calcium ionophores activate human lung mast cells.

59. **What is the least common granulocyte?**
Basophils represent the least common type of granulocyte, constituting < 1% of peripheral blood leukocytes.

60. **Compare mast cells and basophils.**
Like mast cells, basophils are derived from CD34+ progenitor cells, express FcεRI surface receptors, release histamine and Th2 cytokines, and exhibit metachromatic staining. However, basophils differentiate and mature in the bone marrow under the influence of interleukin-3 and circulate in the blood, rather than residing in the tissues.

Also in common with mast cells, basophils store histamine, neutrophil chemotactic factor, and other preformed mediators in secretory granules. The predominant proteoglycan in human basophils is chondroitin sulfate A. Basophils also contain small amounts of Charcot-Leyden crystal protein and major basic protein. Following FcεRI-dependent activation, mature human basophils release IL-4 and IL-13. Activated basophils also generate LTC_4, LTD_4, LTE_4, and PAF. In contrast to mast cells, basophils typically contain negligible or undetectable amounts of tryptase, chymase, carboxypeptidase, and cathepsin G and do not produce LTB_4, PGD_2, or IL-5. However, basophils in some humans have been reported to contain tryptase in levels that approach those in mast cells.

Schroeder JT, MacGlashan DW: New concepts: The basophil. J Allergy Clin Immunol 99: 429–433, 1997.

61. **Identify the eosinophil progenitor cell.**
Eosinophils are produced in the bone marrow from a CD34+ progenitor cell capable of differentiating into basophils and eosinophils. Increased numbers of circulating CD34+ eosinophil-basophil progenitor cells expressing the IL-5 receptor have been identified in atopic subjects.

62. **How do cytokines regulate eosinophilopoiesis?**
Eosinophils differentiate in the bone marrow under the influence of multiple cytokines, including IL-3, IL-5, and granulocyte-macrophage colony-stimulatory factor (GM-CSF), until they mature and are indistinguishable from eosinophils in the peripheral circulation. IL-5 is relatively specific for eosinophils and induces eosinophil-basophil progenitors to differentiate into eosinophils; IL-3 and GM-CSF stimulate eosinophils, basophils, and neutrophils. In contrast, TGF-β and IFN-α inhibit eosinophil proliferation and differentiation.

63. **Discuss the kinetics of the eosinophil life cycle.**
After circulating in the peripheral blood for a short time (average half-life 8–18 hours), eosinophils migrate by diapedesis at endothelial intercellular junctions into epithelial tissues such as the skin, lungs, and gastrointestinal tract, where they are exposed to the external environment. Following migration, most eosinophils remain in the tissues, where their life span typically ranges from 2 to 5 days. IL-3, IL-5, GM-CSF, and TNF-α may prolong eosinophil survival by inhibiting programmed cell death (apoptosis).

Gleich GJ: Mechanisms of eosinophil-associated inflammation. J Allergy Clin Immunol 105:651–663, 2000.

64. **Describe cell adhesion molecules and their role in eosinophil migration.**
Cell adhesion molecules (CAMs) are surface proteins essential for the recruitment of eosinophils and other leukocytes from the circulation to sites of inflammation. Subdivided into discrete groups, including selectins, integrins, and members of the immunoglobulin superfamily, CAMs regulate both cell-cell and cell-extracellular matrix protein interactions. This process occurs in sequential stages: leukocyte rolling and endothelial attachment, activation, firm adhesion, and migration.

Panettieri RA Jr: Cellular and molecular mechanisms regulating airway smooth muscle proliferation and cell adhesion molecule expression. Am J Respir Crit Care Med 158:S133–S140, 1998.

KEY POINTS: MAST CELLS, BASOPHILS, AND CAMs

1. Shared characteristics of mast cells and basophils include derivation from CD34+ progenitor cells, expression of FcεRI surface receptors, release of histamine and Th2 cytokines, and metachromatic staining.

2. The major enzyme in the cytoplasmic granules of mast cells is tryptase: α-tryptase is released constitutively and represents a measure of mast cell mass, whereas β-tryptase is stored in secretory granules and provides an indicator of mast cell activation.

3. Cell adhesion molecules (CAMs), including selectins, integrins, and members of the immunoglobulin superfamily, are surface proteins essential for the recruitment of eosinophils and other leukocytes from the circulation to sites of inflammation.

65. **What is the role of selectins?**
Leukocyte rolling and the initial loose binding to vascular endothelium are mediated primarily by the three selectin glycoproteins: L-selectin is expressed exclusively on the surface of leukocytes; E-selectin is expressed on activated endothelial cells; and P-selectin is present on platelets and endothelial cells. Eosinophils express P-selectin glycoprotein ligand I (PSGL-1), which binds to P-selectin on endothelial cells. Through the combined effects of the cell adhesion molecules PSGL-1/P-selectin and VLA-4/VCAM-1 (see below), eosinophils are tethered to endothelial cells, a requirement for migration into tissues.

66. **Describe the structure and function of integrins.**
Firm adhesion and migration of eosinophils are regulated by integrins and members of the immunoglobulin superfamily. Integrins, glycoproteins composed of noncovalently associated α- and β-subunits, are constitutively expressed on the surface of leukocytes, endothelial cells, and some other cells.

β_1-Integrins, the largest subfamily, represent a group of cellular receptors for extracellular matrix proteins such as collagen, fibronectin, and laminin. The β_1-integrin very late activation antigen-4 (VLA-4) is expressed on eosinophils, basophils, lymphocytes, and monocytes, but lacking on neutrophils. Increased numbers of eosinophils bearing VLA-4 have been reported in sputum from asthmatic patients.

β_2-Integrins are composed of a β subunit called CD18 paired with one of four α subunits (CD11a-CD-11d). Expression of β_2-integrins is limited to leukocytes. Activated eosinophils express the β_2-integrins leukocyte function-associated antigen-1 (LFA-1) and macrophage-1 antigen (Mac-1). Like VLA-4, these integrins are important for the firm adhesion of eosinophils to endothelial cells and their subsequent migration into the tissues.

67. **What are the ligands for integrins?**
    The ligands for integrins include cell surface molecules that are members of the immunoglobulin supergene family, such as intercellular adhesion molecules-1, 2, 3 (ICAM-1, 2, and 3) and vascular cell adhesion molecule-1 (VCAM-1). These proteins are constitutively expressed on endothelial cells, neutrophils, and lymphocytes, among other cells. VCAM-1 binds to VLA-4, promoting adhesion of eosinophils, basophils, lymphocytes, and monocytes, whereas ICAM-1 binds to LFA-1 and Mac-1, enhancing adhesion of eosinophils and neutrophils.

68. **How do cytokines modulate eosinophil recruitment?**
    Proinflammatory cytokines such as IFN-γ, IL-1β, and TNF-α augment the expression of ICAM-1 and VCAM-1, and the Th2 cytokines IL-4 and IL-13 upregulate the expression of VCAM-1 on endothelial cells. This promotes VLA-4/VCAM-1-mediated adherence of eosinophils. Moreover, IL-5 selectively promotes adhesion of eosinophils—the only peripheral blood leukocytes with IL-5 receptors—to unstimulated endothelial cells.

69. **Explain the classification and function of chemokines.**
    Chemokines are cytokines with chemotactic activity. These structurally related proteins are sub-divided into four groups based on the number and appearance of conserved cysteine residues in the primary sequence.
    The two groups that include most identified chemokines are classified on the basis of the position of the first two of these cysteine residues into CC (containing adjacent cysteines) or CXC (containing another amino acid positioned between cysteine residues) subfamilies. The CC subset displays chemotactic activity for eosinophils, T lymphocytes, and monocytes, but not neutrophils. Members of this group include eotaxin (CCL11), macrophage inflammatory protein-1α (MIP-1α or CCL3), monocyte chemotactic protein-1 (MCP-1 or CCL2), and RANTES (regulated activation, normal T cell expressed and excreted, or CCL5). Increased levels of these chemokines have been described in BAL and biopsies from asthmatic patients. Eotaxin and RANTES are especially potent inducers of eosinophil migration. MCP-1 facilitates recruitment of Th1 cells, whereas RANTES promotes recruitment of Th2 cells. Th1 cells selectively express CXCR3; Th2 cells selectively express CCR3, CCR4, and CCR8. The CXC subfamily exerts chemotactic activity primarily toward neutrophils, although its member IL-8 (CXCL8) also expresses chemotactic activity toward activated eosinophils.
    A recently described chemokine subset lacks the first and third cysteine residues and is known as the C subfamily. This group includes the lymphocyte-specific chemotactic peptide XCL1 (lymphotactin). Another chemokine subfamily, known as CX3C, contains three variable amino acids between the two N-terminal cysteine residues.

70. **Describe the intracellular events that follow binding of a chemokine to its receptor.**
    Chemokines regulate activity through interactions with members of the G-protein-coupled receptor superfamily. After binding of a chemokine to its receptor, guanine triphosphate (GTP) associates with the Gα receptor subunit, which leads to disassociation of the G-protein complex from the receptor and separation into Gα and G$\beta\gamma$ subunits. The Gα subunit activates the Src-family tyrosine kinases, which trigger activation of mitogen-activated protein kinases (MAPKs) and protein kinase B (PKB). The G$\beta\gamma$ subunit activates MAPK and PKB through phosphatidylinositol 3 kinase (PI3Kγ), and activates protein kinase C (PKC) through phospholipase C (PLC). Activation of PLC causes influx of calcium and initiates many processes, including degranulation of eosinophils, basophils, and neutrophils.

Nickel R, Beck LA, Stellato C, Schleimer RP: Chemokines and allergic diseases. J Allergy Clin Immunol 104:723–742, 1999.

71. **List other mediators of eosinophil chemotaxis.**
    - Histamine
    - LTD_4 (chemotactic for eosinophils, but not neutrophils)
    - Platelet-activating factor (PAF)
    - Platelet factor 4 (PF4)
    - Anaphylatoxins C3a and C5a
    - Cytokines GM-CSF, IL-2, IL-3, IL-4, and IL-5

72. **Describe the surface receptors on eosinophils.**
    Human peripheral blood eosinophils express receptors for the Fc portion of IgG (FcγRII or CD32), IgA (FcαR), and IgE (FcϵRI and FcϵRII). Fcγ receptors mediate ADCC, degranulation, and phagocytosis. Increased numbers of Fcα receptors have been reported on eosinophils from patients with atopic diseases. Fcϵ receptors mediate killing of schistosomula.
    Surface receptors for cytokines (IL-3R, IL-5R, and GM-CSFR), complement (C3aR, C5aR, C3bR or CR1), chemokines (CCR1 and CCR3), cell adhesion molecules (VLA-4 and α 4 β7 integrin), and CD69 (a marker for eosinophil activation) have also been described.

73. **Characterize eosinophil secretory granules.**
    Eosinophils contain two principal types of secretory granules: specific granules and small granules. Specific secretory granules represent the primary source of major basic protein (MBP), localized to the crystalloid core of the granules, and eosinophil cationic protein (ECP), eosinophil-derived neurotoxin (EDN), eosinophil peroxidase (EPO), and β-glucuronidase, all identified within the matrix of the specific granules. Small secretory granules contain acid phosphatase and arylsulfatase B, among other enzymes. Eosinophils also contain lysophospholipase, neutrophil elastase, and collagenase.

74. **Which protein causes the distinctive staining of eosinophils?**
    Major basic protein binds to acid aniline dyes such as eosin, which stains the granules red.

75. **Define Charcot-Leyden crystals.**
    Charcot-Leyden crystals are hexagonal bipyramidal crystals identified in the sputum of patients with asthma. (They have also been found in cervical smears and elsewhere.) Charcot-Leyden crystal protein is present within eosinophils and basophils and possesses lysophospholipase activity.

76. **Discuss the biologic effects of the major eosinophil peptides.**
    MBP neutralizes heparin and induces the release of histamine from human basophils, lysozyme and superoxide from neutrophils, and serotonin (5-hydroxytryptamine) from platelets. MBP causes bronchoconstriction, impairs ciliary function, induces exfoliation of respiratory epithelial cells, and increases airway responsiveness. ECP neutralizes heparin and kills schistosomula and other parasites. Like MBP, this protein is toxic to airway epithelial cells. EDN damages myelinated neurons. EPO and hydrogen peroxide (H_2O_2), in the presence of halide, kill a variety of microorganisms (including bacteria and protozoa) and tumor cells. In addition, EPO with H_2O_2 and halide trigger mast cell degranulation in an animal model. EPO also releases serotonin from platelets.

77. **Describe the eicosanoids synthesized by eosinophils and their relevance to asthma.**
    Eosinophils represent a major source of LTC_4, the most prevalent lipoxygenase metabolite produced by eosinophils, and its active metabolites LTD_4 and LTE_4, but synthesize only small amounts of LTB_4. Eosinophils also produce the 5-lipoxygenase metabolite 5-HETE. These mediators induce bronchoconstriction, mucus secretion, increased vascular permeability, and chemotaxis of eosinophils and neutrophils.

78. Which cytokines do eosinophils synthesize?

Eosinophils produce a variety of cytokines, including autocrine cytokines, such as IL-3, IL-5, and GM-CSF, which act upon eosinophils themselves. Eosinophils also have the capacity to synthesize IL-1, IL-4, IL-6, IL-8, IL-10, IL-16, MIP-1α, RANTES, TNF-α, TGF-α, and TGF-β1.

79. Summarize the stimuli that induce degranulation/activation of eosinophils.

Degranulation of eosinophils may be triggered by secretory IgA (sIgA), IgA, IgG, IgE, RANTES, MIP-1α, PAF, C3a, C5a, substance P, melittin, and β-integrin ligands. Among immunoglobulins, sIgA is the most potent mediator of degranulation. MBP and EPO also induce eosinophil degranulation, suggesting the presence of an autocrine degranulation pathway. Eosinophils may also be activated by cytokines, including IL-1, IL-3, IL-4, IL-5, GM-CSF, TNF-α, and IFN-γ.

80. What is the population of eosinophils of abnormal density identified in some diseases?

Analysis of circulating eosinophils in patients with eosinophilia has demonstrated a population of eosinophils of lower density than normal. Called hypodense eosinophils, these cells have been identified in subjects with parasitic infections, allergic diseases, and idiopathic hypereosinophilic syndrome. They are believed to represent primed or partially activated eosinophils.

81. Describe the kinetics and CAMs of neutrophil migration.

After release from the bone marrow, neutrophils circulate in the blood for 6–8 hours prior to being sequestered through margination, primarily in the lung capillaries. Migration of neutrophils from blood vessels into tissues requires the expression of cell adhesion molecules. Neutrophils express several adhesion proteins, including the integrins Mac-1 (important for binding to fibrinogen and degranulation) and LFA-1 (important for migration into tissues).

82. Which neutrophil products may contribute to allergic inflammation?

Neutrophils recruited to sites of allergic inflammation generate a number of molecules that may induce tissue damage, including collagenase, elastase, oxygen radicals, LTB$_4$, PAF, and thromboxane A$_2$(TXA$_2$). In contrast to mast cells and eosinophils, neutrophils produce little LTC$_4$.

83. What evidence supports a pathogenic role for neutrophils in asthma?

Both PAF and LTB$_4$ have been identified in human airways following allergen challenge, consistent with neutrophil activation. Increased neutrophils have been reported in sputum during exacerbations of asthma. In patients who died from an acute asthma attack, neutrophils comprised the majority of cells infiltrating the airways, whereas in patients who died from hours to days after an asthma flare, most infiltrating cells were eosinophils.

84. Describe the kinetics of the monocyte life cycle.

Progenitors of monocytes/macrophages differentiate in the bone marrow over a period of about 6 days to form monocytes, which are released into the peripheral blood and circulate with a half-life of approximately 3 days. These cells then migrate into tissues such as the lungs and differentiate into macrophages, which have a life span that ranges from days to months. Monocytes may also differentiate under the influence of local tissue factors into dendritic cells, which display MHC class II antigens and are found in the lungs and other tissues.

Vignola AM, Gjomarkaj M, Arnoux B, Bousquet J: Monocytes. J Allergy Clin Immunol 101:149–152, 1998.

85. Which mediators influence the production of monocytes?

Monocyte production is stimulated by GM-CSF, IL-3, and macrophage-colony-stimulating factor (M-CSF) but inhibited by interferon-α/β and PGE$_2$.

86. **What is the role of monocytes and macrophages in generating an immune response?**

The monocyte-macrophage system—consisting of monocytes in the circulation and macrophages in tissues—plays a key role in generating the immune response by presenting antigen to lymphocytes, as described above. In addition, monocytes are the primary source of IL-12, which acts on T cells and natural killer (NK) cells to induce the production of IFN-γ, thereby promoting the Th1 pattern of differentiation. In contrast, IL-10 secreted by monocytes inhibits the synthesis of IFN-γ, which may counterbalance the effects of IL-12. Monocytes also produce the cytokines IL-1 and TNF-α; chemokines MIP-1α, monocyte chemotactic proteins (MCPs), and RANTES; proinflammatory arachidonic acid metabolites PGD_2, LTB_4, and LTC_4; and PAF.

87. **Identify the major antigen-presenting cells in the lungs.**

Pulmonary dendritic cells are the primary antigen-presenting cells in the lungs. Although alveolar macrophages demonstrate potent phagocytic and antimicrobial properties, they are weak activators of T cells. In fact, alveolar macrophages may function as suppressors rather than inducers of the immune response.

88. **Explain mechanisms by which macrophages may induce airway damage in asthma.**

Macrophages represent potential inducers of airway damage through production of nitric oxide (NO), which may be triggered by either allergic or infectious processes. NO reacts with superoxide anions to form toxic hydroxyl radicals. Alveolar macrophages also synthesize fibroblast growth factors, platelet-derived growth factor, and transforming growth factor-β, which may contribute to irreversible airway remodeling in asthma.

89. **Describe the structure of platelets.**

Platelets contain three types of secretory granules: alpha granules, dense granules, and lysosomes. Alpha granules, the most numerous, contain fibronectin, fibrinogen, platelet factor 4, and β-thromboglobulin. Dense granules contain adenosine diphosphate (ADP), serotonin, calcium, and pyrophosphate. Lysosomes contain acid hydrolases. Resting platelets possess surface receptors for platelet agonists, collagen (gpIa/IIa), and fibrinogen/von Willebrand factor (gpIIb/IIIa).

90. **Which stimuli induce platelet aggregation and activation?**

Platelet aggregation occurs through platelet-platelet interaction and adhesion to fibrinogen, which induces the release of the contents of alpha granules and dense granules. Platelet activation may result from adhesion or soluble agonists such as ADP, epinephrine, serotonin, thrombin, substance P, C-reactive protein, complement components, eosinophil-derived MBP, interferon, and TNF. In addition, platelets possess FcϵRII receptors and are activated by aggregation of these receptors following binding of specific allergen or anti-IgE antibody.

91. **List the mediators released by activated platelets.**

- Adenosine
- β-thromboglobulin
- Factor D
- Free radicals
- 12-HETE
- Histamine
- Histamine releasing factor (HRF)
- Nitric oxide
- PAF
- Platelet-derived growth factor (PDGF)
- Platelet factor 4
- RANTES
- Thromboxane A_2
- Transforming growth factor-β

92. **How is histamine synthesized and metabolized?**

Histamine is synthesized in the Golgi apparatus of mast cells and basophils by decarboxylation of histidine and associates with the acidic residues of the glycosaminoglycan (GAG) side chains of heparin and other proteoglycans. Human mast cells contain 3–6 pg histamine per cell and secrete histamine spontaneously at low levels, producing a normal plasma level of 0.5 to 2 nm. Histamine is rapidly metabolized (usually within 1 or 2 minutes) following extracellular release by either of two mechanisms, methylation by histamine-N-methyltransferase or oxidation by diamine oxidase (histaminase).

93. **Describe the biologic effects mediated by histamine.**
The biologic effects of histamine are mediated by activation of specific cell surface receptors, of which 3 subtypes have been identified. Binding of histamine to H_1-receptors induces contraction of airway and gastrointestinal smooth muscle, mucus secretion, and increased vascular permeability. Stimulation of H_2-receptors inhibits T cell cytotoxicity, IFN-γ production, and release of lysozyme, but increases suppressor T cell activity, expression of complement receptors for C3b (CR1) on human eosinophils, and eosinophil and neutrophil chemokinesis. H_3-receptors are located presynaptically on histaminergic nerves and function as autoreceptors that regulate the synthesis and release of histamine from neurons.

94. **How is arachidonic acid converted to prostaglandins and thromboxane?**
Cyclooxygenase converts arachidonic acid to the intermediate compounds prostaglandin G_2 (PGG_2) and prostaglandin H_2 (PGH_2). PGH_2 is converted to the biologically active prostaglandins PGD_2, PGE_2, and $PGF_{2\alpha}$ by prostaglandin synthases and isomerases, to prostacyclin (PGI_2) by prostacyclin synthase, and to TXA_2 by thromboxane synthase.

95. **Explain the differences between the isoenzymes cyclooxygenase-1 (COX-1) and cyclooxygenase-2 (COX-2).**
COX-1, present in most types of cells, is a constitutive isoenzyme that exerts cytoprotective effects on the gastric mucosa, regulates renal blood flow, and decreases platelet aggregation. In contrast, COX-2, present in mast cells, macrophages, and leukocytes, is an inducible enzyme activated by proinflammatory mediators.

96. **What are the biologic effects of cyclooxygenase metabolites?**
PGD_2, the major cyclooxygenase product generated by human pulmonary mast cells, is 30 times as potent a bronchoconstrictor as histamine in patients with mild allergic asthma. PGD_2 also induces pulmonary and coronary artery vasoconstriction and peripheral vasodilatation, mediates neutrophil chemotaxis, and decreases platelet aggregation. $PGF_{2\alpha}$, a metabolite of PGD_2, exerts similar effects on the airways and blood vessels. TXA_2 mediates vasoconstriction, increases platelet aggregation, and may represent a more potent bronchoconstrictor than PGD_2. In contrast, PGE_2 and prostacyclin induce bronchodilatation.

97. **Describe the lipoxygenase pathway of arachidonic acid metabolism.**
Metabolism of arachidonic acid by lipoxygenase yields unstable hydroperoxyeicosatetraenoic acids (HPETEs). 5-Lipoxygenase converts arachidonic acid to 5-HPETE and then to 5-HETE or leukotriene A_4 (LTA_4). In turn, LTA_4 may be metabolized to LTB_4 or LTC_4. Sequential amino acid cleavage from LTC_4 yields LTD_4 and LTE_4. Collectively known as cysteinyl-leukotrienes (cys-LTs), LTC_4, LTD_4, and LTE_4 comprise the major lipoxygenase products synthesized by mast cells. An alternative metabolic pathway catalyzed by 15-lipoxygenase produces 15-HETE from arachidonic acid but appears to be of lesser importance in mediating allergic reactions.

98. **Explain the relevance of these mediators to allergic diseases.**
Cysteinyl-leukotrienes exert potent bronchoconstrictor effects that are up to 1,000 times more potent than histamine and 100 times more potent than prostaglandins. In addition, cys-LTs increase postcapillary venule permeability, augment bronchial mucus secretion, and attract eosinophils.

LTB$_4$ possesses potent chemotactic activity for neutrophils, eosinophils, monocytes, lymphocytes, and fibroblasts—cells responsible for the late phase response and tissue remodeling. LTB$_4$ also increases vascular permeability and may enhance production of IgE and cytokines.

99. **Bronchoalveolar lavage fluid obtained during the late-phase allergic reaction has been reported to contain cys-LTs without PGD$_2$ or tryptase. What does this finding imply?**
    This finding suggests that the cys-LTs present at this stage are derived from eosinophils or basophils rather than mast cells.

100. **Describe the synthesis and actions of platelet-activating factor (PAF).**
    Platelet-activating factor is an ether-linked phospholipid (alkylacetyl-glycerylether-phosphorylcholine) produced in a two-stage reaction during which phospholipase A$_2$ hydrolyzes membrane phospholipid to form lyso-PAF. Acetylation of lyso-PAF yields PAF, which is inactivated by conversion back to lyso-PAF. Figure 2-2 summarizes the characteristics of PAF and eicosanoid generation.
    Platelet-activating factor is synthesized by activated human lung mast cells, eosinophils, neutrophils, mononuclear phagocytes, platelets, endothelial cells, and epithelial cells. Biologic effects of PAF include platelet aggregation, bronchoconstriction, increased vascular permeability, and chemotaxis for eosinophils and neutrophils.

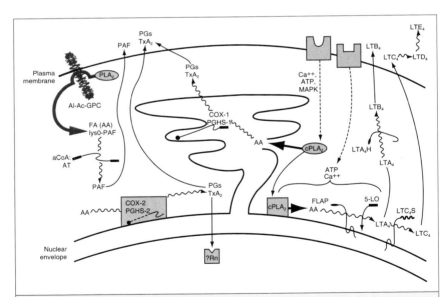

Figure 2-2. Cellular and enzymatic characteristics of eicosanoid and platelet-activating factor (PAF) generation. PGs = protaglandins, TxA$_2$ = thromboxane A$_2$, COX = cyclooxygenase, PGHS = prostaglandin H synthase, LTB$_4$ = leukotriene B$_4$, AA = arachidonic acid, cPLA$_2$ = cytoplasmic phospholipase A$_2$, FA = fatty acid, aCoA = acetyl coenzyme A, AT = acetyltransferase, Al-Ac-GPC = alkyl-acyl-glycerophosphorylcholine, ATP = adenosine triphosphate, MAPK = mitogen-activated protein kinase, FLAP = 5-lipoxygenase-activating protein, Rn = nuclear receptor, thin arrow = intracellular redistribution or secretion, thick arrow = release of AA or PAF precursor, dashed arrow = stimulation by a plasma membrane receptor, wavy arrow = enzymatic conversion. (From Goetzl EJ: Lipid mediators of hypersensitivity and inflammation. In Adkinson NF Jr, Yuninger JW, Busse WW, et al (eds): Middleton's Allergy: Principles and Practice, vol. 1, 6th ed. St. Louis, Mosby, 2003, Fig. 14-1, p 214, with permission.)

101. **How do kinins mediate allergic disorders?**

Kinins are potent vasoactive peptides produced in tissues and airway secretions in patients with inflammatory airway diseases, including allergic rhinitis, viral rhinitis, and asthma. The non-apeptide bradykinin is generated from high-molecular-weight kininogens in plasma by kinino-genases, including kallikrein and tryptase. In the upper airways, kinins stimulate submucosal glands, increase vascular permeability, and activate sensory nerves, producing symptoms of rhinitis such as rhinorrhea, nasal congestion, and pruritus. In the lower airways, kinins induce bronchoconstriction by stimulation of sensory nerve-parasympathetic bronchoconstrictor reflexes and release of neuropeptides, including tachykinins, from sensory nerves.

102. **Describe tachykinins and their effects.**

Tachykinins are peptides with rapid onset of action located in neuronal endings within the skin, mucosa, and viscera, where they may induce vasodilatation, increase vascular permeability, attract inflammatory cells, and produce pain. The tachykinins identified within the mammalian nervous system are substance P, neurokinin A (NKA), neurokinin B (NKB), neuropeptide K (NPK), and neuropeptide (NP).

103. **Define cytokines.**

Cytokines may be defined as low-molecular-weight proteins that regulate immune and inflam-matory responses. They are secreted by lymphocytes, mast cells, macrophages, and airway cells, among others. This diverse group of glycoproteins can modulate both nonspecific inflam-matory and specific immune effects on target cells and may contribute to tissue remodeling in chronic asthma.

104. **Describe the actions of cytokines relevant to allergic and immune responses.**

See Table 2-3.

TABLE 2-3.	ACTIONS OF CYTOKINES RELEVANT TO ALLERGIC AND IMMUNE RESPONSES
Cytokine	**Effects**
GM-CSF	Secreted by activated macrophages, T cells, mast cells, eosinophils, and other cells
	Promotes differentiation of neutrophils and macrophages
	Activates mature eosinophils
	Prolongs eosinophil survival
IFN-γ	Derived mainly from Th1 lymphocytes, cytotoxic T cells, NK cells, but also macrophages
	Represents the most important cytokine activator of macrophages
	Increases expression of class I and II MHC antigens
	Stimulates B cell proliferation and differentiation
	Inhibits IL-4-induced IgE synthesis
	Inhibits Th2 lymphocytes
	Induces ICAM-1 expression
IL-1	IL-1 family contains IL-1α, IL-1β, the IL-1 receptor antagonist (IL-Ira), and IL-18

(continued)

TABLE 2–3.	ACTIONS OF CYTOKINES RELEVANT TO ALLERGIC AND IMMUNE RESPONSES *(continued)*
Cytokine	Effects
	Produced mainly by monocytes and macrophages, but also by lymphocytes and other cells
	Induced by endotoxin, microorganisms, antigens, and cytokines
	Increases proliferation of B cells and antibody synthesis
	Promotes growth of Th cells in response to APCs
	Stimulates production of T cell cytokines and IL-2 receptors
	Without IL-1, tolerance develops or immune response is impaired
	Promotes formation of arachidonic acid metabolites, including PGE_2 and LTB_4
	Induces proliferation of fibroblasts and synthesis of fibronectin and collagen
	Increases ICAM-1, VCAM-1, E-selectin, and P-selectin expression
	IL-1 receptor antagonist (IL-1ra) antagonizes proinflammatory effects of IL-1
IL-2	Induces clonal T cell proliferation
	Enhances proliferation of cytotoxic T cells, B cells, NK cells, macrophages
IL-3	Derived primarily from Th cells, but also from mast cells and eosinophils
	Stimulates development of mast cells, lymphocytes, macrophages
	Activates eosinophils
	Prolongs eosinophil survival
IL-4	Preformed peptide in mast cells and eosinophils
	Also secreted by Th2 cells, cytotoxic T cells, and basophils
	Promotes growth of Th2 cells, cytotoxic T cells, mast cells, eosinophils, basophils
	Initiates IgE isotype switching
	Upregulates expression of high- and low-affinity IgE receptors
	Increases expression of class I and II MHC antigens on macrophages
	Stimulates VCAM-1 expression
IL-5	Produced by Th2 cells and mast cells
	Attracts eosinophils
	Activates eosinophils
	Prolongs eosinophil survival
IL-6	Synthesized primarily by monocytes and macrophages, but also by T, B, and other cells
	Mediates T cell activation, growth, differentiation
	Induces B cell differentiation into plasma cells
	Inhibits TNF and IL-1 synthesis and stimulates IL-Ira synthesis
IL-7	Necessary for development of B and T cells
	Enhances growth of cytotoxic T and NK cells
	Increases tumor killing by monocytes and macrophages

TABLE 2–3.	ACTIONS OF CYTOKINES RELEVANT TO ALLERGIC AND IMMUNE RESPONSES *(continued)*
Cytokine	**Effects**
IL-8	Produced mainly by monocytes, phagocytes, and endothelial cells
	Exerts potent chemoattraction for neutrophils
	Attracts activated eosinophils
	Induces neutrophil degranulation and activation
	Inhibits IL-4-mediated IgE synthesis
IL-9	Produced by Th2 cells
	Promotes mast cell and T cell proliferation
	Stimulates IgE synthesis
	Produces eosinophilia
	Induces bronchial hyperreactivity
IL-10	Secreted primarily by monocytes and B cells
	Inhibits monocyte/macrophage function
	Stimulates growth of mast cells, B cells, and cytotoxic T cells
	Induces permanent tolerance in Th lymphocytes
	Decreases synthesis of IFN-γ and IL-2 by Th1 cells
	Inhibits IL-4-induced IgE synthesis and promotes IgG4 production
	Decreases eosinophil survival
IL-11	Produced in response to respiratory viral infections
	Promotes generation of mast cells and B cells
	Induces bronchial hyperreactivity
IL-12	Synthesized by monocytes/macrophages, dendritic cells, B cells, neutrophils, mast cells
	Induced by IFN-γ and microorganisms
	Promotes Th1 and inhibits Th2 cell development
	Inhibits IL-4 induced IgE synthesis
	Enhances activity of cytotoxic T cells and NK cells
IL-13	Produced by Th1 and Th2 cells, mast cells, and dendritic cells
	Exerts effects similar to IL-4 on B cells and macrophages but does not affect T cells
	Induces IgE isotype switching
	Increases VCAM-1 expression
	Promotes airway hyperreactivity and mucus hypersecretion
	Suppresses production of proinflammatory cytokines and chemokines
	Decreases synthesis of nitric oxide
IL-16	Secreted by CD8+ T cells, eosinophils, mast cells, and epithelial cells
	Promotes growth of CD4+ T cells
	Provides major source of CD4+ T cell chemotactic activity after antigen challenge
	Induces IL-2 receptors and class II MHC expression on CD4+ T cells

(continued)

TABLE 2-3. ACTIONS OF CYTOKINES RELEVANT TO ALLERGIC AND IMMUNE RESPONSES *(continued)*

Cytokine	Effects
IL-18	Produced by lung, liver, and other tissues, but not by lymphocytes
	Stimulates secretion of IFN-γ and GM-CSF
	Enhances IgE synthesis
	Promotes Th1 responses and activates NK cells (similar to IL-12)
	Induces synthesis of TNF, IL-1, Fas ligand
	Decreases IL-10 synthesis
IL-23	Induces secretion of IFN-γ
TGF-α	Synthesized by macrophages and keratinocytes
	Stimulates proliferation of fibroblasts
	Promotes angiogenesis
TGF-β	Secreted by platelets, monocytes, some T cells (Th3), and fibroblasts
	Stimulates monocytes and fibroblasts, inducing fibrosis and extracellular matrix formation
	Attracts mast cells, macrophages, fibroblasts
	Inhibits B cells, T helper cells, cytotoxic T cells, NK cells, mast cells
	Induces IgA isotype switching and secretory IgA synthesis in gut lymphoid tissue
	Inhibits airway smooth muscle cell proliferation
TNF-α	Produced primarily by mononuclear phagocytes; stored preformed in mast cells
	Induced by endotoxin, GM-CSF, IFN-γ, IL-1, and IL-3
	Binds to cell surface receptors TNFR I and TNFR II
	Enhances class I and II MHC expression
	Activates neutrophils, modulating adherence, chemotaxis, degranulation, respiratory burst
	Increases cytokine production by monocytes and airway epithelial cells
	Promotes ICAM-1, VCAM-1, and E-selectin expression
	Stimulates COX-2 expression in airway smooth muscle
	Induces bronchial hyperreactivity
	Mediates toxic shock and sepsis
	Produces cachexia associated with chronic infection and cancer
TNF-β	Synthesized primarily by lymphocytes
	Binds to cell surface receptors TNFR I and TNFR II
	Mediates functions similar to TNF-α

WEBSITE

American College of Allergy, Asthma and Immunology: www.acaai.org

BIBLIOGRAPHY

1. Barnes PJ, Chung KF, Page CP: Inflammatory mediators of asthma: An update. Pharmacol Rev 50:515–596, 1998.

2. Boyce JA. Mast cells: Beyond IgE. J Allergy Clin Immunol 111:24–32, 2003.

3. Busse WW: Respiratory infections: Their role in airway responsiveness and the pathogenesis of asthma. J Allergy Clin Immunol 85:671–683, 1990.

4. Church MK, Levi-Schaffer F: The human mast cell. J Allergy Clin Immunol 99:155–160, 1997.

5. Costa JJ, Weller PF, Galli SJ: The cells of the allergic response: Mast cells, basophils, and eosinophils. JAMA 278:1815–1822, 1997.

6. Escoubet-Lozach L, Glass CK, Wasserman SI: The role of transcription factors in allergic inflammation. J Allergy Clin Immunol 110:553–564, 2002.

7. Gleich GJ: Mechanisms of eosinophil-associated inflammation. J Allergy Clin Immunol 105:651–663, 2000.

8. Hamid QA, Minshall EM: Molecular pathology of allergic disease. I: Lower airway disease. J Allergy Clin Immunol 105:20–36, 2000.

9. Kalish RS, Askenase PW: Molecular mechanisms of CD8+ T cell-mediated delayed hypersensitivity: Implications for allergies, asthma, and autoimmunity. J Allergy Clin Immunol 103:192–199, 1999.

10. Larché M, Robinson DS, Kay AB: The role of T lymphocytes in the pathogenesis of asthma. J Allergy Clin Immunol 111:450–463, 2003.

11. McHugh RS, Shevach EM: The role of suppressor T cells in regulation of immune responses. J Allergy Clin Immunol 110:693–702, 2002.

12. Nel AE: T-cell activation through the antigen receptor. Part 1: Signaling components, signaling pathways, and signal integration at the T-cell antigen receptor synapse. J Allergy Clin Immunol 109:758–770, 2002.

13. Nickel R, Beck LA, Stellato C, Schleimer RP: Chemokines and allergic diseases. J Allergy Clin Immunol 104:723–742, 1999.

14. Panettieri RA Jr: Cellular and molecular mechanisms regulating airway smooth muscle proliferation and cell adhesion molecule expression. Am J Respir Crit Care Med 158:S133–S140, 1998.

15. Romagnani S: The role of lymphocytes in allergic disease. J Allergy Clin Immunol 105:399–408, 2000.

16. Rotrosen D, Matthews JB, Bluestone JA: The immune tolerance network: A new paradigm for developing tolerance-inducing therapies. J Allergy Clin Immunol 110:17–23, 2002.

17. Santeliz JV, Van Nest G, Traquina P, et al: Amb a 1-linked CpG oligodeoxynucleotides reverse established airway hyperresponsiveness in a murine model of asthma. J Allergy Clin Immunol 109:455–462, 2002.

18. Schroeder JT, MacGlashan DW. New concepts: The basophil. J Allergy Clin Immunol 99:429–433, 1997.

19. Stanzani M, Martins SL, Saliba RM, et al: CD25 expression on donor CD4+ or CD8+ T cells is associated with an increased risk of graft-versus-host disease following HLA-identical stem cell transplantation in humans. Blood 2003 [in press].

20. Vignola AM, Gjomarkaj M, Arnoux B, Bousquet J: Monocytes. J Allergy Clin Immunol 101:149–152, 1998.

21. Wardlaw AJ: Molecular basis for selective eosinophil trafficking in asthma: A multistep paradigm. J Allergy Clin Immunol 104:917–926, 1999.

22. Weller PF: Human eosinophils. J Allergy Clin Immuno. 100:283–287, 1997.

23. Zimmermann N, Hershey GK, Foster PS, Rothenberg ME: Chemokines in asthma: Cooperative interaction between chemokines and IL-13. J Allergy Clin Immunol 111:227–242, 2003.

CHAPTER 3

AEROALLERGENS

Christopher Chang, M.D., Ph.D.

1. **What is an allergen?**
    An allergen is a type of material that can produce an IgE-mediated response in a susceptible person. The component of an allergen capable of binding to IgE is generally a protein or a glycoprotein. Most indoor allergens range from 10 to 50 kd in length, and a large number have been cloned and sequenced.

2. **What constitutes an aeroallergen?**
    An aeroallergen is an allergen that is airborne. Aeroallergens usually cause symptoms because they are able to enter the body via the respiratory tract. Aeroallergens may be classified as primarily outdoor or indoor allergens. Examples of outdoor allergens are pollen grains originating from weeds, grasses, and trees. Examples of indoor allergens include dust mite particles, dog and cat dander, and cockroach allergens. Mold spores may be present in both indoor and outdoor air.

3. **Describe the physical characteristics of an aeroallergen.**
    Aeroallergens vary in size, shape, and electrical charge. Pollen and mold allergens are carried on pollen grains and spores, respectively, whereas animal proteins and dust mite proteins may be carried on dust particles in the environmental air and then transported into the human respiratory tract. The size of particles that carry indoor allergen proteins can thus be highly variable (Table 3-1).

TABLE 3-1.   INDOOR ALLERGENS

Allergen	Origin	Mol. Wt. (kd)	Function	Size of Particles on Which Allergen Is Carried (μm)
Der p 1, Der p 2	Dust mite	25, 14	Cysteine protease	10
Der f 1, Der f 2	Dust mite	25,14	Cysteine protease	10
Fel d 1	Cat	35	Isolated from cat hair root sebaceous gland	1–7
Can f 1	Dog	27	Not known	Not known
Bla g 1	Cockroach	20–25	Not known	10
Bla g 2	Cockroach	36	Inactive aspartic protease	10
Mus m 1	Mouse	19	Alpha-2U-globulin	Not known
Rat n 1	Rat	19	Present in urine, saliva	Not known

4. **How do aeroallergens gain access to the human body?**
    Aeroallergens travel through the mouth and nose and deposit onto the mucous membranes of the respiratory tract at various levels.

5. **What determines the extent to which aeroallergens penetrate the respiratory tract?**
   The aerodynamic properties (i.e., size and shape) of the particles and the flow characteristics of the particular airway. Simplistically speaking, smaller particles travel further into the small airways. Particles of 8 μm or less are considered able to penetrate the respiratory tract, whereas particles greater than 20 μm are usually deposited in the naso- or oropharynx or on ocular mucous membranes, leading to symptoms of allergic rhinitis or conjunctivitis, respectively. These particles are subsequently cleared by mucociliary function.

6. **What are the sources of aeroallergens?**
   Aeroallergens can be predominantly indoors or outdoors. Aeroallergens can originate from plant material, as in pollens from trees, weeds, and grasses, or derive from fungal material, as in fungal spores. Aeroallergens may also derive from animals and insects, as in the case of dust mites, cats, dogs, and other pets.

KEY POINTS: THE MOST COMMON AEROALLERGENS

1. Pollens

2. Molds

3. Dust mites

4. Animal danders

5. Insect allergens (cockroaches)

7. **Where are most of the common allergenic pollens found?**
   Allergies are common throughout the world. Most plants contain proteins that can function as allergens. Table 3-2 lists common pollen allergens. The geographical distribution of these allergens and their primary season of pollination are quite complicated and depend on climate and nutrient sources. Many varieties of plants have been transplanted from one region of the world to another with great success, making understanding of the pollination patterns even more difficult.

8. **Describe the physical characteristics of pollen grains.**
   Pollen grains are identified by light microscopy at 400x magnification. Pollen grains range from 10 to 100 μm in diameter. The majority of pollen grains are between 20 and 35 μm. Pollen grains frequently have surface characteristics that assist with buoyancy. Pollen grains are stained with a dye such as phenylsafranin for identification and counted using a stage micrometer.

9. **Describe patterns of cross-reactivity in pollen allergens**
   Cross-reactivity exists between pollens and is strongest between species of the same genus. There may also be cross-reactivity between genera within the same family, but as the relationship between plants becomes more distant, there is progressively less cross-reactivity.

10. **Discuss cross-reactivity among grasses.**
    Cross-reactivity among grasses generally falls into three groups. There is significant cross-reactivity within the Pancoideae family, including Bahia and Johnson grasses, which may exhibit some cross-reactivity with Bermuda grass of the Eragrostoideae family. The Northern pasture

TABLE 3-2. OUTDOOR ALLERGENS

Scientific Name	Common Name	Zone	Range of Mol. Wt. of Allergens (kd)	Size Range of Pollen Grains (μm)
		Trees		
Cryptomeria japonica	Sugi	Japan	41–45	35–46
Parietaria judaica	Pellitory of the wall	Mediterranean basin	10–14	12–14
Acer macrophyllum	Oregon maple	Pacific Coast		36–45
Olea europea	Olive	Warmer western states of U.S.; introduced from Europe	8–19	22–28
Platanus occidentalis	Sycamores	Eastern U.S. river bottoms, Mexico, Canada		22
Quercus alba	Oak	Throughout U.S., Mexico, South America, southern Europe	17	30–40
Betula verrucosa	White birch	Scandinavia, northwest U.S., eastern U.S.	17	28–30
Alnus gultinosa	Black alder	Northwest U.S.: Rocky Mountain region, Scandinavia	17	26–28
Carpinus betulus	European hornbeam	Europe	17	25–31
Acer negundo	Box elder	Eastern agricultural region of U.S., Canada, Mexico		27–36
Juglans californica	Walnut	Western North America		30–40
Corylus avellana	European hazelnut	Introduced from Europe to U.S., Turkey	17	27–31
		Grasses		
Cynodon dactylon	Bermuda grass	Bermuda grass is present in both hemispheres but particularly predominant in Southeast Africa	32	28–30
Agrostis alba	Red top	Canada, U.S., Europe		25–34
Anthoxanthum odoratum	Sweet vernal	Canada, Europe		40–45

(Continued)

TABLE 3-2. OUTDOOR ALLERGENS *(continued)*

Scientific Name	Common Name	Zone	Range of Mol. Wt. of Allergens (kd)	Size Range of Pollen Grains (µm)
Dactylis glomerata	Orchard grass	England, France, Germany, Italy, U.S.–Canadian border provinces	25–32	34–40
Phelum pratense	Timothy	U.S., Canada, Western Europe	25–54	28–42
Lolium perenne	Italian rye	U.S., Canada	11–34	32–45
Poa pratensis	Blue grass	Western Europe, U.S., Canada	26–33	38–40
Secale cereale	Cultivated rye	Eurasia, Canada	33	58–68
		Weeds		
Ambrosia	Ragweed	Eastern U.S.	4–38	18–22
Plantago lanceolata	Plantain	Temperate U.S.		26–34
Salsola kali	Russian thistle	Warm barren soils		27–30
Artemisia gnaphaloides	Mugwort	Mexico, Canada, U.S.	20–35	25–28

grasses, belonging to the family Festucoideae, are different from Bermuda grass, but they may cross-react with Pancoideae.

11. Discuss cross-reactivity among trees.
Conifers cross-react with each other. Examples include cedar, cypress, juniper, and arbor vitae. Pecan and hickory cross-react, and poplar, cottonwood, and aspen in the genus *Populus* cross-react with each other.

12. What other type of cross-reactivity may occur?
In addition to cross-reactivity between pollens, there may also be cross-reactivity between pollens and edible fruits, as in the case of birch pollen and raw potatoes, carrots, apples, hazelnuts, kiwi, or celery. Similarly, people allergic to ragweed may also exhibit allergies to bananas and melons.

13. List the common classes of fungi.
Zygomycetes, Ascomycetes, Basidiomycetes, Oomycetes, and Deuteromycetes

14. How are mold spores identified?
Mold spores are counted using light microscopy. Slides for mold-counting may or may not be stained, and accurate counts are best obtained under oil immersion (1000x). Most mold spores can be identified down to the level of genus.

15. How is species-specific identification made?
Cultures can be done on a number of different media, depending on the type of mold. Mold spores are between 2 μm and 50 μm in diameter. Ascospores are small enough to penetrate the lower airways, whereas large spores such as *Epicoccum* may only penetrate into the large airways or the oropharynx or nasopharynx. Cultures are particularly useful in the speciation of *Aspergillus* and *Penicillium*.

16. What determines the allergenicity of an aeroallergen?
The ability of an allergen to induce sensitivity or allergic symptoms in humans depends on the allergenicity of the proteins contained in the airborne material and on their concentration.

17. How many of the known aeroallergens have been characterized or standardized? How is standardization achieved?
More and more aeroallergens are standardized every year. Standardization is most commonly achieved by skin testing using either intradermal or epicutaneous techniques and measuring the resulting erythema or wheal reaction. Standardization allows calibration of a batch of allergen against a control curve. Currently, most common grass allergens have been fully characterized and standardized. Their activity is expressed in biologic activity units per milliliter (BAU/mL). Dust mite and cat allergen have also been standardized.

18. Describe the characteristic of dust mite allergens.
Dust mite allergens are mostly digestive enzymes, which are excreted along with the feces. The two most commonly seen dust mite species are *Dermatophagoides pteronyssinus* and *Dermatophagoides farinae*. Other species include *Dermatophagoides microceras* and *Euroglyphus maynei*. A mite species that propagates primarily in warmer climates is *Blomis tropicalis*. From these species are derived a number of important dust mite allergens, which are divided into classes based on their chronologic order of discovery and, more importantly, their homology with each other. The most common of these are the group I allergens, Der p 1 and Der f 1, with a similar molecular weight of about 25 kd, and the group II allergens, Der p 2 and Der f 2.

Arlein L, Platts-Mills TAE: The biology of dust mites and the remediation of mite allergens in allergic disease. J Aller Clin Immunol 107:S406–S413, 1999.

19. **How many micrograms of mite allergen does one dust mite contain?**
Approximately 0.02 μg or 20 ng

20. **Describe the characteristics of cat and dog dander.**
The major allergenic determinant of cats is Fel d 1; that of dogs is Can f 1. Fel d 1 is a 35-kd protein that is a component of cat hair root sebaceous gland and sublingual mucous salivary gland. Fel d 1 attaches itself to small dust particles between 2 and 10 μm in diameter. While dog allergenic proteins vary from breed to breed, one of the more common nonspecific dog allergens is Can f 1, derived from the scientific name *Canis familaris*.

21. **Discuss the role of mouse and rat dander in allergies.**
Mice and rats may play a role in occupational asthma in laboratory workers, but also in homes in which children keep them as pets. The major mouse allergenic protein is a 17.8-kd protein produced in salivary glands and in the liver. There are two major rat allergens, designated as Rat n 1.01 and Rat n 1.02. These allergens originate from urine, pelt, and saliva. Rat n 1.01 is about 21 kd in weight, whereas Rat n 1.02 has a molecular weight of about 16 kd.

22. **What is the significance of cockroach allergen?**
In the past 10 years, it has been recognized that cockroach allergen plays a significant role in asthma in urban environments. The most common cockroach encountered in America is *Blatella germanica*. Two proteins of molecular weight 25 kd and 36 kd have been isolated from this species of cockroach and found to be allergenic. They have been designated Bla g 1 and Bla g 2.

23. **How effective are cockroach abatement measures?**
In a recent study, cockroach abatement measures have been successful in decreasing cockroach allergen concentrations below 2U/gm-vacuumed dust in inner city homes. The abatement measures included the use of cockroach insecticide, professional cleaning, and resident education.
Arbes SJ Jr, Sever M, Archer J, et al: Abatement of cockroach allergen (Bla g 1) in low-income, urban housing: A randomized controlled trial. J Aller Clin Immunol 112:339–345, 2003.

24. **How are allergens named?**
Allergens are named according to the first three letters of the genus, followed by a space, the first letter of the species, another space, and a number that is generally representative of the chronologic order of discovery of the allergen. This nomenclature system was developed by the International Union of Immunological Societies (IUIS) Allergen Nomenclature Subcommittee. The scientific name of cat is *Felis domesticus*; thus the nomenclature Fel d 1 for the first cat allergen identified.

25. **How is our environment tested for the presence of fungal aeroallergens?**
Currently many companies advertise services as mold inspectors or mold remediators. Most of these companies have no scientific advisory staff or knowledge of the health concerns of aeroallergens. In addition, many laboratories receive samples from mold inspectors and test for the presence of aeroallergens. Because there is little regulation, the quality of the results varies greatly. Some companies send self-test kits to homeowners or analyze the kits returned by homeowners. This is a new industry, and the knowledge of the health effects of aeroallergens is still an area of fertile research.

26. **What causes indoor allergen particles to become airborne?**
Most aeroallergens settle quickly, depending on the size of the particle. Once settled, particles can become airborne by disturbance of their surroundings, such as vacuuming, changing the bed sheets, use of a ceiling fan, walking on carpeting, keeping windows open, or use of an air conditioner.

27. What are the different types of air samplers?

Samplers currently used fall into one of three categories: passive samplers, rotary-impact samplers, and slit-type volumetric spore traps.

28. How do passive samplers work?

Passive samplers are simply placed in an exposed environment and particles are allowed to collect on the surface. The surface can be a greased microscope slide or a culture plate. Particle deposition is dependent on wind and gravity. Counts are generally not accurate. A current example of such a device is the Durham sampler.

29. How do rotary impaction devices work?

Rotary impaction devices work by spinning a collection surface through ambient air, collecting particles as the surface traverses the surrounding air. Advantages of rotary impaction devices over passive samplers include better reliability of the equipment and unattended operation. Limitations of rotary impaction devices include the generation of turbulence by the rotating arm, lack of correlation with wind direction, absence of periodic sampling, and lack of accuracy in converting deposited numbers of spores or pollen grains with actual volumetric counts.

30. How do slit-type samplers work?

Slit-type samplers are now the most widely used samplers because or the ability to obtain periodic measurements and to convert observed counts to actual volumetric counts in the surrounding air. Slit-type devices rely on a vacuum pump to draw air into a chamber in which a collection surface sits. Because of the aerodynamic characteristic of allergen-containing particles, only particles of interest will be deposited on the slide. The efficiency of collection of slit-type devices is far superior to that of rotary impaction samplers. An example of a slit-type device is the Burkard sampler. An outdoor Burkard sampler is shown in Figure 3-1.

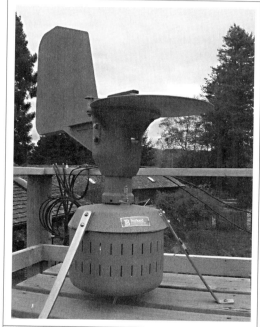

Figure 3-1. Outdoor Burkard sampler.

31. Describe the microscope and accessories used to count pollen grains and mold spores.

A well-illuminated binocular microscope is recommended for counting pollen grains or mold spores. Use the 10x objective to scan for areas of high counts or, preferably, areas that are ideal for counting and will give the most accurate results. The 40x objective is used for counting pollen grains, whereas the 100x objective is used for counting mold spores. For accurate counting, either a Whipple disk (attached to the eyepiece) or a stage micrometer can be used to determine the field of vision at each magnification.

32. **How are indoor air samples analyzed for mold particles?**
     Various sampling devices are available for the collection of viable and nonviable samples.
     Nonviable samples are collected on a greased microscope slide or a spore trap. A vacuum pump
     that runs at 15 L/min is used to sample nonviable mold spores. Viable samples are collected
     using a vacuum pump operating at 28 L/min onto an agar plate containing a medium that facili-
     tates mold growth. Alternatively, a portable Burkard volumetric sampler is a self-contained unit
     with its own timing mechanism.

33. **Where should air be sampled?**
     For pollens, the sampler should be placed on an elevated surface about 16–20 feet above ground.
     The collecting device should be clear of any obstruction and placed away from trees that may
     affect the results. An outdoor sampler such as this can also be used to sample for mold spores.
     When sampling for indoor mold spores, air should be sampled both indoors and outdoors.
     Most mold spores originate outdoors, and if the indoor levels are the same as outdoor levels, a
     problem in the home is unlikely. Indoor air samplers can be placed in areas where problems
     may be suspected and run for 5–15 minutes. Sampling of surfaces and bulk dust samples do
     not necessarily reflect airborne concentrations but may be useful in predicting or forecasting
     future air problems.

34. **In addition to air sampling, what other sampling locations may provide useful
     information into the presence of aeroallergens?**
     Surface sampling and bulk sampling may also yield results that may provide useful information
     about environmental exposure. Bulk sampling involves the collection of dust samples from
     vacuum cleaners for the purposes of analyzing for indoor allergens. Tape or surface swabs are
     useful in studying the presence of mold spores on surfaces that have excess moisture.

35. **How are indoor dust samples analyzed for animal danders and dust mites?**
     Indoor dust samples are collected using any standard vacuum into a small container. Examples
     range from a simple piece of microfiber filter cloth to more sophisticated devices into which
     elution buffer can be directly added. Once eluted, the samples can be analyzed for Der p 1, Der p
     2, Der f 1, Fel d 1, Can f 1, Bla g 1 and Bla g 2, Mus m 1 and Rat n 1 using enzyme-linked
     immunosorbent assay (ELISA). Most ELISA procedures utilize monoclonal antibodies, and stan-
     dard curves are produced with each assay using known concentrations of the allergen under
     investigation. Results are expressed in ng or µg per ml and can be converted into ng or µg per
     gm of dust collected, if the original weight of collected dust is known.

36. **Describe the flow characteristics of airborne particles.**
     Two objects of different masses dropped from an identical height at precisely the same moment
     under the same gravitational influence will reach the ground at the same time only in a vacuum. In
     reality, the aerodynamic and sedimentation behavior of particles depends on their size, density,
     shape, and viscosity of the surrounding air; airflow properties; and interaction with other particles in
     the vicinity. Gravitational sedimentation velocity is proportional to the square of the mass median

KEY POINTS: DIFFERENT TYPES OF AIR SAMPLERS

1. Passive samplers

2. Rotary impact samplers

3. Slit-type volumetric samplers

aerodynamic diameter (MMAD), which is an equivalency measure for a particle of unknown shape or size that produces the same settling velocity as a unit density sphere (1 gm/cc). For example, a particle of MMAD of 16 μm will settle four times quicker than a particle with an MMAD of 4 μm. Most particles greater than 10 μm MMAD will fall to the ground fairly quickly.

37. **What other physical factors can affect the airborne characteristics of particles?**
Brownian diffusion, inertial impaction, interaction with carrier gases, physical agglutination, chemical agglutination, and electrostatic charges.

38. **How is the settling velocity of purely spherical particles calculated?**

$$V_s = gr^2(D_p - D_a)/18\,\mu$$

where V_s = settling velocity, g = acceleration due to gravity (9.8 m/s^2), r = radius of the particle, D_p = particle density, D_a = air density (1.3×10^{-3} gm/cm at 18°C), and μ = viscosity of air (1.8×10^4 gm/sec at 18°C).

39. **List the functions of the nose.**
   - Warming of air
   - Filtering of large particles
   - Olfaction
   - Resonance
   - Speech

40. **How are allergies to aeroallergens assessed?**
The diagnosis of allergic rhinitis or asthma is based on clinical history and physical examination, but identification of specific allergies is also facilitated by allergy testing. Allergy testing can be done by skin testing or by a blood test known as radioallergosorbent (RAST) testing, which is a form of ELISA for IgE. Skin testing is done by epicutaneous (skin prick testing) or intradermal (ID) methods. Costs of skin testing and RAST testing are comparable.

41. **List the advantages of skin versus RAST testing.**
   1. Quicker results
   2. Direct measurement of in vivo allergic responses
   3. Can test a larger range of allergens

42. **List the disadvantages of skin versus RAST testing.**
   1. Patients may not be on certain medications:
      - Beta blockers
      - Antihistamines
   2. More traumatic (especially to pediatric patients)
   3. Cannot be performed if patient has allergic or nonallergic skin pathology or problems

43. **What molds are commonly seen in indoor air environments?**
Most common indoor molds originate from the outside. The outdoor concentration of common molds varies depending on the temperature and moisture. Frequently there are showers of mold spore dispersal as in the case of basidiospores after a rain shower. Table 3-3 lists common molds and their growth patterns.

44. **What media may be used to culture for mold growth?**
Molds grow preferentially in different types of media, which vary in pH, nutrients, and ability to induce sporulation. Common media include Sabouraud's dextrose agar (SDA), potato dextrose agar (PDA), cornmeal agar, inhibitory mold agar (IMA), casein agar for the

TABLE 3-3. COMMON MOLDS AND THEIR GROWTH CHARACTERISTICS

Spore Name	Class	Grows On	Spores	Health Effects
Alternaria	Fungi Imperfecti	Plants	Pear-shaped, 12–50 µm	Allergies
Aspergillus	Fungi Imperfecti	Soil, hay, grain, fruits	Long, columnar conidia	Allergies, ABPA, sinusitis, hypersensitivity alveolitis
Cephalosporium	Fungi Imperfecti	Soil, dust	Conidia are 1–4 µm	Allergies, hypersensitivity pneumonitis
Chaetomium	Ascomycetes	Soil, paper, straw	Ascospores are 5 µm dia	Allergies
Cladosporium (Hormodendrum)	Fungi Imperfecti	Plants, decaying wood products	Spores are 3–7 µm dia	Allergies
Curvularia Drechslera	Fungi Imperfecti	Soil, plants	Conidia have 3–5 cells, brown and septate	Allergies
Epicoccum	Fungi Imperfecti	Soil, vegetables, plants	Conidia are globose and dark	Allergies (summer, fall)
Fusarium	Fungi Imperfecti	Plants, vegetables	Microconidia are 5–6 µm	Allergies
Helminthosporium	Fungi Imperfecti	Cereal grain plants	Bean-shaped, 15–23 by 5–7 µm	Allergies
Mucor	Zygomycetes	Soil, animal waste	Spores are elliptical 5 by 10 µm	Allergies
Penicillium	Fungi Imperfecti	Soil, fruit, cheese, bread	Spores are 2.6–3.2 µm in diameter	Allergies
Phoma	Fungi Imperfecti	Paper, plants	Spores are elliptical 5 by 7 µm	Allergies
Pullularia	Fungi Imperfecti	Soil, decaying vegetation	1 by 3 µm, elliptical	Allergies
Rhizopus	Zygomycetes	Bread, meats, vegetables	Elliptical, 9 to 12 by 8 µm	Allergies
Spondylocladium	Fungi Imperfecti	Decaying wood, plants	Spindle-shaped, amber; contain 3 cells	Allergies
Stemphyllium	Fungi Imperfecti	Damp paper, canvas, cotton fabric	Large spores, 25–40 by 16–20 µm	Allergies
Trichoderma	Fungi Imperfecti	Decaying wood, cotton, wool	Oblong to spherical, 1–3 µm in diameter	Allergies

differentiation of aerobic actinomycetes, V-8 agar for ascospores, malt extract agar, and water agar.

45. **What are some of the effects of mold particles on human health?**
Mold spores can cause allergies. Symptoms may affect the upper airway and eyes in the form of allergic rhinitis and conjunctivitis, respectively, or they may affect the lower airway, causing asthma. In addition to allergic conditions, mold spores have been found to produce mycotoxins, which have been suggested, though not proved, to be harmful to the human body if inhaled.

46. **Can aeroallergens cause other types of nonallergic illnesses?**
Yes. Examples include the following:
   - In the 1970s, *Legionella pneumophila* was found to be associated with a pneumonia-like illness that affected people attending a convention in Philadelphia.
   - Another illness caused by *Legionella anisa* is Pontiac fever, which is characterized by chills, fever, and mylagia and was found in workers in a health department building.
   - *Aspergillus fumigatus* has long been known to be a cause of acute bronchopulmonary aspergillosis, which affects the sinopulmonary tracts of humans, causing inflammation and an asthma-like illness.

47. **What about *Stachybotrys* species?**
More recently, *Stachybotrys* species have been linked to infant pulmonary hemorrhage, although no studies have clearly demonstrated any cause-and-effect relationship between the two. It is believed that trichothecens, a mycotoxin generated by *Stachybotrys chartarum*, is responsible for the illness because of its ability to cause inflammation and to alter surfactant concentration in animals. *Stachybotrys* is a common inhabitant of moist indoor environments, and the isolation of *Stachybotrys* from buildings does not necessarily imply a health risk.

48. **What are the names of some mycotoxin-producing fungi?**
Mycotoxin-producing fungi include *Fusarium, Aspergillus, Cephalosporium, Cladosporium, Penicillium, Stachybotrys,* and *Trichoderma* species.

49. **Are there established exposure standards for aeroallergens?**
Currently there is no consensus about the levels of mold spores in the air that may be dangerous to human health. In contrast to molds, the levels of indoor allergens such as dust mite, animal dander, and cockroach that may cause adverse effects on health have been documented, and the results have been reproducible. The exposure limits on indoor allergens have been expressed in the form of relative risks. High, medium, and low risks for sensitization and exacerbations have been defined for dust mite, dog, cat, and cockroach (Table 3-4). Exposure levels for mold allergy have not been determined.

50. **What is sick building syndrome?**
Sick building syndrome refers to illness linked to buildings and building materials when the illness affects a group of people working in the same environment. In most cases of sick building syndrome, symptoms are vague and difficult to quantify. There is no obvious etiology, and the symptoms may vary from person to person. Common symptoms described in sick building syndrome include, headache, mucous membrane and skin irritation, asthma-like symptoms, dizziness, fatigue, difficulty concentrating, and muscle aches. In most cases, no biochemical or physiologic abnormalities can be detected. No randomized controlled studies have demonstrated any connection between these symptoms and exposure to any single component of a structure or to any biologic agent in the structure. In many cases, mass hysteria may actually be a significant factor in sick building syndrome.

TABLE 3-4.	RISK OF SENSITIZATION AND EXACERBATION OF ALLERGIES		
Allergen	Low Risk	Medium Risk	High Risk
	Sensitization (µg/gm dust)		
Dust mite allergen	< 0.5	2–10	>10
Cat	< 0.5 or > 20	8–20	1–8
Dog	< 0.5 or > 20	8–20	1–8
Cockroach (Bla g1)	< 0.6	1–8	> 8
	Exacerbation (µg/gm dust)		
Dust mite allergen	< 0.5	2–10	> 10
Cat	< 0.5	1–8	8–20
Dog	< 0.5	1–8	8–20
Cockroach (Bla g1)	< 0.6	1–8	> 8

Chang CC, Ruhl RA, Halpern GM, Gershwin ME: The sick building syndrome. I: Definition and epidemiologic considerations. J Asthma 30(4):285–295, 1993.

Ruhl RA, Chang CC, Halpern GM, et al: The sick building syndrome. II: Assessment and regulation of indoor air quality. J Asthma 30(4):297–308, 1993.

51. **What is hypersensitivity pneumonitis?**

Hypersensitivity pneumonitis is a group of conditions that manifest with the same constellation of symptoms, including chills, cough, fever, and dyspnea. Examples of hypersensitivity pneumonitis include farmer's lung, pigeon breeder's disease, and mushroom worker's disease. Other aeroallergens known to be associated with hypersensitivity pneumonitis include thermophilic *Actinomycetes*, *Micropolyspora faenia*, and some viruses.

52. **What is *Stachybotrys*?**

Stachybotrys chartarum is a moderately rapid growing fungus that attains maturity in 7 days. It prefers media with high cellulose content. *Stachybotrys* generally forms dark colonies due to the highly pigmented conidiophores, which are oval-shaped and around 4.5 to 9 µm in dimension. *Stachybotrys* has achieved a status of special interest because of the observation that pulmonary hemorrhage and pulmonary hemosiderosis has occurred in infants in temporal proximity to *Stachybotrys* exposure. A causal relationship has not been proved. *Stachybotrys* is known to produce several mycotoxins, and it is postulated that the fungus may affect humans through ingestion, inhalation, or percutaneous route.

53. **Are aeroallergens responsible for occupational asthma?**

Occupational asthma can be a result of IgE-mediated allergies or may be irritant-induced. IgE-mediated occupational asthma can be a result of development of IgE to high-molecular-weight allergens or to low-molecular-weight chemicals that attach themselves to high-molecular-weight respiratory proteins. Common IgE-mediated occupational asthma occurs in laboratory workers exposed to animal proteins, in workers in the food service industry exposed to cereal proteins or insect allergens, and in farmers or outdoor workers exposed to pollens and mold spores.

54. **Is allergy or anaphylaxis due to latex an airborne allergy?**
Latex allergy had its heyday in the 1990s, when there was a sudden perceived increase in the number of cases of latex allergy and latex anaphylaxis. Common symptoms of a latex allergy include rhinitis, hives, eye symptoms, wheezing, or anaphylaxis. It was subsequently discovered that latex allergy was due to an allergy to natural latex allergens with molecular size between 10 and 67 kd. Latex allergens cross-react with a number of food allergens. Latex allergy occurs when latex allergens become airborne, frequently carried on glove powders such as cornstarch.

    Jaeger D, Kleinhans D, Czuppon AB, Baur X: Latex-specific proteins causing immediate-type cutaneous, nasal, bronchial, and systemic reactions. J Aller Clin Immunol 89:759–768, 1992.

55. **How does one avoid exposure to aeroallergens?**
Avoidance of allergic triggers is one of the main treatment modalities for allergies and asthma. While avoidance of pollen allergies is difficult to achieve due to the ubiquitous nature of pollen grains outdoors, there are a number of measures that one can take with regards to indoor allergen exposure. Keeping pets outdoors and regular bathing of the pet will decrease the concentration of pet allergen inside the house, although cat dander tends to be very buoyant and difficult to clear. It may take up to 6 months to clear cat dander, following removal of the cat.

56. **List measures for avoidance of dust mites.**
Measures that help avoid dust mites include washing bedding once every 2 weeks in hot water, keeping the relative humidity below 50% indoors, using mite-proof encasings, removing stuffed animals, minimizing upholstery and carpeting, using a HEPA filter, and weekly vacuuming. If the person is remodeling, it helps to install hardwood floors or linoleum instead of carpet and to use blinds instead of draperies.

KEY POINTS: AVOIDANCE MEASURES IN DUST MITE ALLERGY

1. Frequent washing of bedding at 130° F

2. Use of a HEPA filter

3. Use of mattress and pillow coverings

4. Frequent vacuuming and use of a HEPA filter–equipped vacuum cleaner

5. Installation of hardwood floors instead of carpeting

6. Removal of stuffed animals and other items that collect dust

57. **How can mold spores be avoided?**
Avoidance of mold spores can be achieved by ensuring that there are no water leaks and by keeping the relative humidity of the home down, as in the case of dust mite avoidance.

58. **How do HEPA filters work?**
High-efficiency particulate air (HEPA) filters were first developed in the 1940s by the United States Atomic Energy Commission. Their initial purpose was to filter out potentially hazardous radioactive particulate matter. After World War II, the technology was declassified, and now

HEPA filters are used in air cleaners and vacuum cleaners for the removal of allergens from indoor air.

59. **How effective are HEPA filters?**
HEPA filters must conform to a strict standard of being able to filter out at least 99.97% of all particles that are greater than 0.3 μm in size. In addition, airflow standards also exist for the functioning of HEPA filters according to their size and the area that the filter is servicing. In-place HEPA filter testing can be conducted by Brookhaven National Laboratories. The formula used to calculate efficiency is as follows:

$$\text{Removal efficiency (\%)} = [(C_u - C_d)/C_u] \times 100$$

where C_u = upstream aerosol concentration and C_d = downstream aerosol concentration. More recently, other devices have been developed that remove aeroallergens from indoor air, including ionic filters that attract dust particles based on the native charge of the particles.
HEPA filters: http://tis.eh.doe.gov/hepa/docs/std3020.pdf

60. **What are some of the other methods of decreasing environmental exposure to indoor allergens?**
For patients who are allergic to animals, avoidance by removal of the pet from the home is the best way of preventing allergic symptoms. However, many people are very emotionally attached to their pets and will not be able to abandon their animals. In fact, many patients deny that the animal is ever in the home, even when high levels of allergen are detectable in the house. Occasionally, frequent bathing of the animal can help decrease allergen exposure load. Cockroach allergen exposure can be diminished by taking steps to improve home hygiene, disposing of waste regularly, and by not leaving food around. These strategies are especially important in overcrowded surroundings. Cockroach allergen is more common in urban environments.

61. **Can aeroallergens be rendered nonallergenic?**
Many chemicals are available commercially that carry the claim of being able to degrade allergens and render them non-allergenic. There is no evidence that any of these substances are effective in reducing an individual's exposure to an allergen, nor are any of these compounds able to reduce clinical symptoms of allergy and asthma in susceptible patients.

62. **What does the future hold with regard to indoor air analysis?**
Indoor air analysis has only recently become a field of much interest. It is in the early phase of evolution, and there has been little standardization or regulation. Most of the early cases in which indoor air analysis was obtained have been in the areas of litigation. These cases have involved tenants lawsuits against landlords for usually very vague symptoms. Although a cause-and-effect relationship is difficult to establish for most of these cases, judgments have unfortunately been made on the basis of poor science. However, when health care issues are not contaminated by litigation, indoor air analysis can be helpful in the treatment of patients with true IgE mediated allergies, because it gives the health care provider, as well as the homeowner or landlord, information that can be beneficial in the removal of allergic agents from susceptible individuals.

63. **Explain the hygiene hypothesis.**
According to the hygiene hypothesis, early exposure to infections and microbial agents can protect against the development of allergic diseases or asthma. The mechanism is thought to be due to a paradigm shift in the development of the immune system from a predominantly Th1 helper cell lineage to a Th2 helper cell lineage. Simplistically speaking, Th1 helper cells are more involved in protection against infections, whereas Th2 helper cells are focused on IgE-mediated allergic diseases. In advanced societies, amenities such as running water, cleaning products, closed sewage system, disinfectants, vaccines, antibiotics and other advantages protect against

and prevent the spread of infections. The belief is that since the load on the immune system in protecting against infection is reduced, there is a shift in the differentiation of cells toward a different lineage, namely Th2 cells, which increase the incidence of allergies and their associated conditions. Although this may indeed be the pattern of evolution of the immune system, it does not mean that exposure to more infectious agents is actually a good thing. Rather, the information gained from the understanding of how the immune system develops may lead to new ideas in the treatment of allergies and asthma.

Apter A: Early exposure to allergen: Is this the cat's meow, or are we barking up the wrong tree? J Aller Clin Immunol 111:938–946, 2003.

WEBSITE

Asthma and Allergy Foundation of America: www.aafa.org

BIBLIOGRAPHY

1. Apter A: Early exposure to allergen: Is this the cat's meow, or are we barking up the wrong tree? J Allergy Clin Immunol 111:938–946, 2003.

2. Arbes SJ Jr, Sever M, Archer J, et al: Abatement of cockroach allergen (Bla g 1) in low-income, urban housing: A randomized controlled trial. J Allergy Clin Immunol 112:339–345, 2003.

3. Arlein L, Platts-Mills TAE: The biology of dust mites and the remediation of mite allergens in allergic disease. J Allergy Clin Immunol 107:S406–S413, 1999.

4. Berstein J: Allergic rhinitis and asthma: The role of allergen avoidance. J Respir Dis 11:572–80, 2002.

5. Burge HA: An update on pollen and fungal spore aerobiology. J Allergy Clin Immunol 110:544–552, 2001.

6. Chang CC, Ruhl RA, Halpern GM, Gershwin ME: The sick building syndrome. I: Definition and epidemiologic considerations. J Asthma 30(4):285–295, 1993.

7. Custovic A, Simpson B, Simpson A, et al: Current mite, cat, and dog allergen exposure, pet ownership, and sensitization to inhalant allergens in adults. J Allergy Clin Immunol 111:402–407, 2003.

8. Eggleston PA, Bush RK: Environmental allergen avoidance: An overview. J Allergy Clin Immunol 107: S403–S405, 1999.

9. HEPA filters: http://tis.eh.doe.gov/hepa/docs/std3020.pdf

10. Jaeger D, Kleinhans D, Czuppon AB, Baur X: Latex-specific proteins causing immediate-type cutaneous, nasal, bronchial, and systemic reactions. J Allergy Clin Immunol 89:759–768, 1992.

11. Kang B: Study on cockroach antigen as a probable causative agent in bronchial asthma. J Allergy Clin Immunol 58:357, 1976.

12. Remes S, Castro-Rodriguez J, Holberg C: Dog exposure in infancy decreases the subsequent risk of frequent wheeze but not of atopy. J Allergy Clin Immunol 108:509–515, 1998.

13. Ruhl RA, Chang CC, Halpern GM, et al: The sick building syndrome. II: Assessment and regulation of indoor air quality. J Asthma 30(4):297–308, 1993.

14. Solomon W, Platts-Mills TAE. Aerobiology and inhalant allergens. In Middleton E Jr, Ellis EF, Yunginger JW, et al (eds) Allergy: Principles and Practice, 5th ed. St Louis, Mosby, 1998, pp 367–403.

CHAPTER 4

DIAGNOSTIC EVALUATION OF ALLERGIC DISEASE

Calvin So, M.D.

1. **When was allergic skin testing introduced?**
   Blackley introduced skin testing as a diagnostic tool for allergy in 1865. It was then modified by Mantoux and subsequently by Lewis and Grant.

2. **What are the historical clues to suggest allergic rhinitis or asthma?**
   Nasal and ocular complaints predominate in patients with allergic rhinitis. Nasal pruritus, clear rhinorrhea, nasal congestion, and sneezing suggest allergic rhinitis. Ocular complaints may include eye pruritus and lacrimation. A seasonal pattern of symptoms suggests allergic rhinitis. Trees tend to pollinate in the spring, grasses in late spring and early summer and weeds in late summer and fall. A history of specific triggers like cat allergy also suggests allergic disease. Patients with allergic disease may also complain of fatigue and may have decreased scores on quality of life questionnaires compared with nonallergic patients.

3. **Which features of the ocular exam are important to allergic patients?**
   Patients with allergic disease may have bilateral conjunctivitis. Infraorbital darkness, known as an "allergic shiner," may be found on examination. It is thought to be due to venous pooling related to chronic nasal congestion.

4. **What features of the nasal and nasopharyngeal examination are important to the allergic patient?**
   Some patients may have a transverse nasal crease that can indicate repetitive nose rubbing, also known as the "allergic salute," from chronic rhinitis. The typical allergic nasal mucosa is pale blue and boggy. The nasal mucosa can also be erythematous and congested. Other features include bridging mucus across opposing surfaces of nasal mucosa. Nasal secretions may be clear and watery or mucoid, cloudy, or yellowish in patients with chronic rhinitis. "Cobblestoning," which is a granular appearance to the oropharynx, may be an indication of postnasal drip.

5. **What other nasal structures seen on physical examination cause symptoms of rhinitis?**
   In evaluating a patient for allergic disease, one must also survey the nasal cavity for septal deviation and nasal polyps, which may predispose a patient to perennial rhinitis. Nasal polyps are located on the lateral wall of the nasal cavity and originate from the sinus cavities. Nasal polyps are glistening, white, semitransluscent, and round structures that appear gelatinous in texture; they are inflammatory growths originating from the mucosa of paranasal sinuses. Patients must also be examined for nasal tumors, which may cause nasal congestion and predispose to sinusitis. Nasal septal perforations may produce sensations of nasal obstruction.

6. **Which tools are important for the examination of the allergic patient?**
   A handheld otoscope or a nasal speculum with headlight may visualize the anterior one-third of the nares; nasal polyps, septal deviation, or masses may be missed. Some patients benefit from fiberoptic nasal endoscopy to evaluate sinus openings, the rest of the nasal cavity, and, occasionally, the vocal cords for possible dysfunction. Spirometry is useful to detect patients with concurrent obstructive lung disease. Acoustic rhinometry and rhinomanometry are mostly used in research settings. Common tools for skin testing are shown in Figure 4-1.

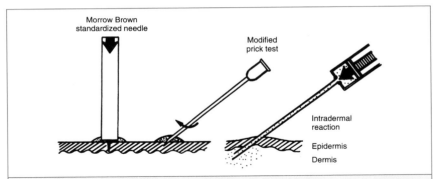

Figure 4-1. Common tools for skin testing. (From Demoly P, Piette V, Bousquet J: In vivo methods for study of allergy. In Adkinson NF Jr, Yunginger JW, Busse WW, et al (eds): Middleton's Allergy: Principles and Practice, vol. 1, 6th ed. St. Louis, Mosby, 2003, Fig. 38-1, p 632.)

7. **Describe the scratch test. What are its limitations?**
A scratch test is the introduction of allergen into skin by a linear abrasion without bleeding. It is not commonly used in allergy practice due to increased pain, decreased reproducibility, and possibility for skin disfiguration compared to skin prick testing.

8. **What precautions are observed in administering the skin prick test (SPT)?**
Both a negative saline or glycerin control and a positive histamine control must be placed. A patient with dermatographism may react to a negative control, thus causing a false-positive result. Alternatively, an anergic patient may not react to the positive histamine control, which would suggest the possibility for false-negative tests to allergen.

9. **What are common mistakes made in the administration of the SPT?**
Insufficient penetration into the skin may lead to a false-negative reaction. The pricks must be placed at least 2 cm away from each other to prevent interference. Bleeding from the testing may induce a false-positive reaction. Spreading of the allergen while blotting it off or during the test may also induce a false-positive reaction due to contamination.

10. **What percentage of the general population has positive skin tests?**
One study showed 34% of patients older than 2 years had one or more positive reactions to a panel of common allergens. Of patients with no personal or family history of rhinitis or asthma, 29% had at least one positive reaction on skin testing. Of patients with a family history of asthma or rhinitis but no personal history of asthma and rhinitis, 46% had at least one positive reaction on skin testing.
  Adinff AD, Rosloniec DM, McCall LL, et al: Immediate skin test reactivity to Food and Drug Administration-approved standardized extracts. J Allergy Clin Immunol 86:766–74, 1990.

11. **What percentage of patients with symptoms of rhinitis, eczema, or asthma have a positive skin test?**
About 80–90% of patients with asthma, rhinitis, or eczema have positive skin tests.

12. **What proportion of patients with poor histamine reactions have negative skin test reactions to given allergens?**
Of patients who reacted only at the highest concentration of histamine, slightly more than half had negative skin tests to all allergens tested.

13. **What proportion of patients with allergic reactions to stinging insects and latex have negative skin test reactions to given allergens?**
Of patients who reacted to the lowest amount of histamine, about 10% had negative skin testing to all allergens.

14. **Are children more likely to have a positive skin test than adults?**
About 20% of children who underwent skin testing had one positive skin test in a panel of five allergens or a mixed panel. However, histamine skin reactivity may be lowest in children aged 9–19 years old compared to older age-groups, but children may have the highest level of total IgE compared to other age-groups. Infants tested against codeine and histamine by skin testing had some reactions by 1 month of age and had very small skin reactions until 6 months of age.

15. **At what age is one at the highest likelihood of having a positive skin test?**
Patients in the first half of their third decade are most likely to have a positive skin test; 52% of 20- to 30-year-old patients have a positive reaction to skin testing. In patients with asthma, those younger than 30 years tended to have more positive skin tests than those who were older than 30.

16. **Does the likelihood of a positive skin test decrease with age?**
Older patients have fewer positive skin tests. Only 16% of patients older than 75 years have a positive skin test.

17. **Does body site make a difference in skin test results?**
The upper back is less reactive than the middle back, which is less reactive than the lower back. The forearm is less reactive than the back. Wheal size may be up to 27% smaller and flare size may also be decreased by up to 14%. One estimate is that 2.7% of positive back skin tests might be negative on the forearm skin.

18. **Does handedness have an effect on skin test results?**
Right-handed patients with a family history of right-handedness may have increased reaction sizes on the left forearm, and patients who are left-handed or ambidextrous may have increased reaction sizes on the right forearm.

19. **How does time of day affect skin testing?**
There is minimal diurnal variation in skin testing; therefore, time of day should not significantly affect results.

20. **Is there a seasonal effect on skin testing?**
Patients with pollen allergy may be more sensitive to skin testing after the pollinating seasons and may have decreased sensitivity until the following pollinating season.

21. **How does gender affect skin testing?**
Men and women do not differ significantly with respect to sensitivity to skin testing.

22. **Does the menstrual cycle affect skin test results?**
There may be increased reactions to histamine during the days of ovulation and increased estrogen secretion of the menstrual cycle.

23. **What is the ideal length of time to withhold antihistamines before skin testing?**
Doxepin may need to be withheld up to 1 week before performing skin testing. In general, patients recovered skin reactivity 2 days after discontinuing fexofenadine, 3 days after discontinuing chlorpheniramine, and 5 days after discontinuing hydroxyzine.

24. **Which standardized extracts have been approved by the Food and Drug Administration?**
Dermatophagoides pteronyssinus, D. farinae, cat, ragweed, and several grasses.

25. **What are the relative potencies of nonstandardized extracts?**
Most nonstandardized pollen extracts are quite potent, whereas dog dander extract and most fungi extract are weakly potent. Cockroach and fungi extract may be more unstable due to their protease content.

26. **What is the minimum age for skin testing?**
Children less than 1 year of age may not be able to mount a positive skin reaction. Some children with seasonal allergic rhinitis may not have a positive response until they have had exposure in two seasons.

27. **What should be recorded on skin testing result sheets for easy interpretability among allergists?**
   - Concentration of extract used
   - Whether SPT or intradermal testing was used
   - If SPT was used, which testing device was used
   - Anatomic site of testing
   - Size of positive and negative reactions
   - Legend for grading system used in interpreting skin test results

28. **What different grading systems may be used in interpreting skin test results?**
   - 0 to 4+ system based on erythema size and wheal size as well as presence of pseudopods
   - Preferred method may be measurement of area or diameters of wheal and erythema

29. **What is the standardized concentration of histamine used in skin testing?**
A concentration of 10 mg/mL of histamine for skin prick testing may be used as a positive control in skin prick testing.

30. **Does the administration device make a difference in determining positive values in skin prick tests?**
Different devices impart different degrees of trauma on the skin tested. Increased trauma to skin may cause increased skin reactivity to the device and not necessarily to the allergen used. Quintest puncture, smallpox needle prick, DuoTip prick, and Lancet puncture devices have a significantly positive wheal at 3 mm. However, DermaPIK prick and twist, DuoTip twist, bifurcated needle prick and puncture, and MultiTest puncture may require a wheal > 3 mm to be significantly positive.

31. **What is the difference in allergen concentration between skin prick tests and intradermal tests?**
Intradermal tests use a concentration that is 1000 times less than that used in prick testing at equivalent threshold doses. Concentrations greater than 1:1000 in intradermal testing may increase sensitivity but are not necessarily clinically relevant.

32. **List the advantages of skin prick testing versus intradermal testing.**
   - Less discomfort
   - Decreased risk of systemic reactions
   - Quicker to perform
   - May perform more tests at one time
   - More stable extracts due to glycerin content
   - Positive tests may correlate better with symptoms
   - Easier to interpret results
   - Decreased cost

33. **List the advantages of intradermal testing versus skin prick testing.**
    - Increased reproducibility of test results
    - Increased sensitivity; especially useful in venom and drug allergy testing

34. **Discuss the usefulness of positive intradermal tests in patients with negative skin prick tests to the same allergen.**
    One study using Timothy grass concluded that positive intradermal testing in patients with negative skin prick testing did not indicate clinically significant symptoms on Timothy grass challenge or natural exposure. A second study arrived at the same conclusion with respect to cat allergy.

    Nelson HS, Oppenheimer JJ, Buchmeier A, et al: An assessment of the role of intradermal skin testing in the diagnosis of clinically relevant allergy to Timothy grass. J Allergy Clin Immunol 97:1193–1201, 1996.

    Wood RA, Phipatanakul W, Hamilton RG, et al: A comparison of skin prick tests, intradermal skin tests and RASTs in the diagnosis of cat allergy. J Allergy Clin Immunol 103:773–779, 1999.

35. **What is a delayed reaction to skin testing?**
    A delayed reaction is an increased wheal and flare that continues after the peaking of the immediate reaction due to the release of mast cell contents. In skin testing, the histamine control usually peaks around 8 minutes and the allergen skin test usually peaks in 15 minutes. However, a reaction of erythema and induration may continue at the allergen skin test site, peaking at 4–6 hours.

36. **Is it possible to predict clinically which patients will have delayed reactions?**
    Usually only patients who have had an immediate reaction of a threshold minimum size will have an IgE-related, delayed reaction.

37. **Do medications prevent delayed reactions?**
    Antihistamines do not prevent delayed reactions. Corticosteroids and immunotherapy may decrease the magnitude of the delayed reaction.

38. **Discuss the safety profile of skin testing.**
    One study at the Mayo Clinic found an incidence of 33 nonfatal systemic reactions per 100,000 skin prick/puncture tests. Some deaths have been reported with skin testing, mostly with potent allergens such as horse serum and almost invariably with intradermal testing.

    Valyaseui MA, Maddox DE, Li JTC: Systemic reactions to allergy skin tests. Ann Allergy 83:132–136, 1999.

39. **Explain the phenomenon of "localized allergy."**
    Some patients may have negative skin testing and negative RAST testing in the presence of clinically suspicious histories for allergic rhinitis. Such patients may have IgE antibodies only in nasal secretions without systemically increased IgE levels. These antibodies may cause symptoms RAST tests may be performed on nasal secretions, and symptoms may improve with anti-IgE therapy.

40. **Which patients may develop non-IgE-mediated late reactions?**
    Most such reactions occur after intradermal testing in patients who have tested positive on skin testing. One hypothesis is that they represent a late reaction due to a delayed-type hypersensitivity, which may also account for symptoms of allergic rhinitis.

41. **Why is total IgE not used in routine evaluation of allergic disease?**
    Total IgE may also be elevated in nonatopic patients and therefore is not necessarily useful in helping to identify atopic patients. In contrast, allergen-specific IgE levels are useful for helping to identify atopic patients.

42. **How does a first-generation RAST test work?**
Serum is incubated with the allergosorbent, which in a first-generation RAST test is a cellulose paper disc onto which the allergen is bound. Antibodies from the serum (both IgE and non-IgE) bind to the antigens on the allergosorbent. After the first buffer wash, ^{125}I-labeled anti-human IgE antibodies bind to IgE in the solution. A second buffer wash removes free anti-IgE antibodies. The bound, radiolabeled anti-IgE/IgE complexes are quantified by a gamma radiation counter. The amount of radiation is in direct proportion to the amount of IgE bound to the original antigen.

43. **Summarize the improvements in the second-generation RAST assay.**
   - Use of cellulose sponges (rather than discs) to help increase binding capacity and decrease nonspecific binding.
   - Better anti-IgE monoclonal and polyclonal antibodies increase specificity and decrease sensitivity.
   - Increased automation increases precision and reproducibility of test results.
   - Nonradioactive reagents are easier to use and easier to store.
   - Improved calibration using a reference curve can quantitate allergen-specific IgE.

44. **What factors may account for the difference in different allergen-specific IgE commercial assays?**
   - Difference in composition of protein mixture
   - Difference in immunogenicity among different preparations
   - Area and season in which the allergens are collected
   - Purity of allergen after extraction
   - Amount of cross-contaminants in sample
   - Allergen stability
   - Differing IgE antibodies used as reference
   Different producers, therefore, may produce different results because different populations of IgE molecules may be collected.

45. **Explain the conversion between allergen-specific IgE antibody units and amount of IgE protein.**
Each international unit (kU/L) is the same as one allergen-specific IgE antibody unit or the equivalent concentration of 2.4 µg/L of IgE protein.

46. **What are the cut-off values for best diagnostic precision in RAST and skin testing?**
A value of 11.7 kU/L in the Pharmacia CAP system and a wheal size of about 6 mm in diameter seem to have the highest accuracy.

47. **What is evaluated in skin testing that is not evaluated by RAST testing?**
   - Mast cell releasability
   - Histamine reactivity
   - IgE-binding affinity

48. **Summarize the relative sensitivities among the skin tests and RAST testing.**
Skin prick tests, as well as RAST tests, are less sensitive than intradermal tests. However, RAST testing is less sensitive than skin prick testing.

49. **How does allergen-specific IgE testing compare with other tests for aeroallergens?**
Allergen-specific IgE tests have been compared to skin testing. Modified RAST testing was found to be equivalent to skin prick testing and better than intradermal testing in predicting clini-

cal reactivity to cat dander. The allergen-specific IgE testing was also found to have a sensitivity of 69%, specificity of 100%, positive predictive value of 100%, and negative predictive value of 73% compared to cat allergen inhalation testing. A correlation was found between the concentration of dust mite–specific IgE and the concentration of dust mite allergen in the patient's bedding. There was a 77% chance of high dust mite allergen exposure when the concentration of dust mite allergen-specific IgE was > 2 kUa/L. In general, allergen-specific IgE testing is comparable to allergic skin prick testing.

Wood RA, Phipatanakul W, Hamilton RG, et al: A comparison of skin prick tests, intradermal skin tests and RASTs in the diagnosis of cat allergy. J Allergy Clin Immunol 102:773–779, 1999.

50. **What is the relationship between RAST testing, skin testing, and graded nasal challenges?**
Nasal challenge symptoms may correlate with skin prick tests but not with RAST testing. This finding may be due partly to histamine and basophil releasability, which is not evaluated by RAST testing.

51. **Summarize the relationship between skin testing and graded bronchial challenge.**
The correlation between skin testing and graded bronchial challenge is poor. This finding may be explained by nonspecific bronchial hyperreactivity.

52. **What is the value of testing a panel of foods in skin testing for food allergy?**
The testing of food panels is discouraged due to the low positive predictive value of skin testing on its own merits.

53. **What is the negative predictive value for IgE-mediated food allergy in skin testing with common food allergens?**
The negative predictive value is greater than 95%.

54. **What is the positive predictive value for IgE-mediated food allergy in skin testing with common food allergens?**
The positive predictive value is less than 50%. A positive skin test alone may indicate the presence of IgE antibodies against a given food but does not necessarily diagnose a food allergy. However, the history of anaphylactic symptoms to a sole food allergen and a positive skin test to that food allergen may be considered diagnostic.

55. **Discuss the role of intradermal skin testing in food allergy.**
Intradermal skin testing is not recommended in food allergy because it has a higher false positive rate than skin prick testing as well as an increased rate of adverse reactions. Skin prick tests, as well as allergen-specific IgE tests, may be used as preliminary tests with double-blinded food challenges used as second-tier tests.

56. **What is the prick-prick test?**
The prick-prick test is a skin prick test in which the fresh food is pricked before pricking the patient's skin. This method may introduce proteins from the fresh food that is not available in the commercial extract. A prick from the fresh food must also be pricked on a patient without the pertinent history as a control. Spices may also be used after the material is ground into a powder and solubilized with diluent.

57. **Summarize the limitations of skin testing in food allergy.**
- Some proteins in food may not be present in commercially prepared extracts due to extraction methods or storage.
- Skin treated with topical steroids may create smaller wheals than they would otherwise.

- Prick-prick tests may be necessary in patients with negative skin prick tests and a higher index of suspicion for food allergy.

58. **What is the value of using allergen-specific RAST testing in the evaluation of food allergy?**
One use of allergen-specific RAST testing is as a substitute in patients who cannot undergo skin testing. It does, however, have a relatively high negative predictive value and lower specificity. In addition, some experts have advocated following quantitative levels of IgE to help determine patients who may have a subsequent negative food challenge.

59. **How does allergen-specific IgE testing compare with other allergy testing for food allergy?**
One study investigated the correlation between allergen-specific IgE antibody levels to cow's milk, chicken egg, peanut, wheat, soy, and fish with the gold standard of double-blind, placebo-controlled food challenge. The authors concluded that, by using positive modified RAST test results, they could predict with 95% certainty a positive food challenge. A subsequent retrospective study confirmed that using allergen-specific antibody levels can help identify greater than 95% of children with food allergy to chicken egg, cow's milk, peanut, and fish. Taken together, the studies suggest that allergen-specific may be as effective as double-blinded placebo controlled food challenges in identifying certain food allergies.
    Sampson HA, Ho DG: Relationship between food-specific IgE concentrations and the risk of positive food challenges in children and adolescents. J Allergy Clin Immunol 100:444–451, 1997.
    Sampson HA: Utility of food-specific IgE concentrations in predicting food allergy. J Allergy Clin Immunol 107:891–896, 2001.

60. **What is the wheal size of a positive skin test in food allergy testing?**
Generally, a positive skin test is 3 mm greater in diameter than the diameter of the negative control. However, in children less than 3 years old, a lower threshold of 8 mm wheal diameter may be needed due to decreased mast cell reactivity or decreased sensitization levels.

61. **What experimental techniques are used in the evaluation of food allergies?**
- Basophil histamine release
- Intestinal mast cell assay
- Lymphocyte stimulation test

62. **What is the gold standard for diagnosis of food allergy?**
The gold standard for the diagnosis of food allergy is a double-blind, placebo-controlled food challenge test.

63. **What is an open food challenge?**
An open food challenge is simply the observation in the clinical setting of a patient consuming a food suspected of causing the patient to have systemic or organ-specific reactions.

64. **What is the value of an open food challenge test in the evaluation of food allergies?**
The open food challenge is useful when the clinician's index of suspicion for a reaction to a given food is low. For example, a patient with a positive skin test but prior consumption without difficulty may be suitable for an open food challenge.

65. **What is a single-blind food challenge?**
A single-blind food challenge is the administration by staff of placebo or a food suspected of causing a reaction to a patient blinded to the contents of the food. The food is given to the patient in progressively larger doses over 1 to 2 hours, and the patient may be observed for 2 to 4 additional hours, depending on symptoms.

66. **Discuss the value of a single-blind food challenge test in the evaluation of food allergies.**
The single-blind food challenge is useful when a patient's attitudes may affect the result of a food challenge. It is less time-consuming than a double-blind, placebo-controlled food challenge, but it is single-blinded to prevent the patient from knowing whether he or she is consuming placebo or the suspect food.

67. **What is a double-blind, placebo-controlled food challenge?**
In a double-blind, placebo-controlled food challenge, neither the physician and clinical staff nor the patient knows whether a given test food is placebo or the suspect food. The placebo and suspect food may be given during the same day in morning and afternoon sessions or on different days.

KEY POINTS: DIAGNOSTIC TESTS USED TO EVALUATE ALLERGIC DISEASE

1. Skin prick test

2. Intradermal testing

3. Serum allergen-specific IgE testing (RAST/modified RAST)

4. Graded allergenic lung challenge

5. Leukocyte histamine release

6. Blinded food/allergen challenge

68. **What is the value of a double-blind, placebo-controlled food challenge test in the evaluation of food allergies?**
The double blind, placebo-controlled food challenge may used when the single-blind food challenge has yielded inconclusive results or in complex situations in which higher diagnostic accuracy is needed to evaluate symptoms or signs attributed to the ingestion of a given food.

69. **List contraindications to oral food challenges.**
- History of anaphylaxis
- Food-related airway compromise

70. **List the important indoor allergens and their sources.**
See Table 4-1.

Allergen	Size	Species	Source
Der f 1	25 kd	*Dermatophagoides pteronyssinus*	Dust mite fecal particles
Der p 1	25 kd	*Dermatophagoides farinae*	Dust mite fecal particles
Fel d 1	35 kd	*Felis domesticus*	Cat sweat gland excretion
Can f 1	25 kd	*Canis familiaris*	Dog sweat gland excretion
Bla g 1		*Blatella germanica*	German cockroach
MUP	19 kd	*Mus musculus*	Mouse urinary excretion

TABLE 4-1. IMPORTANT INDOOR ALLERGENS

71. **How can the clinical laboratory be used to assess the home environment for allergens?**

    A patient may obtain samples of the dust of his or her home via a dust collection device placed on a vacuum cleaner. Areas sampled may include air ducts, flooring, bedding, or furniture. The dust may then be evaluated by solubilizing allergenic proteins in a buffer solution and identifying them via monoclonal antibody immunoassays. The laboratory may report amounts of allergen per gram of dust.

72. **How can the clinical laboratory assist in the evaluation of mold allergies in patients?**

    Air is sampled from an environment and sent for quantitation. Both nonviable and viable spores are assessed by morphology to determine the species of the mold, including *Alternaria, Cladosporium, Aspergillus*, and *Penicillum*. Viable molds are then grown on culture plates. One to two days later, the plates are evaluated for the number and species of mold grown. If a home has above 25,000 colonies per gram of dust, it is in the 75th percentile of homes randomly assessed in the United States. At this point, allergic patients may consider steps to rid mold from their homes.

73. **Is mold allergen level an indicator of mold prevalence in an environment?**

    Immunoassays may be used to identify mold allergens such as Alt a 1 from *Alternaria* species. However, the expression of allergens in molds differs according to the environment in which it is growing. Therefore, indoor molds may express certain allergens to a different degree than the same mold growing under different circumstances. As a result, measuring mold allergen levels may not be a good indicator of actual mold prevalence in a given environment.

74. **Which allergens should be tested in seasonal allergic rhinitis?**

    Weeds, trees, and grasses.

75. **Which allergens should be tested in perennial allergic rhinitis?**

    Dust mites, fungi, and pet or animal dander.

76. **In what situations is immunoassay testing preferable to skin testing?**

    - Atopic dermatitis
    - Dermatographism
    - Inability to discontinue antihistamines
    - Increased risk of anaphylaxis with skin testing
    - Noncompliance with skin testing

77. **Are any lung challenge tests available for the evaluation of allergic disease?**

    Two lung provocation tests exist for evaluation of allergic lung disease: (1) graded challenge to allergen and (2) provocative test using a general irritative agent such as histamine or methacholine. The graded challenge is administered by progressively increasing amounts of inhaled allergen until there is evidence of obstructive disease by physical examination or spirometry. Methacholine or histamine challenges can be used with high sensitivity in evaluating a patient with asthma; methacholine has fewer systemic side effects than histamine and is usually preferred. Although such patients may not necessarily have allergic asthma, reactivity of the airways can be evaluated with this approach.

78. **Is serum eosinophil count used for allergy screening?**

    No. Eosinophilia has low sensitivity as a screening test in allergy diagnosis.

79. **What diagnostic tests are available for evaluation of drug allergy?**

    The evaluation of drug allergies in patients can be difficult. Before using diagnostic tests, one must be sure that the reaction is truly due to an IgE-mediated event. This may be difficult since many reactions are caused by nonallergic mechanisms. The prototypical drug that has been well studied for true drug allergy is penicillin. Skin test and allergen-specific IgE tests are available for penicillin but usually do not exist for other drugs.

80. **What are the major and minor antigenic determinants of penicillin and their importance in skin testing?**
The major antigenic determinant of penicillin is the degradation product penicilloyl (Fig. 4-2). The minor antigenic determinants of penicillin are penicilloate and penilloate. Skin testing only with penicilloyl, which is commercially available as Pre-Pen, and penicillin G may miss as many as 10–20% of patients with an IgE-mediated reaction to penicillin.

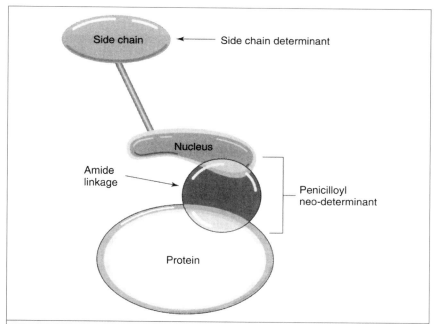

Figure 4-2. The immunodominant major penicilloyl eptitope contains constituents from bicyclic nucleus, amide linkage, and adjacent carrier protein. (From Adkinson NF Jr: Drug allergy. In Adkinson NF Jr, Yunginger JW, Busse WW, et al (eds): Middleton's Allergy: Principles and Practice, vol. 2, 6th ed. St. Louis, Mosby, 2003, Fig. 92-5, p 1683.)

81. **What are contraindications to skin testing for penicillin or drug allergy?**
Patients who have had serum sickness or Stevens-Johnson reaction to penicillin should not be skin tested and should not use penicillin in the future.

82. **How can IgE competitive assay studies help in choosing extracts for venom immunotherapy?**
Vespid insects, which include the yellow jacket and the white-faced and yellow hornet insects, cross-react with *Polistes* wasp venom. Some allergists give immunotherapy with all allergens that provide positive skin tests. A competitive inhibition RAST test can be used to find IgE antibodies that cross-react with both vespids and *Polistes*. If yellow jacket venom cross-reacts with *Polistes* wasp venom, the patient may need only yellow jacket venom or mixed vespid venom for immunotherapy rather than *Polistes* wasp venom as well.

83. **How can IgG monitoring help in determining duration of venom immunotherapy?**

In Hymenoptera venom allergy, specific IgG levels may be used to assist in determining chance of remission of symptoms with immunotherapy. One study evaluated 109 patients with a history of systemic allergic symptoms from an insect sting and positive intradermal testing to Hymenoptera. Two years later, of patients with greater than 3 μg/ml anti-Hymenoptera IgG, 1.6% had systemic symptoms, and of patients with less than 3 μg/ml 16% had systemic symptoms. The study suggests that those with higher amounts of Hymenoptera-specific IgG may have less risk of subsequent systemic allergic reactions to stings than those with lower amounts of Hymenoptera-specific IgG.

Golden DBK, Lawrence ID, Hamilton RG, et al: Clinical correlation of the venom-specific IgG antibody level during maintenance venom immunotherapy. J Allergy Clin Immunol 90:386–393, 1992.

84. **What is the gold standard for diagnosing allergic contact dermatitis?**

Patch testing is the gold standard for diagnosing allergic contact dermatitis. This test involves the adhesion of a chamber containing the suspected allergen against the skin and evaluating that area of skin for an allergic reaction.

85. **List contraindications for patch testing.**
- Immunodeficient patients
- Patients with uncontrolled dermatitis
- Use of topical steroids on skin to be tested
- Testing with an unknown substance

86. **Which laboratory tests are useful in evaluating a patient with urticaria?**

The history and physical exam are used to make the diagnosis of urticaria and to evaluate for nonallergic causes of urticaria. Levels of thyroid-stimulating hormone (TSH) and antithyroid antibodies are obtained to evaluate for hypothyroidism. A white blood cell count with differential is obtained to evaluate for hematopoietic abnormalities. Serologies for hepatitis B and hepatitis C may be useful to evaluate for chronic viral hepatitis. If the diagnosis is unclear, one may need to obtain a skin biopsy to evaluate for vasculitis. Finally, the patient's serum can be reintroduced to the patient via skin testing, looking for wheal and flare to evaluate for autoimmune-related chronic idiopathic urticaria.

87. **What physical examination diagnostic tests are useful in evaluating a patient with urticaria?**

A scratch test with a tongue blade or fingernail can be used to elicit dermatographism. Ice cube tests can be used to evaluate for cold-induced urticaria. Application of a warm test tube can be used to evaluate for local heat urticaria. Placing a sling with a 5- to 15-pound weight attached to a forearm or shoulder for 10–15 minutes can be used to evaluate for pressure-induced urticaria.

88. **What is tryptase?**

Tryptase is a four-subunit serine esterase protein. Tryptase degrades into four inactive monomers when it dissociates from heparin. The protein is important because it is released during anaphylaxis from activated mast cells along with histamine and other mediators of anaphylaxis. Unlike histamine, it can be measured in a clinical setting.

89. **What is the difference between alpha tryptase and beta tryptase?**

Alpha tryptase is useful as a marker of mast cell number. However, beta tryptase is a marker for the amount of activation of mast cells. The alpha-tryptase level can be approximated by subtracting the beta-tryptase level from the total tryptase level.

90. **How is tryptase measured in serum?**
Alpha and beta tryptase are first converted by the laboratory into inactive enzymes and then are separately measured. A monoclonal assay binds both alpha prototryptase and beta tryptase. Beta tryptase is further quantified by a noncompetitive, solid-phase immunoassay.

91. **What are normal levels of tryptase?**
In a normal person, tryptase levels should range from 1 to 10 ng/ml. Patients who have had recent anaphylaxis may have a beta-tryptase level greater than 1 ng/ml due to mast cell activation. Baseline tryptase levels greater than 20 ng/ml may suggest systemic mastocytosis.

92. **Explain the importance of the half-life of tryptase.**
The half-life of tryptase is about 2 hours. It is useful in autopsies for evaluation of possible death by anaphylaxis with a postmortem peak of beta tryptase exceeding 10 ng/ml. The ideal collection time of serum beta tryptase is within one-half to 4 hours after an episode of anaphylaxis. Histamine is also released in anaphylaxis but has a short half-life and is more difficult to assay than tryptase.

93. **What is the basophil histamine release assay?**
In a histamine release assay, peripheral leukocytes are obtained from the patient and then incubated in a solution with different concentrations of the allergen under evaluation. Histamine released from the leukocyte is assayed within 30 minutes and quantified. The basophil is one of the principal cells involved in the release of histamine in an allergic reaction. Limitations to this test are its expense and need for fresh blood. Basophil histamine release assay results do correlate with skin testing and brochoprovocation studies.

94. **How can diagnostic laboratory tests help with the diagnosis of hypersensitivity pneumonitis?**
Hypersensitivity pneumonitis (HSP) is an inflammatory lung disease causing fever and chills, malaise, cough, and dyspnea hours after heavy exposure to certain organic allergens such as molds and bird droppings. In most patients with HSP, evidence of IgG directed toward the causative antigen is detectable by the double diffusion technique. A positive test occurs when a single line is formed from the precipitation of the patient's serum with known antigen extract. However, as many as half of asymptomatic patients with organic dust exposure may have a positive double diffusion test.

95. **What antigens are evaluated in an IgG double diffusion assay for HSP?**
The antigens include those of pigeon serum, thermophilic *Actinomyces*, *Aspergillus fumigatus*, and the droppings of parakeets and pet parrots such as the Amazon, cockatiel, and blue front varieties.

96. **What tests are not well studied and are of unknown validity in the evaluation of allergic disease?**
See Table 4-2.

TABLE 4-2. UNPROVEN TESTS OF ALLERGIC DISEASE	
Test	Deficiency
Cytotoxic test	Results not reproducible and do not correlate with clinical allergy
Provocation-neutralization procedure	Results not reproducible and do not correlate with clinical allergy
Electrodermal diagnosis	Not evaluated for efficacy
Applied kinesiology	Not evaluated for efficacy
"Reaginic" pulse test	Not validated as allergy test
Analysis of body tissues of exogenous chemicals	Not validated as allergy test

WEBSITE

American Academy of Allergy, Asthma and Immunology: www.aaaai.org

BIBLIOGRAPHY

1. Bernstein IL, Storms WW: Practice parameters for allergy diagnostic testing. Ann Allergy Asthma Immunol 75:543–615, 1995.
2. Kemp SF, Lockey RF: Diagnostic Testing of Allergic Disease. New York, Marcel Decker, 2000.
3. Leung DYM, Sampson HA, Geha RS, Szefler SJ: Pediatric Allergy: Principles and Practice. St. Louis, Mosby, 2003.
4. Li JT: Allergy testing. Am Fam Physician 66:621–624, 2002.
5. Lieberman PL, Blaiss MS: Atlas of Allergic Diseases. Philadelphia, Current Medicine, 2002.
6. Lieberman PL, Anderson JA: Allergic Disease Diagnosis and Treatment, 2nd ed. Totowa, NJ, Humana Press, 2000.
7. Middleton E, Reed CE, Ellis EF: Allergy Principles and Practice, 5th ed. St. Louis, Mosby, 1998.
8. Ownby DR: Skin tests in comparison to other diagnostic methods. Immunol Allergy Clin North Am 21:355–367, 2001.
9. Rich RR, Fleischer TA, Shearer WT: Clinical Immunology Principles and Practice, 2nd ed. London, Mosby International, 2001.
10. Rose NR, Hamilton RG, Detrick B: Manual of Clinical Laboratory Immunology, 6th ed. Washington, DC, ASM Press, 2002.
11. Shearer WT, Li JT (eds): Primer on Allergic and Immunologic Diseases. J Allergy Clin Immunol 111:S441–S774, 2003.

CHAPTER 5

ALLERGIC RHINITIS

Gordon Garcia, M.D.

1. **Define rhinitis.**
   Generally, rhinitis is defined as inflammation of the mucous membranes of the nose. The term includes a heterogeneous group of disorders characterized by one or more of the following symptoms: sneezing, rhinorrhea, congestion, or nasal itch.

2. **Classify the types of rhinitis.**
   - Allergic rhinitis: accounts for approximately 50% of all cases of chronic rhinitis
   - Idiopathic nonallergic syndromes: nonallergic rhinitis with eosinophlia syndrome (NARES), perennial nonallergic rhinitis (vasomotor), cholinergic syndromes (e.g. gustatory rhinitis, cold air rhinitis)
   - Infectious: viral, bacterial
   - Occupational: allergic, nonallergic
   - Endocrinologic: menstrual cycle/pregnancy, hypothyroidism
   - Drug-induced: topical decongestants (rhinitis medicamentosa), antihypertensive agents, oral contraceptives, aspirin or nonsteroidal anti-inflammatory drugs (NSAIDs) in aspirin-sensitive rhinosinusitis, cocaine abuse
   - Other: atrophic conditions, gastroesophageal reflux

3. **What is the differential diagnosis of rhinitis?**
   - Granulomatous diseases: sarcoidosis, Wegener's granulomatosis, midline granuloma, rhinoscleromatosis, relapsing polychondritis
   - Anatomic or mechanical obstruction: septal deviation, nasal polyps, hypertrophic turbinates, tumors, foreign bodies, adenoidal hypertrophy, choanal atresia
   - Miscellaneous: ciliary dyskinesis, cerebrospinal fluid (CSF) leak

4. **Distinguish beween intermittent and persistent allergic rhinitis.**
   Intermittent: Symptoms occur on fewer than 4 days/week *or* for less than 4 weeks.
   Persistent: Symptoms occur on at least 4 days a week *and* for more than 4 weeks.

5. **How common is allergic rhinitis?**
   Most studies estimate the cumulative prevalence of allergic rhinitis in the United States to be between 10 and 20%; however, one study documented that 42% of 6-year-old children had doctor-diagnosed allergic rhinitis.

6. **Describe the natural history of allergic rhinitis.**
   The mean age at onset is 10 years old, with 80% of cases starting before age 20. In childhood, males are more frequently affected than females; however, the gender-specific prevalence equalizes in adulthood. Once established, the disease generally persists for many years.

7. **Name major risk factors for developing allergic rhinitis.**
   - Family history of allergy
   - Serum IgE > 100 IU/ml before age 6 years
   - Higher socioeconomic status

- Exposure to indoor allergens, such as animals and dust mites
- Presence of a positive allergy skin test

8. **List the physiologic functions of the nose and summarize its basic anatomy.**
   - Provides a conduit for airflow.
   - Warms, humidifies, and filters air. By the time it reaches the larynx, nasally inspired air is warmed to 35–37° C and humidified to 75–95% saturation. Airborne particles 10 μ or greater are completely filtered.
   - Antimicrobial defense. Innate or natural immunity includes the presence of the antibacterial proteins lysozyme and lactoferrin. Phagocytic cells enter the mucosa in response to invasion by foreign organism. Acquired immunity is provided by secretory IgA and, to a lesser extent, IgG.
   - Olfaction

   The basic anatomy of the nose is summarized in Figure 5-1.

9. **What is the nasal cycle?**
   Approximately 80% of people have a cyclic, reciprocal alteration in blood content of the turbinate vasculature (Fig. 5-2). This cycle averages 1 to 4 hours in length and results in reciprocal increasing and decreasing of nasal airway caliber. The sympathetic, alpha-adrenergic nervous system is believed to be integral to this process by reducing blood pooling in the venous sinusoids of the submucosa.

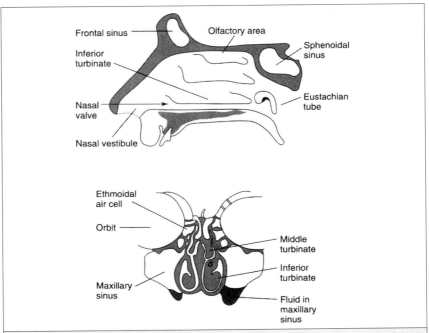

Figure 5-1. Anatomy of the nasal cavity with a view of the lateral wall *(top)* and a coronal section through the middle of the nasal cavity *(bottom)*. (From Eccles R: Anatomy and physiology of the nose and control of nasal airflow. In Adkinson NF Jr, et al (eds): Middleton's Allergy: Principles and Practice, 6th ed. St. Louis, Mosby, 2003, Fig. 47-1, p 776.)

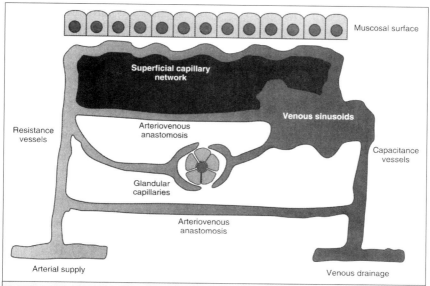

Figure 5-2. The nasal vasculature, with resistance and capacitance vessels as well as differing layers of arteriovenous anastomosis. (From Howarth PH: Allergic and nonallergic rhinitis. In Adkinson NF Jr et al (eds): Middleton's Allergy: Principles and Practice, 6th ed. St. Louis, Mosby, 2003, Fig. 76-3, p 1396.)

10. **List several factors that affect turbinate size.**
    - **Increases** turbinate size: lying supine, chilling skin, cold air, sexual stimulation
    - **Decreases** turbinate size: exercise, warming skin, fear

11. **What is the primary physiologic method of controlling nasal secretions?**
    Cholinergic nerves innervate the submucosal glands, arterial vessels, and sinusoids. The primary effect of cholinergic stimulation is to increase glandular secretion.

12. **Explain the role of the mast cell in the pathophysiology of allergic rhinitis.**
    Mast cells in the nasal epithelium are coated with allergen-specific IgE. Contact with airborne allergen crosslinks surface IgE, causing mast cell degranulation of preformed mediators, such as histamine. Leukotrienes C_4, D_4, and E_4 and prostaglandin D_2 are newly produced and secreted also. These, along with several other mediators lead to the **early-phase** symptoms of sneezing, itching, rhinorrhea, and congestion.
    Additionally, some of these mediators, including chemokines and cytokines, upregulate adhesion molecules on vascular endothelium and attract inflammatory cells such as eosinophils, basophils, neutrophils, and T-lymphocytes to migrate into the mucosa, leading to the **late-phase** response, 4–8 hours after the initial reaction.

13. **Summarize the physiologic effects of histamine release in the nose.**

Symptom	Mechanism
Sneeze, itch	Direct sensory nerve stimulation
Rhinorrhea	Direct and reflex stimulation of glandular mucus secretion
Congestion	Vascular engorgement and increased plasma transudation

14. **Explain the priming effect.**

With repeated nasal allergen challenges, the dose of allergen required to induce symptoms decreases. This effect is thought to be due to the influx of inflammatory cells into the nasal mucosa, resulting in repeated and prolonged late-phase responses.

15. **Discuss the utility of measuring total IgE level and allergen-specific IgE in the evaluation of chronic rhinitis.**

While a clear association exists between elevated serum IgE level and allergic rhinitis, no single dividing line can adequately differentiate the allergic from the nonallergic person. Assessment of allergen-specific IgE by skin testing or in vitro technique, by contrast, is the defining test for the confirmation of allergy in a patient suffering from chronic rhinitis.

Importantly, the results of the test must be correlated with the history. Positive allergy tests alone do not prove a cause-and-effect relationship. In studies of teenaged and college students, 15–25% of the group who had no symptoms had at least one positive skin test. In vitro testing has a greater incidence of false-negative result compared to skin testing but fewer false positives.

16. **List common triggers for seasonal and perennial allergic rhinitis.**

Seasonal
- Pollen: Trees pollinate earliest in the season in most areas of the country, with the specific start month determined by climate and tree type. Grass usually pollinates later in spring and early summer, and weeds may pollinate from spring through fall.
- Mold: Certain species also are released into the air in a seasonal fashion. Common examples include *Alternaria* and *Cladosporium*.

Perennial
- Dust mites are prevalent throughout much of the country and live in bedding, carpeting, and upholstered furniture.
- Indoor pets.
- Perennial molds.
- Pollens may also be present perennially in certain areas of the country (e.g., grass pollen in Florida).

KEY POINTS: DIAGNOSTIC CRITERIA FOR ALLERGIC RHINITIS

1. Presence of one or more typical symptoms (e.g., sneeze, rhinorrhea, nasal itch, congestion)

2. Pattern of seasonal or persistent perennial symptoms

3. Positive skin or blood test for specific allergens

4. Allergen test results correlate with patient history

17. **What is vasomotor rhinitis? How is it differentiated from NARES and allergic rhinitis?**

Vasomotor rhinitis, also known as nonallergic or idiopathic rhinitis, describes a perennial condition with nasal congestion and/or rhinorrhea as the predominant symptoms. Typical symptom triggers include fumes/odors, temperature or humidity changes, alcohol ingestion, emotion, and bright light.

Patients with NARES and allergic rhinitis have elevated eosinophils in the nasal mucosa, which is not true for vasomotor rhinitis. In contrast to allergic patients, patients with vasomotor rhinitis and NARES have negative allergen skin tests.

18. **How can nasal cytology be evaluated? What purpose does it serve?**
Material for cytologic staining may be obtained by blowing the nose into plastic wrap, taking a cotton swab of the mucosa, or using a flexible plastic curette (Rhino-Probe). The presence of eosinophils suggests allergic rhinitis or NARES, both of which respond well to treatment with topical intranasal steroids.

19. **Give examples of some occupations and allergens associated with IgE-mediated occupational rhinitis.**

Occupation	Allergen
Baker	Flour
Lab worker	Animals
Spray painter	Isocyanates
Plastics/resin worker	Anhydrides
Woodworker	Western red cedar
Health care provider	Latex

20. **List some of the main points to be reviewed in obtaining a rhinitis history.**
1. Symptoms
   - What? (sneeze, itch, or drip; clear versus purulent discharge; bilateral versus unilateral congestion; associated ocular symptoms)
   - When? (seasonality, age at onset)
   - Where? (indoors versus outdoors, effect of travel out of the home area)
2. Triggering or exacerbating factors, including:
   - Allergens (animals, pollen, house dust)
   - Irritants (smoke, odors, fumes)
   - Miscellaneous (weather, emotion, food/alcohol)
3. Home and occupational environmental exposures
4. Other medical history including medications
5. Response to current and prior medications
6. Personal or family history of other atopic conditions (asthma, eczema, conjunctivitis)

21. **How valuable is the nasal exam in differentiating allergic rhinitis from other causes of rhinitis?**
No features of the nasal exam are found exclusively in allergic patients. Classically, the mucosa is pale and edematous in allergic patients; however, this picture may also be found in nonallergic patients. Conversely, the mucosa may appear hyperemic in both types of rhinitis. Mucus, when apparent, is typically clear and thin. Mucopurulent discharge suggests infection. An external transverse nasal crease may be seen at the point where the nasal septal cartilage attaches to the bone. This finding results from chronically rubbing the nose upward (termed the "allergic salute") in childhood. Perhaps the most important role of the exam is to look for structural causes of obstruction, such as septal deviation, polyps, tumors, or hypertrophied turbinates.

22. **What are nasal polyps?**
Nasal polyps are smooth, pale, semitranslucent structures composed of edematous stroma infiltrated with inflammatory cells, including activated eosinophils, lymphocytes, plasma cells, mast cells, and, in some cases, neutrophils. Few mucous glands are present. They most commonly arise from the ethmoid sinuses and are seen in the area of the middle meatus.

Edematous turbinates are sometimes confused with polyps on exam; however, if a topical decongestant such as phenylephrine is applied to the mucosa, the turbinate will shrink, unlike the polyp. Additionally, polyps are mobile and insensitive to touch.

23. **What is the association between allergic rhinitis and nasal polyps?**
While nasal polyps do occur in patients with allergic rhinitis, allergy does not appear to predispose to polyp formation. In fact, nasal polyps are considerably more common in nonallergic patients.

24. **When nasal polyps are seen in a child, what disease should be suspected?**
Polyps rarely occur in children under 10 years old. Cystic fibrosis should be considered in these patients; the prevalence of polyps in CF is at least 20%.

25. **Discuss the treatment of nasal polyps.**
Medically, systemic and topical corticosteroids are used to shrink polyps. Large polyps respond more consistently to a 10- to 14-day burst of prednisone, followed by long-term corticosteroid nasal spray. If the polyps are severe or do not respond well to corticosteroid treatment, endoscopic polypectomy should be considered. Despite therapy, recurrence of polyps is common.

26. **Describe the typical presentation of a patient with a nasal CSF leak. What screening test should be performed?**
Typically, such a patient presents with copious unilateral or bilateral watery nasal discharge. Often flow increases with leaning forward or straining. A history of head trauma or surgery is suggestive, but spontaneous leaks may occur. The presence of glucose in the fluid (>30 mg/dl) suggests a CSF leak, but measuring beta$_2$-transferrin in the fluid is more sensitive and specific.

27. **What is rhinitis medicamentosa? How is it treated?**
Rhinitis medicamentosa results from prolonged use of nasal decongestant sprays. Tachyphylaxis occurs rapidly with this class of medication; therefore, it is common for patients to use increasing doses to maintain nasal patency. The nasal exam classically shows erythematous, swollen turbinates. Intranasal steroids are recommended as the patient weans off the decongestant spray. In more severe cases, a 5- to 10-day course of prednisone may be required.

28. **Review the role of environmental control measures in treating patients with allergic rhinitis.**
All patients with allergic rhinitis should be encouraged to reduce their exposure to relevant allergen and irritant triggers. Environmental control measures (Table 5-1) are usually combined with appropriate pharmacologic treatment, since most allergens are difficult to avoid completely.

29. **True or False: The use of allergen-impermeable mattress and pillow encasings has been proved to reduce symptoms in patients with house dust mite-sensitive allergic rhinitis.**
False. While it is hoped that the use of impermeable encasings as part of a comprehensive environmental control program (as listed in question 26) will be effective, the use of encasings alone has not been shown to improve clinical symptoms.

Terreehorst I, et al: Evaluation of impermeable covers for bedding in patients with allergic rhinitis. N Engl J Med 349:237–246, 2003.

30. **Explain the pharmacologic and clinical actions of antihistamines.**
All antihistamines competitively bind to the H$_1$ histamine receptor, blocking histaminic effects. In addition, many antihistamines inhibit the release of mast cell mediators in response to a

TABLE 5-1.	ENVIRONMENTAL CONTROL OF ALLERGENS
Allergen	**Control Measures**
Pollen	Close home and car windows in season and use air conditioning
	Shower after outdoor activities
	Wear dust mask if yard work is performed
Mold (outdoor)	Similar to pollen; avoid leaf raking and working with compost
Mold (indoor)	Keep indoor humidity below 50%
	Avoid indoor plants
	Clean mold with commercial fungicide or 10% bleach in water
Animals	Remove allergenic pet from home, then thoroughly clean (even with extensive cleaning, allergen may remain for months)
Dust mite	Cover mattress, boxspring and pillows with mite-proof encasings
	Wash all bedding in hot (130° F) water at least biweekly
	Remove items that collect dust from the bedroom
	Use a high-quality vacuum (e.g., HEPA) to decrease dust dispersal
	Consider removal of carpeting, especially in the bedroom
	Keep indoor humidity below 50%

variety of triggers. The clinical relevance of this mast cell effect is uncertain. Clinically, antihistamines reduce sneeze, itch, and rhinorrhea but have little effect on nasal congestion. Taking an antihistamine prior to contact with an allergen enhances the effectiveness of the drug.

31. **List the six chemical classes for the first-generation antihistamines and provide specific examples of each class.**
   1. Ethylenediamines (pyrilamine, tripelennamine): generally lower incidence of sedative and anticholinergic effects
   2. Ethanolamines (diphenhydramine, clemastine, carbinoxamine): generally higher incidence of sedation, especially diphenhydramine
   3. Alkylamines (chlorpheniramine, brompheniramine, triprolidine): most common class used in over-the-counter products
   4. Piperazines: hydroxyzine, meclizine
   5. Piperidines (cyproheptadine, azatadine)
   6. Phenothiazines (promethazine): marked sedative effects

32. **What are the advantages and disadvantages of the second-generation antihistamines compared to their predecessors?**
   The primary advantage of most newer antihistamines is that they do not cross the blood-brain barrier and hence do not cause sedation or reduce psychomotor performance. Desloratadine (Clarinex), loratadine (Claritin), and fexofenadine (Allegra) have side-effect profiles indistinguishable from placebo, while cetirizine (Zyrtec) has a mild potential for sedation. It is now standard practice to recommend the use of nonsedating or minimally sedating antihistamines in preference to the first-generation antihistamines. The primary disadvantage of most newer antihistamines is their much higher cost; however, inexpensive generic, nonprescription loratadine is now available.

33. **Discuss the safety and performance issues associated with use of first-generation antihistamines.**

Approximately one-third of patients using a first-generation antihistamine report drowsiness to a variable degree. However, many studies have demonstrated the potential for psychomotor impairment even when no sedation is reported. Specific techniques used to document this impairment have included measures of sleep latency period, reaction time, driving performance, memory, learning, and visual-motor coordination. Epidemiologic studies have linked first-generation antihistamines to fatal automobile accidents as well as occupational injuries. In many states, people taking sedating antihistamines are legally considered to be "under the influence of a drug" while driving.

34. **What symptoms may be seen with overdose of first-generation antihistamines? Contrast the toxic effects in young children and adults.**

Overdose in adults typically causes severe lethargy. Coma and death may occur. Anticholinergic effects may include dry mucous membranes, urinary retention, tachycardia, and decreased intestinal motility. The QTc interval may be prolonged, predisposing the patient to torsade de pointes.

In contrast, infants and young children may show paradoxical central nervous system stimulation with irritability, hyperactivity, hallucinations, and seizures.

35. **Discuss the pharmacokinetics of antihistamines.**

Antihistamines are rapidly absorbed from the gastrointestinal tract, and most reach their peak plasma concentration within 1 to 3 hours. All oral antihistamines except cetirizine, acrivastine, and fexofenadine are metabolized predominantly by the hepatic cytochrome P450 system. Cetirizine and acrivastine are excreted predominantly in the urine, while 80% of fexofenadine is found unchanged in the feces. Terminal half-lives range from 2 to > 24 hours for currently available products, with children having more rapid rates of clearance. Tissue half-life is greater than serum half-life, as demonstrated by suppression of histamine-induced wheal-and-flare reactions on skin testing.

36. **What is unique about the antihistamine azelastine?**

Azelastine (Astelin) is the first antihistamine nasal spray in the United States. It is approved for the treatment of allergic and nonallergic rhinitis. It is dosed twice daily and has an onset of action of 2–3 hours compared with placebo. Side effects include bitter taste in 20% of users, and despite its topical formulation 11% of patients report drowsiness.

37. **What are the two basic classes of decongestants?**

Oral decongestants include pseudoephedrine and phenylephrine; **topical** decongestants include oxymetazoline, xylometazoline, naphazoline, tetrahydrozoline, and phenylephrine.

38. **Describe the actions and side effects of oral and topical decongestants.**

Decongestants are alpha-adrenergic agonists that cause nasal vasoconstriction, thus reducing blood volume in the venous sinusoids. The most common side effects of oral decongestants are nervousness, palpitations, loss of appetite, insomnia, and urinary hesitancy. Caution should be used in patients with hypertension, glaucoma, hyperthyroidism, and coronary artery disease. Topical products should be limited to 3–5 days of continuous use, because tachyphylaxis develops rapidly and may lead to rebound nasal congestion (rhinitis medicamentosa).

39. **Describe the mechanism of action of cromolyn sodium nasal spray. What is its role in the treatment of allergic rhinitis?**

Cromolyn sodium (Nasalcrom) inhibits mediator release from mast cells, reducing the allergic reaction rather than alleviating symptoms once they have begun. The protective effect of a single dose of cromolyn lasts for 4–8 hours. It is best to start cromolyn before the onset of the allergy season (e.g., spring) because the onset of sustained benefit takes several days to 2 weeks.

Suggested dosing is 1 spray in each nostril every 4 hours during the day. Cromolyn may also be used as an intermittent medication to pretreat infrequent exposures to the patient's known allergic triggers. Like antihistamines, cromolyn is more effective for reducing sneeze, itch, and rhinorrhea than it is for nasal congestion. In general, cromolyn is less effective than antihistamines and nasal steroids.

40. **What is the role of leukotriene receptor antagonists in the treatment of allergic rhinitis?**
Montelukast (Singulair), originally released for the treatment of asthma, is now FDA-approved for allergic rhinitis. Cysteinyl leukotrienes are among the allergic mediators released from mast cells; they increase local vascular permeability, thereby causing nasal congestion. Overall, montelukast appears equal in efficacy to loratadine in the treatment of allergic rhinitis. Combining montelukast with an antihistamine may have additive benefit, but the studies examining this question give conflicting results.

41. **What is the most effective class of medication used to treat allergic rhinitis?**
A meta-analysis of 16 studies comparing intranasal steroids sprays to antihistamines showed a highly significant superiority of nasal steroids in controlling sneeze, itch, congestion, nasal discharge, and total nasal symptom score. In addition, compared to antihistamines, nasal steroids were equally effective at controlling ocular symptoms. The authors' conclusion based on efficacy, safety, and cost was that intranasal steroids are preferred as first-line therapy for allergic rhinitis. Nasal steroids have also been shown to be more efficacious than cromolyn and montelukast.

  Weiner JM, Abraham MJ, Puy RM: Intranasal corticosteroids versus oral H$_1$ receptor antagonists in allergic rhinitis: Systematic review of randomised controlled trials. BMJ 317:1624–1629, 1998.

42. **List the currently available intranasal steroid sprays and their dose range in the average adult patient.**
See Table 5-2.

TABLE 5-2. COMMONLY AVAILABLE INTRANASAL STEROID SPRAYS		
Generic Name	**Trade Name**	**Dose Range (Per Nostril)***
Beclomethasone	Beconase AQ	1–2 sprays twice daily
Budesonide	Rhinocort Aqua	2–4 sprays daily
Flunisolide	Nasalide, Nasarel	1–2 sprays twice daily
Fluticasone	Flonase	1–2 sprays daily
Mometasone	Nasonex	2 sprays daily
Triamcinolone	Nasacort AQ	1–2 sprays daily

*With all products, once control of nasal symptoms has been attained, the dose is weaned to the lowest effective.

43. **How do intranasal steroid sprays work?**
Topical intranasal steroids have multiple physiologic effects, including:
- Reduction of the inflammatory cellular infiltrate in the nasal mucosa

- Reduced vascular permeability and mucus secretion
- Reduced early- and late-phase allergen responses with chronic use
  Some nasal steroids have shown statistically significant symptom reduction within 12 hours, although peak benefit may take up to 2 weeks.

KEY POINTS: TREATMENT OPTIONS FOR ALLERGIC RHINITIS (IN ORDER OF INCREASING EFFICACY)

1. For all patients: allergen avoidance

2. Cromolyn nasal spray

3. Antihistamine (preferably nonsedating), +/− decongestants or leukotriene receptor antagonist

4. Intranasal steroid spray

5. Allergen immunotherapy

44. **Discuss potential local side effects of intranasal steroid sprays.**
The most common adverse effects are nasal stinging or burning, sneeze, mild epistaxis, and rarely nasal septal perforation. In order to reduce the chance of septal perforation, the patient should be instructed to direct the spray slightly away from the septum. Additionally, patients who develop nosebleeds should be instructed to discontinue the spray until a nasal exam can be performed. Mucosal thinning has not been reported, even in biopsy specimens from patients using beclomethasone spray for 5 years.

45. **Do intranasal steroid sprays reduce growth rates in children?**
One study of beclomethasone spray dosed at 168 µg twice daily in children showed a 0.9-cm decrement in growth rate over a 1-year period compared to the placebo control group. Neither fluticasone, dosed at 200 µg daily, nor mometasone, dosed at 100 µg daily, showed any effect on growth rate when studied over a 1-year period. There are no multiyear studies of the effect of nasal steroids on growth, but in children with asthma long-term inhaled budesonide has not been shown to affect final height.
   Allen DB et al: No growth suppression in children treated with fluticasone. Allergy Asthma Proc 23:407–413, 2002.
   Schenkel EJ et al: Absence of growth retardation in children with perennial allergic rhinitis after 1 year treatment with momentasone. Pediatrics 105:22, 2000.
   Skoner D et al: Detection of growth retardation in children during treatment with beclamethasone. Pediatrics 105:23, 2000.

46. **What is the preferred therapy for a patient complaining of isolated watery rhinorrhea?**
Ipratropium bromide (Atrovent) nasal spray is an anticholinergic agent that is indicated to treat rhinorrhea only. With its quaternary amine structure, it is poorly absorbed and has few potential side effects other than excessive nasal drying. It is available in 0.03% and 0.06%. The lower strength is used for allergic and nonallergic rhinitis, while the higher strength can be used to reduce rhinorrhea associated with the common cold. Dosing is usually 2–3 sprays in each nostril 2 or 3 times/day. Atrovent is particularly useful for patients with gustatory or cold air–induced rhinorrhea, because the spray can be administered prophylactically.

47. **Design a rational stepwise therapeutic approach for the managing rhinitis.**
For all levels of severity, allergen avoidance should be instituted to the degree possible. Other treatment options are outlined in Table 5-3.

TABLE 5-3.   MANAGEMENT OF RHINITIS

Severity	Treatment Options
Mild intermittent	Oral antihistamines and/or decongestants as needed
	Topical decongestants and saline sprays may also help
Mild persistent	Daily use of antihistamines with/without decongestant
	Cromolyn nasal spray
	Low-dose intranasal steroid spray
Moderate persistent	Intranasal steroid spray as first line therapy
	Add antihistamine with/without decongestant if needed
	Immunotherapy may be considered
Severe persistent	Intranasal steroid spray plus antihistamine-decongestant
	Consider adding a leukotriene receptor antagonist
	Possibly burst of oral or intramuscular steroid
	Immunotherapy

48. **List possible complications of allergic rhinitis.**
    - Abnormal facial development in childhood, leading to elongated midface ("adenoid facies") and high-arched palate with dental malocclusion. Chronic mouth-breathing, which results in the lack of normal tongue contact with the palate, is the presumed mechanism of these abnormalities.
    - Otitis media and sinusitis due to eustachian tube and sinus ostia obstruction, respectively.
    - Decreased sense of smell
    - Sleep disturbance

49. **What are the preferred medications to treat allergic rhinitis in pregnancy?**
    1. **Antihistamine:** first generation: chlorpheniramine (FDA class B); second generation (if first generation not tolerated): loratadine, cetirizine (class B)
    2. **Decongestant** (avoid all decongestants in first trimester): pseudoephedrine (class C)
    3. **Nasal sprays:** saline and cromolyn (class B); budesonide or beclomethasone (class C) preferred when an intranasal steroid is required.

50. **Discuss the role of rhinoscopy and computed tomography (CT) in the evaluation of rhinitis.**
    Upper airway endoscopy (rhinoscopy) is used to examine the middle and superior meatal areas for polyps or mucopurulent sinus discharge, structures in the more posterior portion of the nasal airway, and the nasopharynx. Anatomic problems, which would otherwise not be visible with routine anterior nasal examination, may be diagnosed with this technique. It is particularly valuable in evaluating nasal obstruction.
    CT scanning also provides detailed information about the nasal and sinus anatomy and can detect pneumatization of the turbinates (concha bullosa).

WEBSITE

American College of Allergy, Asthma and Immunology: www.acaai.org

BIBLIOGRAPHY

1. Bousquet J, van Couwenberge P, Khaltaev N, et al: Allergic rhinitis and its impact on asthma (ARIA), Workshop Report. J Allergy Clin Immunol 108:S147–336, 2001.

2. Dykewicz MS, Fineman S (eds): Diagnosis and management of rhinitis: Complete guidelines of the Joint Task Force on Practice Parameters in Allergy, Asthma, and Immunology. Ann Allergy Asthma Immunol 81:478–518, 1998.

3. Eccles R: Anatomy and physiology of the nose and control of nasal airflow. In Adkinson NF Jr et al (eds): Middleton's Allergy: Principles and Practice, 6th ed. St. Louis, Mosby, 2003, pp 775–787.

4. Howarth PH: Allergic and nonallergic rhinitis. In Adkinson NF Jr et al (eds): Middleton's Allergy: Principles and Practice, 6th ed. St. Louis, Mosby, 2003, p 1391.

5. Joint Committee of the American College of Obstetricians and Gynecologists and the American College of Allergy, Asthma and Immunology. Position Statement: The use of newer asthma and allergy medications during pregnancy. Ann Allergy Asthma Immunol 84:475–480, 2000.

6. Lieberman P: Rhinitis. In Slavin RG, Reisman RE (eds): Expert Guide to Allergy and Immunology. Philadelphia, American College of Physicians, 1999, pp 23–40.

7. Settipane RA, Lieberman P: Update on nonallergic rhinitis. Ann Allergy Asthma Immunol 86:494–508, 2001.

8. Simons FER: Antihistamines. In Adkinson NF Jr. et al (eds): Middleton's Allergy: Principles and Practice, 6th ed. St. Louis, Mosby, 2003, pp 834–869.

CHAPTER 6

ASTHMA

Nicholas J. Kenyon, M.D., and Samuel Louie, M.D.

1. **Define asthma.**

   Understanding of asthma has suffered from the lack of a definition that is easily applicable both in the clinic and research laboratory. This reflects the complex nature of the disease and the different perspectives gained by asthma researchers, primary care physicians, and specialists. The best definition, formulated by the National Institutes of Health (NIH), has several components. Asthma is a chronic inflammatory airways disease that manifests as a syndrome with episodic symptoms of wheezing, dyspnea, and cough. Patients also should have evidence of reversible airflow obstruction and airways hyperreactivity, both of which are key to making the proper clinical diagnosis.

2. **Who devised the guidelines for determining the severity of asthma?**

   In 1997 and 2002, the National Asthma Education and Prevention Program (NAEPP), sponsored by NIH, published comprehensive guidelines to help physicians classify the severity of asthma and focus treatment. Their recommendations are available at the following website: http://www.nhlbi.nih.gov/guidelines/asthma/asthgdln.htm. An important update on selected topics is included with a useful guideline tool for the Palm OS.

3. **Summarize the NAEPP guidelines for determining severity.**

   Patients with **mild intermittent** asthma experience symptoms once or twice per week and have near-normal spirometry and peak expiratory flow rates (PEFR). Their infrequent symptoms can often be treated with as-needed bronchodilators. Patients with regular daytime and nocturnal symptoms are classified as having **mild, moderate, or severe persistent asthma,** depending on the degree of variability in PEFR or forced expiratory volume in one second (FEV_1) and frequency of exacerbations. The majority of asthmatics have moderate and severe persistent asthma, and the frequency of nocturnal symptoms often classifies them at these levels.

4. **What is status asthmaticus?**

   Status asthmaticus is defined as a severe asthma exacerbation that does not respond readily to aggressive bronchodilator therapy. Descriptive terms for a status asthmaticus attack include "life-threatening asthma" or "near-fatal asthma," but a more specific definition with physiologic and gas exchange parameters is lacking. Patients in status asthmaticus are on the verge of acute respiratory failure and are at risk for mechanical ventilatory support and respiratory arrest.

5. **Who is susceptible to status asthmaticus?**

   Most asthma deaths and episodes of status asthmaticus occur in patients with prolonged, poorly treated exacerbations. All asthmatics are potentially at risk, and patients and physicians must treat exacerbations earlier and promptly.

6. **Does the physical examination aid in the evaluation of asthmatic patients in the emergency department?**

   Physical findings in patients with exacerbations of asthma do not correlate well with the degree of airflow obstruction. Diffuse expiratory wheezing is a nearly ubiquitous finding, but the most severely impaired patients may have dramatically decreased breath sounds that limit auscultatory wheezing, often termed the "quiet chest." Simple observation of the respiratory pattern and recording of the vital signs provide much of the relevant physical exam in status asthmaticus patients.

7. **What signs and symptoms are most helpful?**

Distressed patients are tachypneic, sit upright, and use accessory muscles of respiration. Heart rates typically exceed 110 beats/minute, but blood pressure can fluctuate significantly, depending on the degree of hemodynamic embarrassment secondary to high intrathoracic pressures. The **pulsus paradoxus,** a reflection of high intrathoracic pressures, may prove the most helpful finding in status asthmaticus patients. An exaggerated pulsus paradoxus, defined as the difference in systolic blood pressure between expiration and inspiration of > 15 mmHg that does not improve after initial therapeutic efforts, has been suggested as a parameter for intensive care monitoring.

8. **Describe the natural history of wheezing in infancy and development of asthma.**

This issue has not been fully resolved, but longitudinal data from several large population studies provide important evidence. Children less than 3 years of age who develop respiratory illnesses with wheezing appear to have worse adult lung function than children who do not have wheezing illnesses. It is unclear, however, whether this relationship is causal or whether infants with wheezing illnesses were predisposed to such episodes because of diminished airway function at birth. An Arizona population study has shown that most infants with wheezing viral respiratory infections before the age of 3 years do not develop asthma by the age of 6 years. A significant minority of infants (25–40%) with wheezing is diagnosed ultimately with asthma, and identification of this subset is difficult. Such apparently contradictory epidemiologic data make firm conclusions difficult to draw. Factors associated with an increased risk of developing persistent asthma include maternal smoking and a history of maternal asthma or atopy.

9. **When should spirometry be performed in asthmatic patients?**

Office spirometry is an important tool in evaluating and managing persistent asthma. First, spirometry is used to gauge the severity of airways obstruction by measuring FEV_1 (L/sec), forced vital capacity (FVC), $FEV_1\%$, and forced expiratory flow at 25–75% of FVC (FEF_{25-75}). Patients frequently minimize their symptoms, and spirometry may be the only indicator of significant impairment. Recent evidence suggests that most asthmatics have moderate or severe persistent asthma, and regular spirometry is a vital part of their assessment. Secondly, spirome-

---

KEY POINTS: OVERVIEW OF ASTHMA

1. Status asthmaticus is defined as a severe asthma exacerbation that does not respond to aggressive therapy.

2. Physical examinations in patients with asthma exacerbations do not correlate well with the degree of airflow obstruction.

3. An asthma action plan should be provided to patients with chronic asthma.

4. High doses of short-acting β_2 agonists are associated with increased morbidity and mortality.

5. Death from asthma is 25-fold higher for those over 75 years of age and is also a major problem for teenagers living in inner cities.

try provides a sound objective method to follow disease progression over years. It is more accurate and reliable than home peak flow rate meters, which measures the PEFR or extrapolated peak airflow in 1 minute (L/min). Home FEV_1 devices are available, albeit expensive.

10. **What should the evaluation of an asthmatic patient include?**
In addition to lung function testing, the evaluation should include an investigation for disease triggers and concomitant conditions. In patients suspected of having allergies to indoor or environmental allergens, skin testing should be performed and serum immunoglobulin E measured according to a common allergen panel. In 30–80% of asthmatics, allergic rhinosinusitis, gastroesophageal reflux disease, or both may complicate management. Approximately 20–30% of asthmatics smoke cigarettes—a habit that complicates the distinction between asthma and chronic obstructive pulmonary disease in adults. Because of the link between asthma and obstructive sleep apnea, patients should be questioned about excessive daytime hypersomnolence, snoring, and sleeping patterns. Establishing the proper diagnosis of asthma is important but often not sufficient for treating a patient's symptoms appropriately.

11. **Is airway challenge testing useful in diagnosing asthma?**
Pulmonary function testing, including spirometry, detects airway expiratory flow obstruction, not asthma. As such, both are insensitive in screening for asthma. While routine spirometry may show impairment in expiration (i.e., decreased FEV_1 and FEV_1/FVC) and indicate obstruction, these parameters commonly are normal in patients with intermittent and mild-to-moderate persistent asthma. In patients with symptoms worrisome for asthma and an unclear diagnosis, bronchoprovocation testing should be performed. Airway hyperresponsiveness is shown by a 20% reduction in FEV_1 with serial increases in doses of methacholine or histamine. Provocation testing via treadmill or ergometer for patients with symptoms of exercise-induced bronchospasm may also be beneficial. The absence of hyperreponsiveness with challenge testing is highly specific (>9 5%) in ruling out asthma. Monitoring airway hyperresponsiveness may offer an additional guide for long-term control of asthma in addition to FEV_1 measurements and symptoms.

12. **Are certain demographic populations at increased risk of asthma-related death?**
While all asthmatics are at risk of dying from the disease, certain disturbing demographic trends in asthma deaths have been noted. A correlation between age and death from asthma appears clear. The likelihood of dying from asthma is 25 times higher for those greater than 75 years of age compared to younger adults. Likewise, mortality rates from asthma are 2–3 times higher in African-Americans compared to whites. Recently, an unexplained increase in mortality was observed during a 28–week safety study in asthmatics who added salmeterol to usual asthma treatments (e.g., inhaled corticosteroids). Subgroup analysis suggested the risk may be higher in African-American compared to Caucasian patients. This finding underscores the importance of clinical monitoring in chronic asthma once pharmacotherapy is begun in each patient.

13. **Does gender affect mortality?**
Women 55 years of age and older are currently at the highest risk for death from asthma. A large cohort study of severe asthmatics—The European Network for Understanding Mechanisms of Severe Asthma (ENFUMOSA)—found that there were 2.5 times as many women as men. Furthermore, the age-adjusted mortality rates are significantly higher for women (2.5 versus 1.9/100,000 population). Why women make up 60–80% of adult patients with severe asthma is unclear. Postmenopausal hormone use is associated with an increased rate of newly diagnosed asthma.
    Barr RG, Wentowski CC, Grodstein F, et al. Prospective study of postmenopausal hormone use and newly diagnosed asthma and chronic obstructive pulmonary disease. Arch Int Med 164:379–386, 2004.

14. **Can demographic trends be explained?**
    Insight into demographic trends is lacking, but many contend that some of these populations have poor access to medical care. Misinformed patients frequently underestimate the severity of their asthma, and physicians are often guilty of similar misjudgments. Together, misunderstanding and misdiagnosis may contribute to undue morbidity and mortality from asthma.

15. **Define refractory asthma. Is it common?**
    Refractory asthma was defined by the American Thoracic Society in 1999 to describe a subpopulation of severely asthmatic patients who are difficult to treat and poorly responsive to therapy. They represent approximately only 1–3% of all asthmatics and should be cared for by asthma specialists. The definition of refractory asthma can be made in patients who require daily treatment with high-dose inhaled corticosteroids (> 880 μg/day fluticasone or equivalent) or oral corticosteroids > 50% of the year and have at least 2 of 7 minor criteria, including (1) the need for additional controller therapy, (2) daily β-agonist usage, (3) persistent airway obstruction, (4) one or more urgent care visits per year, (5) three or more prednisone bursts/year, (6) prompt clinical deterioration with a < 25% reduction in steroid dose, and (7) a history of near-fatal asthma. It is much more likely that a difficult-to-control asthmatic patient may be misdiagnosed or have untreated concomitant conditions that exacerbate their asthma than fit the definition of refractory asthma.

16. **Name and describe the key effector cells in asthma.**
    Eosinophils, T-lymphocytes, mast cells, and antigen-presenting cells (e.g., dendritic cells, alveolar macrophages) play key roles in the pathogenesis of asthma. Recently, both airway epithelial and smooth muscle cells have been implicated as active participants in the inflammatory events in asthma. Identifying a single effector cell that governs the airway inflammation in all asthmatics is not possible since a host of native cells and foreign leukocytes contribute to the pathogenesis.

17. **Give specific examples of effector cell mechanisms in asthma.**
    Th-2 differentiated lymphocytes release specific cytokines, such as interleukin-4 (IL-4), IL-5, and IL-13, which promote the recruitment and activation of eosinophils as well as differentiation and migration of helper lymphocytes from regional lymph nodes into the airway. Activated eosinophils characteristically infiltrate bronchioles and release granule enzymes that promote airway edema and stimulate repair mechanisms. Mast cells, through the release of histamine and leukotrienes, further trigger airway inflammation as well as microvascular leak in both early and late phases of asthma, which occur 6–24 hours later. All effector cells, smooth muscle cells, and goblet cells in the airways of asthmatic patients can adversely affect airway function through various mediators. The complexity of this cascade clearly hampers efforts to target a single cell or mediator for therapeutic means.

18. **How can airway inflammation be assessed in the clinics?**
    Severity of asthma and treatment in clinical practice are not based on an objective assessment of the airway inflammation in individual patients. We rely on clinical symptoms and spirometry, which are poor surrogate markers of inflammation. A semiquantitative assessment of airway inflammation can be made from lung biopsies, sputum, and exhaled nitric oxide. Endobronchial and transbronchial biopsies obtained via fiberoptic bronchoscopy can be helpful but are not often obtained outside the research realm. Analyses of induced sputum samples for eosinophil counts and eosinophil cationic protein levels have been shown to gauge airway inflammation and asthma severity effectively. These tools will become more commonplace in the next 10 years.

19. **How is measurement of exhaled breath nitric oxide levels used in clinical practice?**

    The American Thoracic Society has published standards for the measurement of exhaled nitric oxide, and in May 2003 a device was approved by the Food and Drug Administration (FDA) to measure such levels in the clinical setting. An elevated exhaled breath nitric oxide level > 15 ppb is indicative of airway inflammation; levels increase and decrease with disease flares and remissions. As with other tests, clinical correlation is necessary since other types of inflammation and infection can also raise nitric oxide levels.

20. **Explain the statement, "Asthma is a Th-2 lymphocyte-mediated disease."**

    Atopic asthmatics produce an overabundance of CD4+ T-helper lymphocytes in response to repeated allergen stimulation. These terminal lymphocytes are termed Th-2 cells because they resemble a previously defined subpopulation of mouse lymphocytes that secrete specific cytokines, including IL-4, IL-5, IL-9, IL-10, and IL-13. Bronchial biopsies of atopic asthmatics have shown a marked influx of such CD4+ cells, and lymphocytes isolated from bronchoalveolar lavage fluid of asthmatics generate increased levels of Th-2 cytokines compared to normal controls.

21. **Discuss the role of Th-2 cytokines in asthma.**

    Th-2 cytokines play key roles in the airway inflammation of asthma (Fig. 6-1). IL-5, for example, stimulates proliferation and differentiation of eosinophils from bone marrow progenitor cells and promotes eosinophil degranulation in the lungs. IL-4, in turn, triggers B-cell differentiation and IgE production, thereby reinforcing the atopic phenotype. Recent evidence suggests that IL-13 helps sustain airway inflammation without eosinophil recruitment and encourages subepithelial matrix deposition. While it is clear that Th-2 cytokines are fundamentally important to the allergic asthma phenotype, their role in nonatopic asthmatics and elderly asthmatics, among others, is less well understood. Results from preliminary human studies using a competitive receptor to IL-4 and an anti-IL-5 antibody have shown modest benefit but inability to induce a permanent remission.

22. **What is airway remodeling in asthma? How does it correlate with lung function decline?**

    Many chronic asthmatics experience a decline in lung function (i.e., decline in FEV_1) faster than the general population, and a subset of this group develops irreversible airways obstruction that is refractory to treatment with bronchodilator and anti-inflammatory therapy. Remodeling of the airways is seen in mild-to-severe persistent asthmatics and is characterized by airway wall thickening, subepithelial fibrosis, smooth muscle hypertrophy, increased vascularity, and mucous metaplasia. The relationship between these structural changes and lung function decline is unclear since the majority of patients with mild-to-moderate disease remain healthy overall despite microscopic evidence of airway remodeling. There is strong interest in altering the remodeling response through inhibition of various growth factors and other mediators, yet this research is in its infancy. This area may represent a focus of future therapy.

23. **How is asthma differentiated from allergic rhinosinusitis?**

    Allergic rhinitis is four-fold more prevalent in the United States than asthma, yet the pathogenesis of both disorders shares much in common. What prompts differentiation to the allergic rhinitis, the asthma phenotype, or both is unclear. Up to 78% of asthmatics have a component of allergic rhinitis. Similarities between the two diseases include the effector cells (eosinophils, T- and B-lymphocytes, and mast cells), inflammatory mediators (histamine, prostaglandins, leukotrienes), epithelial and subepithelial matrix remodeling, and cytokine profiles. Relative differences in the upregulation of certain cytokines, the role of bronchial airway smooth muscle tone, and the lack of nasal epithelial disruption and denudation may help distinguish these diseases. Further understanding of the programmed cellular events in the airway may reveal a

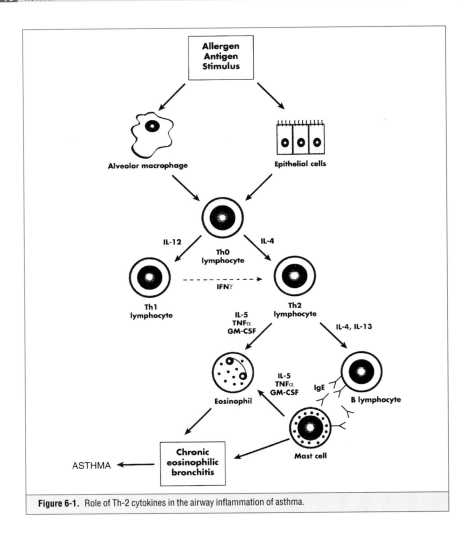

Figure 6-1. Role of Th-2 cytokines in the airway inflammation of asthma.

key mediator that serves as a specific marker for asthma. Such a biochemical marker would be very useful clinically and remains an important focus of research.

24. **Is there an association between asthma and chronic obstructive pulmonary disease (COPD)?**
Lung disease specialists have long noted similarities between asthma and COPD, defined as both chronic bronchitis and emphysema from cigarette smoking. Indeed, the outdated term *asthmatic bronchitis* reflects this overlap clinically. Pathologically, COPD develops from neutrophil infiltration with resultant airway epithelial metaplasia and alveolar destruction from the neutrophil's proteolytic enzymes. As with asthma, however, one histologic description does not uniformly characterize the spectrum of COPD. Overlapping phenotypic and pathologic features in a subset of patients with asthma and COPD is well recognized (Fig. 6-2). Future investigation of the cellular and physiologic mechanisms involved in asthma and COPD may uncover further similarities between these most common lung diseases.

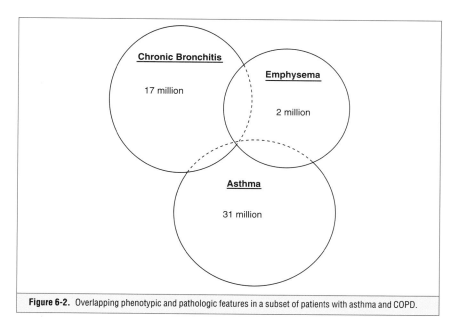

Figure 6-2. Overlapping phenotypic and pathologic features in a subset of patients with asthma and COPD.

U.S. Department of Health and Human Services, The Global Initiative for Chronic Obstructive Lung Disease (GOLD): NHLBI/WHO Workshop Report. Executive Summary. NIH Publication No. 2701A, 2001.

25. **What current evidence supports the association between asthma and COPD?**
    Recent evidence suggests that a subset of asthmatic patients lose lung function, as measured by reduction in FEV_1 (mL/yr), at a rate more comparable to patients with COPD than to normal controls. Furthermore, in patients with severe persistent asthma and $FEV_1 < 60\%$ predicted, Gelb and colleagues found a marked loss of lung elastic recoil at 80% of total lung capacity that accounted for an estimated 35% reduction in maximal airflow. This degree of lung elastic recoil loss is commonplace in COPD and suggests that some asthmatics may have lung parenchymal changes indicative of "pseudo-emphysema."

26. **How common is bronchial asthma?**
    Approximately 31 million people (including 9 million children in the United States) or 10–15% of the population have asthma as of 2001, according to the CDC. In 1996 the National Center for Health Statistics reported an increase in self-reported asthma of nearly 80% since 1980. The prevalence of asthma increased from 30.7 per 1000 persons in the United States to 55.2 per 1000 persons, and hospitalization rates increased 120% between 1978 and 1994. Although deaths from asthma have averaged 5000 to 6000 annually for over a decade, mortality rates remain unacceptably high in African-Americans and the elderly. While boys have more asthma difficulties than girls do, women have more frequent and severe exacerbations than men.

27. **Why is the prevalence increasing?**
    These alarming statistics have emerged despite unprecedented public health initiatives to better manage asthma. Factors that may account for the increase in asthma prevalence and incidence include more accurate diagnosis, outdoor air pollution, obesity, dietary habits, and more concentrated exposure to indoor allergens (e.g., dust mites and cockroaches.)

KEY POINTS: MIMICS OF ASTHMA

1. COPD
2. Bronchiectasis
3. Bronchiolitis
4. Congestive heart failure
5. Pulmonary embolism
6. Vocal cord dysfunction
7. Airway tumor
8. Foreign body

KEY POINTS: CONCOMITANT DISEASES ASSOCIATED WITH ASTHMA

1. Gastroesophageal reflux disease
2. Rhinosinusitis
3. Allergic bronchopulmonary aspergillosis
4. Churg-Strauss syndrome
5. Vocal cord dysfunction
6. Obstructive sleep apnea syndrome

28. **Are short-acting β_2-agonists a factor in asthma deaths?**

High doses of short-acting β_2-agonists have been associated with increased morbidity and mortality due to asthma. Tolerance to frequent β_2-agonist administration may result from downregulation of airway receptors, and overreliance on these agents for symptom management at the expense of controller medications places the patient at increased risk for fatal asthma. A particular polymorphism of the β_2-receptor gene may be associated with a diminished response to β_2-agonists, both short- and long-acting. Patients homozygous for Gly-16 polymorphism on the β-receptor undergo desensitization and downregulation of the β-receptor response, and this genotype is more prevalent in populations with severe asthma. Despite several concerning studies correlating β_2-agonist usage with increased risk of asthma death, many clinicians do not believe that there is a causal relationship between the two. Care must be exercised here. Recent evidence suggests that chronic short-acting β_2-agonist usage may potentiate airway adrenergic receptor activity and bronchoconstriction. Smooth muscle dysfunction in asthma is an area of intense research.

McGraw DW, Almoosa KF, Paul RJ, et al: Antithetic regulation of β-adrenergic receptors of G_q receptor signaling via phospholipase C underlies the airway β-agonist paradox. J Clin Invest 112: 619–626, 2003.

29. **How is occupation-associated asthma diagnosed?**

Asthma is the most common occupational lung disease. The diagnosis requires the temporal association of symptoms and evidence of airway obstruction with exposure to the workplace environment. A host of agents have been shown to trigger asthma, including isocyanates, latex, and baker's yeast. The low-molecular-weight compound toluene diisocyanate, commonly found in paints and adhesives, may promote asthma in up to 5–30% of chronically exposed workers.

Patients with apparent occupational asthma should be asked to keep a symptom diary. Episodes of dyspnea, cough, and wheezing that begin during or soon after work and improve while away from this environment, as on the weekend, are suggestive of occupational asthma. In addition, serial PEFR measurements that consistently worsen during and soon after work and improve at other times provide strong evidence for this condition. Treatment obviously consists of patient removal from the offending work environment.

30. **Define reactive airways dysfunction syndrome.**

    Clinicians often group patients who have asthma, COPD, or other airways disease with a compo-
    nent of bronchospasm under the term *reactive airways disease*. It is an imprecise term and
    should be avoided. In addition, it can be confused with the term *reactive airway dysfunction
    syndrome* (RADS), which is a separate entity from asthma. This condition is defined by persis-
    tent airway hyperreactivity after massive exposure to offending irritants such as acid, ammonia,
    and other fumes. Despite removal from the irritant, symptoms may persist for years and metha-
    choline challenge testing may remain abnormal. Treatment with inhaled steroids and bron-
    chodilators is routinely recommended, but evidence of efficacy is slim.

31. **Can inhaled corticosteroid drugs cause systemic effects?**

    Patients and physicians are concerned about the potential prolonged effects of chronic inhaled
    steroid use in asthmatic patients. A host of pharmacologic studies have shown that regular daily
    intake of high-dose inhaled corticosteroids (e. g., > 840 μg beclomethasone, > 600 μg budes-
    onide, > 660 μg fluticasone, or > 2000 μg triamcinolone) may have systemic effects such as
    pituitary-adrenal axis suppression, bone mineral loss, skin bruising, and growth retardation. For
    example, children aged 6–16 years who receive doses of 400–800 μg/day of beclamethasone
    experience significantly slower annual growth (0.3–1.8 cm/yr). By adulthood, however, there is
    no difference in height between the general population and asthmatics treated with lifelong
    inhaled steroids. Adult asthmatics are affected subclinically by doses of inhaled steroids of 1500
    μg or less per day. Significant adrenal suppression as measured by overnight plasma cortisol
    suppression may occur after daily doses are increased beyond medium dose beclomethasone
    and low-dose fluticasone.

32. **Are high-dose steroids necessary to treat asthma?**

    Exceeding the aforementioned doses did not further improve FEV_1 and PC_{20} in a recent NIH-
    sponsored study by the Asthma Clinical Research Network. Maximum FEV_1 response occurred
    with low-dose fluticasone MDI and medium-dose beclomethasone MDI and was not further
    increased with fluticasone DPI at 2000 μg/day. Higher doses of drug failed to increase the effi-
    cacy of the inhaled corticosteroids studied.

33. **Are low-dose inhalers safer than higher-dose oral steroids?**

    Isolated patients may suffer accelerated bone mineral loss or adrenal gland suppression, but, in
    general, the risk of deleterious side effects with inhaled agents is significantly less than with
    long-term, higher-dose oral steroids. Once disease control is achieved, inhaled steroids should
    be reduced to lowest effective dose (Table 6-1).

34. **Is asthma associated with vocal cord dysfunction?**

    Vocal cord dysfunction (VCD) is a condition of unclear etiology in which patients paradoxically
    adduct the true vocal cords with inspiration. Failure to fully open the cords causes inspiratory
    stridor and a sensation of choking or an asthma-like attack. Approximately 50% of patients with
    VCD have asthma, but the two diseases are not causally related. It is frequently difficult to differ-
    entiate VCD from asthma when faced with a distressed patient with apparent compromised air-
    flow in the emergency department. Despite their distress, patients with VCD should have normal
    gas exchange and airway resistance. A flow-volume loop showing truncation of the inspiratory
    limb of a flow-volume loop suggests the diagnosis of VCD, but definitive diagnosis requires
    direct visualization of the abnormal vocal cord movement via rhinoscopy or bronchoscopy (Fig.
    6-3). Treatment consists of speech therapy but is variably successful. Asthmatic patients with
    VCD require standard treatment for asthma as well.

35. **When should patients be referred to an asthma consultant?**

    Referral to an asthma consultant is a treatment option in all patients with moderate and severe per-
    sistent asthma. Recurrent emergency department visits or failure to control symptoms despite

TABLE 6-1. ESTIMATED COMPARATIVE DAILY DOSAGES FOR INHALED CORTICOSTEROIDS

Drug	Low Dose	Medium Dose	High Dose
Adults			
Beclomethasone dipropionate	168–504 µg	504–840 µg	> 840 µg
42 µg/puff	(4–12 puffs: 42 µg)	(12–20 puffs: 42 µg)	(> 20 puffs: 42 µg)
84 µg/puff	(2–6 puffs: 84 µg)	(6–10 puffs: 84 µg)	(> 10 puffs: 84 µg)
Budenoside Turbuhaler 200 µg/dose	200–400 µg (1–2 inhalations)	400–600 µg (2–3 inhalations)	> 600 µg (> 3 inhalations)
Flunisolide 200 µg/puff	500–1000 µg (2–4 puffs)	1000–2000 µg (4–8 puffs)	> 2000 µg (> 8 puffs)
Fluticasone MDI: 44, 110 220 µg/puff DPI: 50, 100, 250 µg dose	88–264 µg (2–6 puffs: 44 µg) or (2 puffs: 110 µg) (2–6 inhalations: 50 µg)	264–660 µg (2–6 puffs: 110 µg) (3–6 inhalations: 100 µg)	> 660 µg (> 6 puffs: 110 µg) or (> 3 puffs: 220 µg) (> 2 inhalations: 250 µg)
Triamcinolone acetonide (Azmacort) 100 µg/puff	400–1000 µg (4–10 puffs)	1000–2000 µg (10–20 puffs)	> 2000 µg (> 20 puffs)
Children			
Beclomethasone dipropionate 42 µg/puff 84 µg/puff	84–336 µg (2–8 puffs: 42 µg) (1–4 puffs: 84 µg)	336–672 µg (8–16 puffs: 42 µg) (4–8 puffs: 84 µg)	> 672 µg (> 16 puffs: 42 µg) (> 8 puffs: 84 µg)
Budenoside Turbuhaler 200 µg/dose	100–200 µg	200–400 µg (1–2 inhalations: 200 µg)	> 400 µg (> 2 inhalations: 200 µg)
Flunisolide 200 µg/puff	500–750 µg (2–3 puffs)	1000–1250 µg (4–5 puffs)	> 1250 µg (> 5 puffs)
Fluticasone MDI: 44, 110 220 µg/puff DPI: 50, 100, 250 µg dose	88–176 µg (2–4 puffs: 44 µg) (2–4 inhalations: 50 µg)	176–440 µg (4–10 puffs: 44 µg) or (2–4 puffs: 110 µg) (2–4 inhalations: 100 µg)	> 440 µg (> 4 puffs: 110 µg) or (> 2 puffs: 220 µg) (> 4 inhalations: 100 µg) (> 2 inhalations: 250 µg)
Triamcinolone acetonide (Azmacort) 100 µg/puff	400–800 µg (4–8 puffs)	800–1200 µg (8–12 puffs)	> 1200 µg (> 12 puffs)

moderate-dose combination therapy is an indication for referral to an allergist, pulmonologist, or any physician with expertise in treating asthma. Cytotoxic drugs (e.g., methotrexate, cyclosporine), allergen immunotherapy, and anti-IgE therapy should be prescribed by asthma consultants only. In addition, a consultant should see any patient in whom the diagnosis of asthma is in doubt.

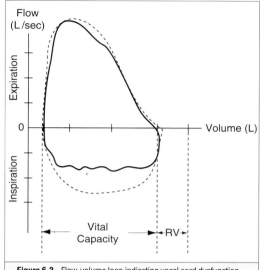

Figure 6-3. Flow-volume loop indicating vocal cord dysfunction.

36. **In an outpatient clinic visit, what patient education objectives should be stressed in asthmatics?**
Patient education is key to successful management of chronic asthma. As time for outpatient visits has been significantly curtailed, three important aspects must be stressed:
   1. Patients must be instructed in the proper method of metered-dose inhaler (MDI) use with a spacer device. Studies repeatedly show that as little as 10% of the dose administered via MDI may reach the constricted bronchioles, which may be further compromised by mucus plugging. Without proper technique, any prescribed inhaler therapy will be ineffective.
   2. Patients must have a clear written "action plan" to follow when signs of deterioration become evident.
   3. Avoidance and control of triggers, especially in strongly atopic patients, is very important. For example, asthmatics allergic to common dust mite antigens must learn to clean their household regularly and, at times, cover their pillowcases in readily washable fabrics. Controlling exposure to known triggers can afford patients the opportunity to reduce the doses of controller drug(s) and protect patients from unwanted adverse side effects of treatments.
Patient education remains an integral part of asthma clinics and should be stressed in follow-up visits in all settings.

37. **What is an asthma action plan?**
An asthma action plan is a document written by the health care provider and agreed upon by the patient. It outlines a strategy for managing the patient's asthma. It is usually based on the patient's measurements of peak expiratory flow rate (PEFR). The 2002 NAEPP guidelines recommend that action plans be written to encourage disease self-management and minimize emergencies. Typically, patients are instructed to gauge their disease by PEFR and match these readings with a simple green (PEFR: 80–100% of personal best), yellow (40–80%), and red zone (< 40%) scale. Readings in the yellow zone are worrisome and prompt an increase in controller therapy (either inhaled or oral corticosteroids), while red zone numbers require urgent intervention with higher dose steroids and notification of the treating physician. The action plan can improve the delivery of care of asthmatics significantly (Fig. 6-4). In a recent case-control study, a written asthma action plan reduced the risk of death from asthma by 70%. Incorporation of oral corticosteroids into the written asthma action plan reduced the risk of death from asthma by 90%.

UC Davis Asthma Network

ASTHMA ACTION PLAN

24-HOUR CONTACT NUMBER: 123-1234

Personal best peak flow _____   Date_____

GREEN   Peak flow is between _____ & _____ (80-100% of personal best)

Treatment Plan:

1.   Anti-inflammatory steroid medication: _____

_____ times/day. Rinse mouth.

2.   Maintenance medication: Long-acting β-agonist _____puffs _____ per day.

3.   Combination maintenance medication_____ puff _____ times/day. Rinse mouth.

4.   Antileukotriene: Singulair/ Accolate _____ mg _____ daily in the morning/evening.

5.   Rescue medication _____as needed.

6.   Other medications: _____

_____

_____

YELLOW   Peak flow is between _____ & _____ (50 - 80% of personal best)

Treatment Plan: **Continue with all GREEN ZONE medications _and_**

1.   Increase/add steroid medication _____ to _____ times/day.

2.   Use your rescue medication _____puffs every ½ hour up to three times **OR**

Use your nebulizer with _____ every ½ hour up to three times.

3.   Prednisone:

If your peak flow is less than (60%) _____, immediately take _____ mg Prednisone one time only.

OR

If your peak flow is between (60%) _____ & (70%) _____. and using your rescue medicine three times

has not helped, take _____ mg prednisone once.

4.   _____.

RED   Peak flow is _____ or less (≤ 50%)

Treatment plan:

1.   Take _____mg Prednisone immediately

2.   Use your rescue medication _____puffs every ½ hour up to three times **OR**

Use your nebulizer with _____ every ½ hour up to three times.

_____

M.D. signature

Figure 6-4. Asthma Action Plan of the University of California at Davis Asthma Network.

38. **Summarize the current approach to emergency treatment for a severe asthma attack.**

Acute, severe asthma refractory to home treatment must be treated in a critical care setting. The treatment is both supportive and therapeutic with critical care respiratory monitoring, supplemental oxygen, early institution of systemic corticosteroids, nebulized or MDI-delivered albuterol and ipratropium bromide, and, in certain young and refractory adult patients, parenteral β_2 agonists such as subcutaneous epinephrine.

39. **Which drugs are considered front-line therapy?**

Aerosolized levalbuterol, racemic albuterol, or albuterol with ipratropium bromide is first-line therapy. Nebulized therapy is preferred over MDI in status asthmaticus because of ease of administration. Doses of 2.5 mg of nebulized albuterol repeated 2 or 3 times per hour or 0.4 mg/kg/hr continuously are routinely prescribed in this situation. The difference between continuous and intermittent aerosol treatments is controversial. Any patient older than 40 years should have close cardiac monitoring for tachyarrhythmias (HR > 120 /min) and chest pain when high doses of albuterol are given (2.5 mg and higher). Levalbuterol, 1.25 mg every 8 hours, is associated with significantly fewer cardiac side effects and may provide better bronchodilator effect than racemic albuterol, 2.5 mg every 4–6 hours.

40. **What is the best predictor of a good outcome?**

An early improvement in PEFR or FEV_1 after 30 minutes of treatment is the most important predictor of a good outcome. If patients do not respond to inhaled β_2 agonist, subcutaneous epinephrine 0.3 ml of 1:1000 solution subcutaneously every 20 minutes for 3 doses or terbutaline 0.25 to 0.5 mg subcutaneously every 4 hours may be given. Airway obstruction from bronchial inflammation and mucus plugging may prevent adequate delivery of aerosolized β_2 agonists and ipratropium bromide in acute severe asthma. Intravenous montelukast has been reported to be of benefit in recent clinical trials but awaits FDA approval.

41. **When is endotracheal intubation indicated?**

Endotracheal intubation with mechanical ventilation is indicated when acute respiratory failure ensues with acute respiratory acidosis (pH < 7.35), hypercarbia ($PaCO_2$ > 45 mmHg), and hypoxemia (PaO_2 < 60 mmHg) that does not readily improve with bronchodilator therapy. The place for noninvasive positive-pressure ventilation in acute severe asthma is unclear but may in selected cases obviate the need for invasive ventilatory support. Clearly, prevention of attacks is the best remedy of all.

KEY POINTS: TOP TEN KEY CLINICAL ACTIVITIES FOR LONG-TERM ASTHMA CARE

1. Establish asthma diagnosis
2. Classify severity of asthma
3. Schedule routine follow-up care
4. Assess for referral to specialty care
5. Recommend measures to control asthma triggers
6. Treat or prevent comorbid conditions
7. Prescribe medicines according to severity
8. Monitor use of β_2 agonists
9. Develop written management plan
10. Provide routine education about patient self-management

42. **Should all severe persistent asthmatics be treated with the same doses of inhaled corticosteroids?**

The NAEPP guidelines, updated in 2002, make specific recommendations for starting doses of inhaled corticosteroid controller therapy in mild, moderate, and severe persistent asthma. For example, doses of 800–1200 µg/ day of fluticasone or the equivalent is recommended for initial therapy for severe persistent asthma. The stepwise guideline was designed to assist clinicians in developing an appropriate initial regimen for specific groups of patients and to minimize undertreatment of patients. This algorithm was designed to assist physicians in initiating therapy in untreated patients. Therapy must be individualized once symptoms and lung function have improved. A recent NIH-sponsored study by the Asthma Clinical Research Network revealed highly variable response to inhaled corticosteroids in persistent asthma. Near maximal improvement in FEV_1 and PC_{20} occurred with low to medium doses of inhaled corticosteroids. Higher doses of inhaled corticosteroids may be necessary to control severe persistent asthma and its frequent exacerbations. A primary goal in all asthmatics is to reduce the dose of inhaled corticosteroids to the lowest effective dose that controls disease. Patients with severe persistent asthma should not remain on high-dose inhaled steroids indefinitely if a combination controller regimen of low-to-moderate dose inhaled corticosteroids plus a long-acting β_2 agonist proves to be equally efficacious.

43. **What should be considered first-line controller therapy for patients with moderate and severe persistent asthma?**

The updated 2002 NAEPP guidelines stress that the combination controller regimen of low-to-moderate dose inhaled corticosteroids plus a long-acting β_2 agonist is equally or more efficacious in maintaining asthma control than high-dose inhaled steroids alone. This statement is supported by several recent clinical trials showing that the combination regimen best improves quality of life and symptoms and most effectively diminishes the number of exacerbations. This recommendation agrees with the recommendation to minimize dosing of inhaled steroids because of the possible, but as yet unproven, long-term side effects of high-dose inhaled steroids.

44. **What are the strongest indications for leukotriene inhibitors?**

The antileukotriene receptor antagonists, montelukast and zafirlukast, and the 5-lipoxygenase inhibitor, zileuton, have advanced asthma therapy significantly. These anti-inflammatory agents block the deleterious effects of specific leukotrienes. The strongest indications for these drugs are aspirin-sensitive asthma and exercise-induced asthma.

45. **In what other scenarios may be leukotriene-blocking drugs be used?**

Difficult-to-control asthmatics who need to decrease their steroid dose or require increased β_2 agonist therapy while on appropriate steroids may benefit from the addition of a leukotriene inhibitor. In addition, the few patients who are unable to cooperate with MDI therapy may also benefit from these oral drugs. In general, leukotriene-blocking drugs alone are not as efficacious as inhaled corticosteroids in the treatment of moderate persistent asthma. Recently, leukotriene antagonists were approved for the treatment of allergic rhinosinusitis. These medications may be considered in atopic asthma or mild persistent asthma and as adjuncts to inhaled steroids for moderate and severe persistent asthma.

46. **Explain the benefit of dry-powder inhalers (DPIs).**

Dry-powder, breath-activated delivery devices are available for both inhaled steroid and bronchodilator medications, and combination formulations will soon be manufactured. They have gained favor among patients and physicians because of their ease of use and the elimination of CFC-containing MDIs. DPIs may benefit patients unable to master the hand-breath coordination of an MDI and improve airway deposition of drug in many patients with poor MDI technique. In addition, the automatic doses counter and simple packaging of DPIs make them appealing to patients and physicians. However, as with MDIs, the success of DPI delivery to the lower respiratory tract is still heavily dependent on patient effort.

47. What causes nocturnal awakenings in asthmatic patients?

Nocturnal symptoms of sleep wakefulness, cough, and wheezing are signs of poorly controlled asthma. The chronobiology of asthma in adults and children is well documented. Typically, PEFRs decrease significantly between 2 AM and 6 AM because of a natural diminution in circulating catecholamines and corticosteroids and a rise in vagal tone.

48. How can nocturnal awakenings be better controlled?

Since many medications lose their effect at these hours, nocturnal symptoms often become challenging to control. Moving the dose of inhaled corticosteroids to the afternoon hours, adding an inhaled long-acting β_2 agonist or anticholinergic bronchodilator, or offering a trial of a leukotriene inhibitor or theophylline before the patient retires to sleep are appropriate measures. A stepwise approach is often needed, and if one intervention does not ameliorate the symptoms, another agent should be added to the regimen.

49. What are the effects of pregnancy on asthma?

Asthma is the most commonly encountered lung disease during pregnancy. Approximately 1% of pregnancies are complicated by asthma, and 1 of 500 pregnant women experience life-threatening consequences. In general, approximately one-third of pregnant women experience worsening of asthma during gestation, one-third remain the same, and one-third actually improve.

50. Should any particular medications be avoided during pregnancy?

Drugs commonly used to treat asthma are generally classified as Category B (no evidence of risk in humans) or Category C (risk cannot be ruled out). Three exceptions are triamcinolone and subcutaneous epinephrine, which are both Category D (evidence of risk), and methotrexate, which is category X (absolutely contraindicated in pregnancy) (Table 6-2). Of importance, despite a known association between chronic moderate-dose systemic steroid use and premature delivery and low birth weight, pregnant asthmatics suffering an exacerbation should be treated with systemic corticosteroids. Morbidity and mortality from asthma are far greater risks to the mother and fetus than a short course of oral steroids.

51. When should antibiotics be prescribed in acute exacerbations of asthma?

Common triggers of acute exacerbations of asthma include allergen exposure (e.g., dust mite, mold, pollens, cats), viral infections, and exercise. Evidence suggests that viral upper respiratory tract infections, namely rhinovirus, cause > 80% of asthma exacerbations in adults. The need for diagnostic chest radiographs or antibiotics for treatment of exacerbations is very uncommon. The 2002 NAEPP guidelines state that antibiotics are not indicated for the treatment of acute asthma exacerbations except when comorbid conditions dictate such use. Indications for antibiotic use include concomitant acute pyogenic sinusitis or acute bacterial bronchitis in patients with underlying COPD. In general, treatment focus is on appropriate steroid and bronchodilator therapy and trigger avoidance. Recent trials, however, have shown the benefits of macrolide therapy (clarithromycin, 1000 mg/d for 6 weeks or equivalent) in some severe asthmatics who have serologic evidence of *Chlamydia pneumoniae* or *Mycoplasma pneumoniae* infection.

52. What future therapies may be useful in targeting mediators of inflammation?

Future therapies will target specific mediators that govern portions of the inflammatory cascade that is seen with chronic airway inflammation. Two examples of this type of therapy include the recent development of a soluble interleukin-4 (IL-4) receptor that competes for the binding of IL-4 and anti-IL-5. The most promise has been seen with subcutaneous anti-IgE therapy. A monoclonal antibody against the Fc fragment of immunoglobulin-E molecule, anti-IgE, has been

TABLE 6-2. FDA INTRAUTERINE PREGNANCY CATEGORY RATINGS FOR ASTHMA DRUGS

Drug	Category		Category
		Inhaled	
Bronchodilator		**Corticosteroid**	
Albuterol	C	Beclomethasone	C
Metaproterenol	C	Budesonide	C
Salmeterol	C	Flunisolide	C
Terbutaline	B	Fluticasone	C
Theophylline	C	Triamcinolone	D
Epinephrine	D	Prednisone	C
Nonsteroidal		**Antileukotriene**	
Cromolyn	B	Montelukast	B
Nedocromil	B	Zafirlukast	B
		Zileuton	C
Cytotoxic drugs		**Anticholinergics**	
Methotrexate	X	Ipratropium	B
Cyclosporine	C	Tiotropium	C

A: controlled studies show no risk to fetus; B: no evidence of risk in humans; C: risk cannot be ruled out; D: positive evidence of risk to fetus; X: absolute contraindication during pregnancy.

approved for the treatment of moderate and severe asthma in other countries and, recently, in the United States. Randomized, controlled trials have shown that patients treated with anti-IgE have reduced serum IgE levels, decreased steroid controller requirements, and improved symptoms. In addition, inhibitors targeting key inflammatory cell adhesion molecules, central transcription factors, and chemokine receptors are being developed. The proper role of these agents is unclear, but some, particularly anti-IgE, are likely to serve as effective adjuncts to corticosteroids in allergic asthma patients.

Busse W, Corren J, Lanier BQ, et al: Omalizumab, anti-IgE recombinant humanized monoclonal antibody for the treatment of severe allergic asthma. J Allergy Clin Immunol 108:184–190, 2001.

53. Is immunotherapy efficacious in asthma?

In many atopic asthmatics exacerbations are triggered by common environmental allergens. NAEPP2 recommends immunotherapy in patients whose asthma is triggered by unavoidable allergens and whose symptoms are not fully controlled by medication. This treatment plan should be pursued by a consulting allergist only and should not be considered until standard therapy has failed.

54. What nonpharmacologic approaches to asthma treatment should be emphasized?

A comprehensive approach to the treatment of asthma includes recommendations for nonpharmacologic interventions. Nonpharmacologic interventions should be directed at a few specific disease precipitants discovered during the evaluation. For example, allergen skin testing or radioallergosorbent (RAST) testing may uncover a strong allergic response to house dust mite in a particular patient. In such a patient, treatment should include recommendations to minimize exposure to dust mite by encasing pillows and mattresses in plastic covers and vacuuming the home frequently. Similarly, if a patient has concomitant gastroesophageal reflux disease, recommendations should include avoidance of spicy foods and late night snacking and elevating the head of the bed on blocks. As with all chronic disease management programs, lifestyle revision is often required to adequately manage persistent asthma.

WEBSITES

1. Allergy and Asthma Network/Mothers of Asthmatics: www.aanma.org

2. Asthmamoms: www.asthmamoms.com

BIBLIOGRAPHY

1. Abramson MJ, Bailey MJ, Couper F, et al: Are asthma medications and management related to deaths from asthma? Am J Respir Crit Care Med 163:12–18, 2001.

2. American Thoracic Society: Guidelines for methacholine challenge and exercise challenge testing. Am J Respir Crit Care Med 161:309–329, 2000.

3. Barnes PJ: Mechanisms of glucocorticoids in asthma. Am J Respir Crit Care Med 154:S21–S26, 1996.

4. Bousquet J, Jeffrey PK, Busse WW, et al: State of the Art. Asthma: From bronchoconstriction to airways inflammation and remodeling. Am J Respir Crit Care Med 161:1720–1745, 2000.

5. Brightling CE, Bradding P, Symon FA, et al: Mast-cell infiltration of airway smooth muscle in asthma. N Engl J Med 346:1699–1705, 2002.

6. Busse W, Corren J, Lanier BQ, et al: Omalizumab, anti-IgE recombinant humanized monoclonal antibody for the treatment of severe allergic asthma. J Allergy Clin Immunol 108:184–190, 2001.

7. Camargo CA, Smitline HA, Malice M-P, et al: A randomized controlled trial of intravenous montelukast in acute asthma. Am J Respir Crit Care Med 167:528–533, 2003.

8. Centers for Disease Control and Prevention: Key clinical activities for quality asthma care: Recommendations of the National Asthma Education and Prevention Program. MMWR 52(RR-6):1–8, 2003.

9. Corbridge TC, Hall JB: The assessment and management of adults with status asthmaticus. Am J Respir Crit Care Med 151:1296–1316, 1995.

10. Doerschug KC, Peterson MW, Dayton CS, et al: Asthma guidelines. An assessment of physician understanding and practice. Am J Respir Crit Care Med 159:1735–1741, 1999.

11. Drazen JM, Israel E, O'Byrne PM: Treatment of asthma with drugs modifying the leukotriene pathway. N Eng J Med 340:197–206, 1999.

12. Israel E, Drazen JM, Liggett SB, et al: The effect of polymorphisms on the β2 adrenergic receptor on the response to regular use of albuterol in asthma. Am J Respir Crit Care Med 162:75–80, 2000.

13. Nelson HS, Bensch G, Pleskow WW, et al: Improved bronchodilation with levalbuterol compared with racemic albuterol in patients with asthma. J Allergy Clin Immunol 102:943–952, 1998.

14. Soler M, Matz J, Townley R, et al: The anti-IgE omalizumab reduces exacerbations and steroid requirement in allergic asthma. Eur Respir J 18: 254–261, 2001.

15. Sont JK, Willems LNA, Bel EH, et al: Clinical control and histopathologic outcome of asthma when airway hyperresponsiveness as an additional guide to long-term treatment. Am J Respir Crit Care Med 159:1043–1051,1999.

16. Szefler S, Martin RJ, King TS, et al: Significant variability in response to inhaled corticosteroids for persistent asthma. J Allergy Clin Immunol 109:410–418, 2002.

17. Truitt T, Witko J, Halpern M: Levalbuterol compared to racemic albuterol. Efficacy and outcomes in patients hospitalized with COPD or asthma. Chest 123:128–135; 2003.

18. U.S. Department of Health and Human Services, National Asthma Education and Prevention Program: Management of asthma during pregnancy. Bethesda, MD. NHLBI/NIH Publication No. 93–3279A, 1993.

19. U.S. Department of Health and Human Services, The Global Initiative for Chronic Obstructive Lung Disease (GOLD): NHLBI/WHO Workshop Report. Executive Summary. NIH Publication No. 2701A, 2001.

20. U.S. Department of Health and Human Services, National Asthma Education and Prevention Program: Executive Summary of the NAEPP Expert Panel Report. Guidelines for the Diagnosis and Management of Asthma. Update on Selected Topics. Bethesda, MD, NIH Publication No. 02–5075, 2002.

21. Wenzel SE, Schwartz LB, Langmack EL, et al: Evidence that severe asthma can be divided pathologically into two inflammatory subtypes with distinct physiologic and clinical characteristics. Am J Respir Crit Care Med 160:1001–1008, 1999.

CHAPTER 7

RHINOSINUSITIS

E. Bradley Strong, M.D.

1. What are the nasal turbinates? Where are they located?

The turbinates are bony projections from the lateral nasal sidewall that are covered with pseu-dostratified, ciliated columnar epithelium. There are three nasal turbinates: inferior, middle, and superior (Fig. 7-1). It is not uncommon to find a fourth turbinate located posterosuperiorly to the superior turbinate. When present, it is called the "supreme turbinate."

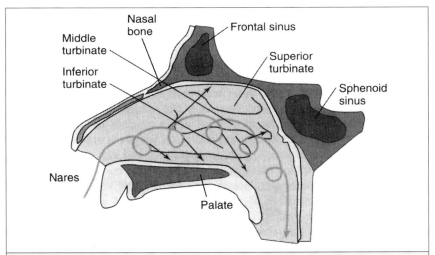

Figure 7-1. Nasal turbinates and related structures. (From Howarth PH: Allergic and nonallergic rhinitis. In Adkinson NF Jr, Yunginger JW, Busse WW, et al (eds): Middleton's Allergy: Principles and Practice, vol. 2, 6th ed. St. Louis, Mosby, 2003, Fig. 76-2, p 1395.)

2. Explain the function of the nasal turbinates.

The turbinates act to warm, humidify, and clean the inspired air. Each turbinate contains a venous plexus that periodically engorges, resulting in an increase in nasal resistance. Engorgement occurs on alternating sides of the nose at varying frequencies (hours to days). This "nasal cycle" is thought to allow one side of the nose to "rest" while the contralateral side "works." Patients can often sense these changes and may perceive them as abnormal. A brief explanation generally alleviates any anxiety.

3. What are the superior, middle, and inferior meatuses?

The superior, middle, and inferior meatus are air passageways located beneath the turbinate of the same name.

4. Which sinuses drain into the superior meatus?

The superior meatus drains the posterior ethmoid air cells.

5. **Which sinuses drain into the middle meatus?**
The middle meatus contains the ostia of multiple sinuses. The maxillary sinus ostium is located on the lateral nasal side wall and is generally less than 2 mm in diameter. The normal maxillary ostium is not visible with nasal endoscopy because the uncinate process obscures it. Accessory maxillary sinus ostia may be located posterior to the true ostia and usually can be visualized. The frontal sinus also drains into the middle meatus via the nasofrontal recess or duct. Finally, the anterior ethmoid air cells are honeycomb-shaped sinuses that drain into the middle meatus. Each ethmoid air cell has an individual drainage pathway to the middle meatus. The openings are too numerous and variable to detail anatomically.

6. **Which sinuses drain into the inferior meatus?**
The inferior meatus drains the nasolacrimal apparatus. The nasolacrimal duct runs from the lacrimal fossa, through the maxillary bone, and exits into the anterior third of the inferior meatus. Obstruction of the inferior meatus can result in epiphora (watery eyes).

7. **What is the osteomeatal complex (OMC)?**
The OMC (also called the osteomeatal unit) is located in the anterior third of the middle meatus. It is the final common drainage pathway from the frontal, anterior ethmoid, and maxillary sinuses.Therefore, it is important to examine this area when nasal endoscopy is performed. Mucosal edema, nasal polyps, and postoperative scarring can obstruct the OMC and result in rhinosinusitis.

8. **Where does the sphenoid sinus ostia drain?**
The sphenoid sinus drains into the spheno-ethmoidal recess located on the sphenoid rostrum, lateral to the septum and medial to the superior turbinate.

9. **Where is the olfactory bulb located?**
The olfactory bulb is located in the anterior cranial fossa, just above the bony nasal roof (cribriform plate). The sensory fibers of the olfactory bulb traverse the cribriform plate to enter the nasal cavity. Odorant molecules enter the nostrils and stimulate the olfactory bulb. Nasal polyps can obstruct normal nasal airflow and result in a decreased or absent sense of smell (hyposmia/anosmia). Because the sense of smell is integral to taste, patients with hyposmia/anosmia often have complaints of poor taste sensation.

10. **Define the terms *acute*, *subacute*, and *chronic* as they apply to rhinosinusitis.**
Acute rhinosinusitis: a sinus infection lasting less than 4 weeks.
Subacute rhinosinusitis: a sinus infection lasting 4 weeks to 3 months.
Chronic rhinosinusitis: a sinus infection lasting 3 months or more.

11. **What other terms are less commonly used to describe rhinosinusitis?**
Recurrent acute rhinosinusitis: greater than four episodes of acute rhinosinusitis per year, each lasting 7–10 days, with an absence of intervening symptoms.
Acute exacerbations of chronic rhinosinusitis: a sudden worsening of chronic rhinosinusitis symptoms with return to baseline symptoms after treatment.
   Baroody FM: Rhinosinusitis. In Lichtenstein LM, Busse WW, Geha RS (ed): Current Therapy in Allergy, Immunology, and Rheumatology, 6th ed. St. Louis, Mosby, 2004, pp 25–30.

12. **How is rhinosinusitis diagnosed?**
A thorough and accurate history of symptoms is extremely important in the diagnosis of rhinosinusitis because the physical examination can be unremarkable even in the face of active infection.
   Hadley JA, Schaefer SD: Clinical evaluation of rhinosinusitis: History and physical examination. Otolaryngol Head Neck Surg 117(Suppl):S8–S11, 1997.

KEY POINTS: OVERVIEW OF SINUSITIS

1. Viral upper respiratory infections are the most common cause of acute bacterial rhinosinusitis.

2. Rhinitis medicamentosa is secondary to overuse of topical vasoconstrictors.

3. The normal sinuses are air-filled cavities with ostia only 1–2 mm in diameter.

4. The most common organism causing chronic bacterial rhinosinusitis is coagulase-negative staphylococcus.

13. **What symptoms are strongly indicative of rhinosinusitis?**
    - Facial pressure/pain
    - Nasal obstruction
    - Purulent nasal discharge
    - Hyposmia/anosmia
    - Fever (acute rhinosinusitis)
    - Dental pain (acute rhinosinusitis)

14. **Discuss the differential diagnosis of facial pressure/pain.**
    While the symptoms of facial pressure/pain are *consistent* with rhinosinusitis, the differential diagnosis of facial pressure/pain is very broad. It also includes intracranial lesions (e.g., tumors, hematoma, infection), peripheral cranial nerve neuralgia, migraine, hypertension, muscle tension headache, orbital abnormalities (eye strain, glaucoma), ear lesions (otitis media, mastoiditis), temporomandibular joint dysfunction, and myofacial syndrome. However, when facial pressure/pain is present in combination with the other major symptoms of rhinosinusitis, it becomes a strongly suggestive historical finding.

15. **What characteristics of nasal obstruction are important to clarify?**
    Nasal obstruction is a common complaint in rhinosinusitis patients, but the nature and timing of nasal obstruction must be clarified. Nasal obstruction secondary to infection is most often bilateral and relatively symmetric. It occurs during an active infection and resolves when the infection clears. Other types of obstruction are more constant. Septal deviation usually results in a unilateral, fixed obstruction. Nasal polyps are generally bilateral and slowly progressive. Dynamic nasal valve collapse can be unilateral or bilateral but is relieved by lateralization of the nasal ala with a Q-tip or by lateralizing the ala with digital pressure on the cheek.

16. **Discuss the role of purulent nasal discharge in the diagnosis of rhinosinusitis.**
    Purulent nasal discharge from the middle meatus is highly suggestive of rhinosinusitis. Foreign bodies can result in purulent nasal discharge in children, but the discharge is usually localized to one nostril. Purulent secretions should be cultured whenever possible. Unfortunately, "blind" nasal cultures with a headlight are notoriously unreliable. Endoscopic guidance is required to obtain reliable cultures from the middle meatus.

17. **How are hyposmina and anosmia helpful in clarifying the differential diagnosis?**
    Hyposmia and anosmia are most commonly seen with nasal polyposis. But mucosal edema due to rhinosinusitis may result in diminished airflow and obstruct odorant molecules from reaching the olfactory bulb located above the nasal roof (cribriform plate).

18. **What symptoms are moderately suggestive of rhinosinusitis?**
    The symptoms listed below support the diagnosis of rhinosinusitis only when they are present in association with other major symptoms.
    - Generalized headache can be a sign of rhinosinusitis, but it is uncommon when other symptoms of rhinosinusitis are lacking (see facial pressure/pain above).
    - Halitosis. Purulent nasal secretions can result in halitosis. Patients more commonly complain of a foul nasal smell.
    - Fatigue
    - Cough. Purulent nasal discharge and postnasal drainage can result in cough. Patients with underlying asthma or bronchitis are at risk for exacerbations of pulmonary disease.

19. **What are the most common symptoms of pediatric rhinosinusitis?**
    Pediatric rhinosinusitis is more difficult to evaluate. Children often give a less detailed history with more atypical symptoms. The most common complaints include chronic cough, rhinorrhea, and nasal congestion.

20. **What are the two most common causes of acute bacterial rhinosinusitis in the children?**
    Viral upper respiratory tract infection and nasal foreign body.

21. **What are the most common disease processes that predispose adults to rhinosinusitis?**
    - Viral upper respiratory tract infections (probably the most common cause of acute bacterial rhinosinusitis. Viral infections result in diffuse nasal mucosal edema, obstruction of sinus ostia, poor mucociliary clearance, and bacterial overgrowth.)
    - Allergic rhinitis (results in mucosal edema, obstruction of ostia, and predisposition for bacterial rhinosinusitis)
    - Rhinitis medicamentosa (secondary to overuse of topical vasoconstrictors)
    - Genetic disorders (e.g., cystic fibrosis, immotile cilia syndrome)
    - Immunologic diseases (e.g., IgA deficiency)
    - Anatomic abnormalities (e.g., septal deviation or concha bullosa [aerated middle turbinate])
    - Neoplastic diseases (e.g., benign polyps, inverted papilloma)

22. **Discuss the pathophysiology of bacterial rhinosinusitis.**
    Normal sinuses are air-filled cavities with small ostia (1–2 mm) for drainage. The nasal lining secretes mucus and IgA. The mucus absorbs any particulate matter or bacteria and the IgA offers an initial barrier to bacterial infection. The cilia beat toward the natural ostia and move any foreign material into the nasal cavity.
    When ostial obstruction occurs, an infectious cycle begins. The mucus stagnates and becomes thick, the pH drops, ciliary function decreases, mucosal edema occurs, and bacterial overgrowth results. The local immune response may exacerbate the ostial obstruction by further increasing mucosal edema.

23. **Summarize the differential diagnosis of patients presenting with sinus complaints.**
    - Viral upper respiratory tract infection
    - Allergic rhinitis
    - Nonspecific rhinitis

- Rhinitis medicamentosa
- Nasal septal deviation
- Bacterial rhinosinusitis

24. **Why should unilateral maxillary rhinosinusitis be of particular concern?**
Rhinosinusitis is generally a mucosal disease that affects all of the sinuses. While some isolated sinus cavities may be spared, it is uncommon to have unilateral maxillary rhinosinusitis. When this occurs, a neoplastic process must be considered. The differential diagnosis includes both benign and malignant lesions. Therefore, isolated maxillary rhinosinusitis should be considered the result of an obstructing malignant lesion until proved otherwise.

25. **What are three common causes of nonrhinogenic headache?**
Temporomandibular joint (TMJ) dysfunction, migraine headache, and muscle tension headache. While TMJ pain and headache pain can be mistaken for rhinosinusitis, they are not associated with other symptoms of rhinosinsusitis, and the timing is not consistent with an infectious etiology.

26. **Describe the symptoms of TMJ dysfunction.**
TMJ dysfunction is a very common cause of facial pain that can be mistaken for sinus pain. TMJ pain is usually localized to the joint or ear, but it can be referred to the maxilla, orbit, temple, vertex, mastoid, and neck. Patients may present with isolated maxillary sinus discomfort masquerading as rhinosinusitis. Therefore, facial pain without other major symptoms of rhinosinusitis must raise suspicion for TMJ dysfunction.

27. **Describe the classic symptoms of migraine headaches.**
Classic migraine symptoms include a brief prodromal period with irritability, visual changes, or paraesthesias. Severe headache, nausea, and photophobia follow. Cluster headaches are a migraine variant. They include severe, sharp periorbital pain associated with ipsilateral pupillary constriction, local vasodilation, rhinorrhea, and lacrimation.

28. **Describe the symptoms of muscle tension headaches.**
Muscle tension/stress headaches are very common. They often begin at the occiput or shoulders and radiate to the fronto-orbital area.

29. **List four common causes of nasal obstruction besides rhinosinusitis.**
Rhinitis medicamentosa, allergic rhinitis, nonallergic vasomotor rhinitis, and nasal septal deviation.

30. **What causes rhinitis medicamentosa? How is it treated?**
Rhinitis medicamentosa results from long-term use of topical vasoconstrictor sprays (oxymetazoline, phenylephrine). These sympathomimetic agents result in marked vasoconstriction of the venous plexuses in the nasal turbinates. While they provide a short-term increase in nasal airflow, the ultimate result is rebound vasodilation and nasal obstruction. Continuous use for greater than 7–10 days can result in chronic inflammation and addiction. The mainstay of therapy is nasal steroid spray. The nasal steroid spray should be applied daily for 1 week, and then the topical decongestant should be stopped. Discontinuing the use of the topical decongestant in one nostril at a time may be easier for some patients. Systemic steroids may be indicated in the most severe cases.

KEY POINTS: FIVE MOST COMMON CAUSES OF NASAL OBSTRUCTION

1. Rhinosinusitis
2. Rhinitis medicamentosa
3. Allergic rhinitis
4. Vasomotor rhinitis
5. Nasal septal deviation

31. How is allergic rhinitis treated?
Allergic rhinitis is a common cause of nasal obstruction. Inhaled allergens result in chronic turbinate hypertrophy and reduced nasal airflow. Common treatments include topical nasal steroids, topical and systemic antihistamines, cromolyn sodium, and immunotherapy. Surgical reduction of the inferior turbinates can increase nasal airflow in refractory cases. Unfortunately, the turbinate hypertrophy may slowly recur in a minority of patients (months to years).

Howarth PH: Allergic and nonallergic rhinitis. In Adkinson NF Jr, Yunginger JW, Busse WW, et al (eds): Middleton's Allergy: Principles and Practice, vol. 2, 6th ed. St. Louis, Mosby, 2003, pp1391–1411.

32. What causes nonallergic vasomotor rhinitis?
Nonallergic vasomotor rhinitis is a poorly defined term referring to chronic nasal obstruction and rhinorrhea. Common causes include pregnancy, temperature-induced rhinitis, and idiopathic rhinitis. Treatment is generally symptomatic and includes nasal steroid sprays or ipratropium nasal spray.

33. What are the symptoms of nasal septal deviation? How is it treated?
Nasal septal deviation generally results in a unilateral, fixed nasal obstruction. However, it is not uncommon to see an S-shaped septal deviation that results in fixed, bilateral nasal obstruction. Initial treatment includes a trial of nasal steroid spray. Significant obstruction that is refractory to nasal steroids may require surgery.

34. What is the most common cause of anosmia/hyposmia?
The most common definable cause of anosmia/hyposmia is paranasal sinus disease (e.g., nasal polyps, rhinosinusitis). An equal number of patients will have an idiopathic etiology. Head trauma is also a common cause.

35. Which organisms most commonly cause acute bacterial rhinosinusitis?
Streptococcus pneumoniae (20–35%), *Haemophilus influenzae* (6–26%), and *Moraxella catarrhalis* (2–10%) are traditionally taught as the most common organisms causing acute bacterial rhinosinusitis. Anaerobes and *Staphylococcus aureus* account for 0–8% of cases. Viral cultures are difficult to obtain, and the exact incidence of viral rhinosinusitis is not clearly defined.

36. Which organisms most commonly cause chronic bacterial rhinosinusitis?
- Coagulase-negative staphylococcus: 24–80%
- Staphylococcus aureus: 9–33%
- Anaerobes: 0–8 %
- Streptococcus pneumoniae: 0–7%

Gram-positive and anaerobic organisms are more common in chronic rhinosinusitis. However, anaerobes are difficult to culture, and the exact incidence is difficult to quantify.

37. **Which sinuses are most commonly involved in acute bacterial rhinosinusitis?**
    The maxillary sinuses are most commonly involved, followed by the frontal and ethmoid
    sinuses. Isolated sphenoid rhinosinusitis is uncommon.

38. **Is there a causal relationship between allergic rhinitis and rhinosinusititis?**
    The evidence to support a direct causal relationship is conflicting. However, there is an increased
    association of allergic rhinitis in patients with chronic rhinosinusitis, and acute bacterial rhino-
    sinusitis is more common in adults with allergic rhinitis. The concordance of allergy and chronic
    rhinosinsitis ranges from 25% to 50%. There is a greater association in the pediatric population,
    with pediatric studies reporting a higher incidence.

39. **Which fungal pathogen most commonly results in rhinosinusitis?**
    Aspergillus fumigatus.

40. **How is fungal rhinosinusitis classified?**
    As acute fulminant fungal rhinosinusitis or chronic indolent fungal rhinosinusitis.

41. **Discuss the characteristics and treatment of acute fulminant fungal
    rhinosinusitis.**
    Acute fulminant fungal rhinosinusitis is a rapidly invasive, life-threatening, fungal infection seen
    in immunocompromised hosts. Mucoraceae is the most common fungal family causing this
    disease. Acute fulminant fungal rhinosinusitis requires aggressive surgical debridement with a
    margin of normal tissue and systemic antifungal therapy (amphotericin B). Mortality rates have
    dropped from greater than 90% before 1970 to less than 20% today.

42. **What is chronic indolent fungal rhinosinusitis? How is it treated?**
    Chronic indolent fungal rhinosinusitis occurs in an immunocompetent, nonatopic host.
    Aspergillus is the species most commonly involved. Tissue invasion can occur. The most
    appropriate treatment is conservative surgical debridement and systemic antifungal therapy
    (e.g., fluconazole).

43. **What is a fungus ball?**
    A fungus ball results from a long-standing fungal infection in an immunocompetent, nonatopic
    host. The most common fungal pathogen is *Aspergillus* species. The fungus ball is usually uni-
    lateral and located in the maxillary sinus. Tissue invasion does not occur. The most appropriate
    therapy is surgical debridement and aeration of the sinus cavity.

44. **What is allergic fungal rhinosinusitis?**
    Allergic fungal rhinosinusitis results from an inflammatory response of the nasal mucosa to a
    fungal allergen (most commonly *Aspergillus* and *Bipolaris* species). The host is immunocompe-
    tent and atopic. Generally no fungal overgrowth or invasion is seen. The most appropriate treat-
    ment is not clearly defined but probably includes surgical debridement and systemic antifungals,
    as well as topical and systemic steroids. The role of immunotherapy is unclear.

45. **What are the key components to an anterior rhinoscopic examination?**
    While the history is extremely important in the diagnosis of rhinosinusitis, anterior rhinoscopy is
    probably the most important part of the physical examination. Anterior rhinoscopy can be per-
    formed with either an otoscope or a nasal speculum and head mirror. The otoscope offers a nar-
    rower field of view but provides magnification of the posterior nasal vault. The nasal speculum
    offers a more thorough examination of the anterior nasal cavity. The structures that can usually
    be visualized include (1) the inferior and middle turbinates; (2) the inferior and middle meatus;
    and (3) the nasal septum. Any evidence of nasal polyposis, turbinate hypertrophy, nasal bleed-
    ing, mucosal lesions, or mucopurulent discharge should be documented.

46. **How does transillumination work? Is it efficacious?**

Transillumination works on the assumption that fluid-filled sinuses transmit less light than air-filled sinuses. The maxillary sinuses can be transilluminated by instructing the patient to purse the lips around a light source placed in the mouth. The left and right side of the frontal sinus can be evaluated by placing the light source on the inferomedial aspect of each supraorbital rim. Unfortunately, not all sinuses are symmetric, and it has been shown that transillumination does not correlate well with other diagnostic studies.

47. **Is fiberoptic rhinoscopy superior to standard anterior rhinoscopy?**

Yes. Fiberoptic nasal endoscopy allows the physician to closely examine the entire nasal vault. Rigid or flexible fiberoptic endoscopes can be passed from the nasal vestibule to the choana. While the examination is monocular, a more complete examination of the turbinates, meatuses, choana, and septum can be performed. After endoscopic sinus surgery, direct visualization into the ethmoid, maxillary, frontal, and sphenoid sinuses is often possible.

48. **Are nasal cultures efficacious?**

Yes. However, the cultures are highly technique-dependent and must be properly obtained. Cultures taken blindly or with anterior rhinoscopy are unreliable and often contaminated by flora from the nasal vestibule. Accurate cultures require endoscopic placement of a culturette swab directly into the middle meatus without touching other areas of the nasal mucosa.

49. **Are plain sinus radiographs efficacious?**

In some cases. A thorough history and physical examination can usually make the diagnosis of acute rhinosinusitis. Plain radiographs are usually not required. Plain films can be ordered to confirm a diagnosis that is in question, but once the diagnosis has been made, the x-rays rarely change the treatment plan. The maxillary sinuses can be evaluated on a Water's view, and the frontal sinus can be visualized on a lateral skull film. Evaluation of the ethmoid sinuses, sphenoid sinus, and osteomeatal complex is difficult. Classic radiographic findings indicative of rhinosinusitis include mucosal thickening, air-fluid levels, and sinus opacification.

50. **When is a computed tomography (CT) scan of the sinuses indicated?**

CT is now considered the gold standard for diagnosing rhinosinusitis. It is generally reserved for patients with chronic rhinosinusitis due to cost and radiation exposure. Sinus CT scans provide both diagnostic and therapeutic information about the sinuses. Diagnostically, the CT scan precisely documents the degree of mucosal thickening, sinus opacification, and polypoid disease. Therapeutically, preoperative CT scans document the anatomy of the skull base, orbital wall, and osteomeatal complex.

51. **Discuss the timing of a sinus CT scan.**

The timing of a sinus CT scan should be considered carefully. A limited sinus CT scan is often ordered to initially document chronic sinus disease. A repeat CT scan after maximal medical therapy (i.e., an aggressive attempt to treat the chronic sinus symptoms) will reveal whether the patient responds to medical therapy or is a surgical candidate. Persistent sinus disease in the face of maximal medical management is an indication for surgical intervention.

52. **Of what does maximal medical therapy consist?**

Maximal medical management generally entails 4–6 weeks of oral antibiotics, a nasal steroid spray, brief treatment with a topical decongestant, oral steroids, and antihistamines (when indicated).

53. **How does maximal medical therapy before a follow-up CT scan simplify the treatment algorithm for chronic rhinosinusitis?**

There are four options:

1. If the patient remains symptomatic and has significant sinus disease on the follow-up CT scan, he or she is a likely candidate for sinus surgery.
2. If the CT scan is normal and symptoms have improved, no further intervention is necessary.
3. If symptoms persist despite a normal CT scan, the diagnosis of rhinosinusitis must be questioned.
4. If there is significant disease on the CT scan but the patient is asymptomatic, observation is generally indicated.

54. **What CT scan findings are indicative of sinus disease?**
    - Obstruction of the osteomeatal complex
    - Circumferential sinus mucosal thickening
    - Complete sinus opacification
    - Nasal polyps or masses
    - Anatomic abnormalities (e.g., concha bullosa, paradoxical turbinate, septal deviation)

55. **What radiographic findings are suggestive of chronic indolent fungal rhinosinusitis or fungus ball?**
    A sinus cavity with peripheral mucosal edema and central radiopacity (metallic-appearing).

56. **When should antibiotics be prescribed for acute rhinosinusitis?**
    Antibiotic treatment of acute rhinosinusitis is controversial. Some studies conclude that oral antibiotics reduce the severity and duration of symptoms, while others have found no effect. Consequently, some authors advocate supportive treatment with decongestants, mucolytics, nasal irrigations, and hydration. Other authors advocate first-line antibiotic therapy. A conservative approach is to treat routine rhinosinusitis symptomatically for 7–10 days. If there is no improvement or if symptoms worsen, the antibiotic therapy should be started. Commonly used first-line agents include amoxicillin, trimethoprim-sulfamethoxazole, or erythromycin plus a sulfonamide.

57. **What is the most appropriate length of antibiotic treatment for acute rhinosinusitis?**
    The duration of antibiotic therapy for acute bacterial rhinosinusitis is also controversial. Historically, patients have been treated for 10–14 days. Few clinical data refute or support this approach. Recently, several studies have shown a 3-day course of oral antibiotics to be as efficacious as 10 days of therapy. Unfortunately, the literature remains unclear, and the majority of clinicians continue to treat for 10–14 days.

58. **What antibiotic choices are most appropriate for chronic rhinosinusitis?**
    Patients with chronic rhinosinusitis have had symptoms for longer than 3 months and have usually failed multiple courses of first-line antibiotic agents. There is a greater incidence of gram-positive cocci and beta lactamase-producing organisms with chronic rhinosinusitis. Therefore, second-line antibiotics such as amoxicillin clavulanate, cefuroxime, levofloxacin, and clindamycin are indicated.

59. **What is the most appropriate length of antibiotic treatment for chronic rhinosinusitis?**
    Chronic rhinosinusitis requires prolonged treatment for complete eradication of the disease. Short courses of antibiotics often provide only temporary symptomatic relief. A prolonged course lasting 4–6 weeks in combination with steroids and decongestants is often required to completely clear the infection.

60. **What is maximal medical management of chronic rhinosinusitis?**
    Maximal medical management implies the maximal *medical* treatment short of surgical interven-
    tion. For patients with refractory sinus disease it often consists of (1) 4–6 weeks of a second-
    line antibiotics, (2) 4–6 weeks of topical nasal steroids, (3) 2 weeks of a topical decongestant
    (with brief breaks to avoid rebound nasal congestion), (4) 2 weeks of oral prednisone, and
    (5) antihistamines as indicated. If symptoms persist despite maximal medical management,
    surgical intervention should be considered.

61. **What risks are associated with topical and systemic decongestants?**
    Prolonged use of **topical** decongestants (oxymetazoline, phenylephrine) results in rebound
    nasal congestion and rhinitis medicamentosa. **Systemic** sympathomimetic agents (pseu-
    doephedrine, phenylephrine, and phenylpropanolamine) can significantly increase the heart rate
    and blood pressure. Caution must be used when prescribing these agents to patients with
    hypertension and coronary artery disease.

62. **Are antihistamines efficacious for nonallergic bacterial rhinosinusitis?**
    No. Antihistamines, particularly the first-generation agents, can thicken mucosal secretions and
    reduce mucociliary transport. Antihistamines are primarily indicated when there is an allergic
    component to the rhinosinusitis.

63. **What role do topical nasal steroids play in the treatment of acute and chronic
    rhinosinusitis?**
    Topical nasal steroids play an important role in the treatment of chronic rhinosinusitis. They
    reduce mucosal edema, open the natural sinus ostia, and increase mucociliary drainage.
    Nasal steroids have a slow onset of action and therefore may be less efficacious for acute
    rhinosinusitis.

64. **Discuss the role of systemic steroids in the treatment of chronic
    rhinosinusitis.**
    Patients whose chronic rhinosinusitis is treated with short courses of antibiotics (1–2 weeks)
    may have persistent infection and mucosal edema despite therapy. Short-term antibiotic therapy
    may briefly reduce the bacterial load, but the infection "rebounds" after the antibiotics are dis-
    continued. Systemic steroids act to reduce mucosal edema in the paranasal sinuses. The combi-
    nation of systemic steroids, prolonged antibiotic administration (4–6 weeks), and topical
    therapy (nasal steroids and decongestants) gives the patient the greatest opportunity to clear a
    chronic infection.

65. **List relative contraindications to the use of systemic steroids for treatment of
    chronic rhinosinusitis.**
    - Diabetes mellitus
    - Psychiatric history
    - Active tuberculosis
    - Pregnancy
    - Seizure disorder
    - Osteoporosis
    - Congestive heart failure

66. **What are the common sinus-related indications for otolaryngologic referral?**
    - Rhinosinusitis refractory to maximal medical management.
    - Impending complications of rhinosinusitis (orbital cellulitis, meningitis, or brain
      abscess)
    - Fixed nasal obstruction (septal deviation, polyp, tumor)
    - Rhinosinusitis associated with an underlying systemic disease

67. **List the common indications for functional endoscopic sinus surgery.**
    - Recurrent acute rhinosinusitis with a defined site of obstruction
    - Chronic rhinosinusitis refractory to medical management
    - Nasal polyposis
    - Nasal obstruction
    - Fungal rhinosinusitis
    - Sinus mucocele
    - Complications of rhinosinusitis

68. **What are the most common complications of rhinosinusitis?**
    - Facial cellulitis
    - Mucopyocele
    - Orbital cellulitis/abscess/blindness-particularly in the pediatric population
    - Meningitis
    - Cavernous sinus thrombosis
    - Brain abscess

    Pediatric patients are at an increased risk for orbital and intracranial complications. Symptoms suggestive of impending complications include periorbital swelling, progressive headache, meningeal signs, and mental status changes. An urgent work-up including a contrast-enhanced CT scan of the brain and sinuses should be performed if there is any suggestion of potential complications.

69. **List the symptoms most commonly associated with orbital cellulites.**
    - Eyelid edema
    - Eyelid erythema
    - Chemosis

    Progression of the disease can result in diplopia, ophthalmoplegia, blindness, meningitis, and death.

70. **How does rhinosinusitis affect asthma?**
    Bronchial asthma can be exacerbated by a variety of stimuli, including allergens, exercise, temperature changes, chemical irritants, stress, and infection. Rhinosinusitis results in an increased upper respiratory tract bacterial load. Purulent postnasal drainage may result in bronchial irritation and exacerbation of asthma.

71. **What is Samter's syndrome?**
    Samter's syndrome is a triad of symptoms, including nasal polyposis, bronchial asthma, and aspirin sensitivity. Aspirin blocks the cyclooxygenase pathway and preferentially shunts arachidonic acid into the lipoxygenase pathway. This results in an overproduction of leukotrienes, bronchoconstriction, and asthma exacerbations. It may also promote polyp formation. The nasal polyps are often refractory to medical management and may require multiple polypectomies.

WEBSITES

1. American College of Allergy, Asthma and Immunology: www.acaai.org
2. National Library of Medicine: www.nlm.nih.gov

BIBLIOGRAPHY

1. Baroody FM: Rhinosinusitis. In Lichtenstein LM, Busse WW, Geha RS (ed): Current Therapy in Allergy, Immunology, and Rheumatology, 6th ed. St. Louis, Mosby, 2004, pp 25–30.

2. Benninger MS, Anon J, Mabry RL: The medical management of rhinisinusitis. Otolaryngol Head Neck Surg 117(Suppl):S41–S49, 1997.

3. Hadley JA, Schaefer SD: Clinical evaluation of rhinosinusitis: History and physical examination. Otolaryngol Head Neck Surg 117(Suppl):S8–S11, 1997.

4. Howarth PH: Allergic and nonallergic rhinitis. In Adkinson NF Jr, Yunginger JW, Busse WW, et al (eds): Middleton's Allergy: Principles and Practice, vol. 2, 6th ed. St. Louis, Mosby, 2003, pp 1391–1411.

5. Kennedy DW: Medical management of sinusitis: Educational goals and management guidelines. Ann Otol Rhinol Laryngol 104(Suppl 167):22–30, 1995.

6. Lanza DC, Kennedy DW: Adult rhinosinusitis defined. Otolaryngol Head Neck Surg 117(Suppl):S1–S7, 1997.

7. Osguthorpe JD, Hadley JA: Rhinosinusitis: Current concepts in evaluation and management. Med Clin North Am 83:27–41, 1999.

1. **What are the clinical features of urticaria?**
   Urticaria is characterized by red edematous plaques surrounded by a clear or red halo. The lesions are round or oval and may become polycyclic when confluent. They are usually multiple and vary from 1 mm to several centimeters in diameter. They can occur at any site of the body and are typically associated with itching and sometimes burning. Skin returns to its normal appearance usually within 1–24 hours. Urticaria is sometimes accompanied by angioedema, in which the edematous process extends into the deep dermis and/or subcutaneous tissues. While patients with urticaria usually have symptoms confined to the skin, they may have concomitant systemic manifestations.

2. **Distinguish between acute and chronic urticaria.**
   Urticaria is termed acute when episodes last less than 6 weeks; it is termed chronic when episodes persist longer. Most cases of chronic urticaria eventually resolve (about 50% within 1 year) but some may continue for over 20 years.

3. **List some forms of physical urticaria.**
   - Dermographism
   - Delayed pressure urticaria
   - Cold urticaria
   - Solar urticaria
   - Aquagenic urticaria
   - Heat contact urticaria
   - Vibratory urticaria

4. **Describe symptoms that may be associated with delayed pressure urticaria.**
   The swellings tend to be deeper and more painful than those of ordinary urticaria and last 24 hours or more. Patients may have flulike symptoms and arthralgia.

5. **Describe the spectra of light that induce solar urticaria.**
   They vary according to patients and can include ultraviolet A (UVA) and ultraviolet B (UVB) as well as visible light. Visible light alone can cause solar urticaria.

6. **What are the possible systemic manifestations of cold urticaria?**
   Cold urticaria may sometimes accompany underlying diseases associated with cryoglobulin, cold agglutinin, or cryofibrinogen.

7. **Define cholinergic urticaria.**
   Cholinergic urticaria presents with multiple wheals, 2–3 mm in diameter, surrounded by a pink flare. It is caused by a rise in the core temperature and develops within minutes after exercising, sweating, or hot bathing and lasts for 20–90 minutes. It can be brought up by anxiety. Lesions are extremely pruritic and may affect the entire body except the palms, soles, and axilla. The condition may occasionally be accompanied by diarrhea, increased salivation, bronchospasm, or hypotension. It often remits within several years but can last for more than 20 years. It is

termed cholinergic because the cholinergic sympathetic innervation of sweat glands is involved. The lesions can be reproduced by intradermal injection of methacholine.

8. **Define adrenergic urticaria.**
Adrenergic urticaria occurs during emotional stress and presents as wheals surrounded by a white halo.

9. **What are the histologic features of urticaria?**
   - Edema in the upper and mid dermis.
   - Dilation of postcapillary venules and lymphatic vessels of the upper dermis.
   - The presence of a mixed perivascular infiltrate, consisting of neutrophils, eosinophils, macrophages, and lymphocytes.

10. **Describe the pathogenesis of urticaria.**
The edema is caused by plasma transudation resulting from increased blood vessel permeability. The erythema is due to vasodilatation resulting from cutaneous neural stimulation and release of neural mediators. The itching is caused by stimulation of free nerve endings by chemical mediators.

11. **What is the major cell type responsible for urticaria?**
Mast cells are the major effector cell in most forms of urticaria, although other cell types may be involved (Fig. 8-1).

12. **How do mast cells contribute to the development of urticaria?**
Histamine released by mast cells causes vasodilatation and increased vasopermeability, resulting in leakage of plasma. It also stimulates nerve endings, causing pruritus. Other mediators, including leukotrienes, prostaglandins, and platelet-activating factor, may contribute to the subsequent inflammatory response. Mast cell–derived cytokines and chemokines also contribute to urticaria.

13. **Is there any difference in mast cells in people with and without urticaria?**
Some studies showed that mast cell numbers are comparable in lesional and uninvolved skin of patients with chronic urticaria and are not different from those in the skin of normal individuals. However, other studies showed increased numbers of mast cells (> twofold) in lesional as well as uninvolved skin. In addition, it has been shown that mediators are more easily released from mast cells in patients with chronic urticaria.

14. **Describe immunologic mast cell stimuli.**
The most common type activates IgE receptor (FcɛRI), which typically involves IgE against certain antigens. When mast cells sensitized with the antigen-specific IgE encounter the antigen, they can become activated. These antigens include chemicals found in foods, insect stings, inhalants, infections, and therapeutic agents. Acute urticaria is often IgE-mediated, while chronic urticaria seldom involves IgE. Other immunologic stimuli include products of complement activation, such as C3a and C5a, and neuropeptides. Cytokines, including histamine releasing factors, can also activate mast cells.

15. **Describe nonimmunologic mast cell stimuli.**
Nonimmunologic stimuli include radiocontrast media, opiates, antibiotics, curare, and dextran. They also include physical stimuli, such as pressure, temperature changes, ultraviolet light, vibration, and contact with water. All of these stimuli contribute to the mast cell activation in various forms of physical urticaria.

16. **What is the role of late-phase reactions in urticaria?**
After an immediate response of mast cells to antigens, a late-phase reaction slowly develops at the antigen challenge site. This reaction is due to a perivascular infiltrate, consisting primarily of

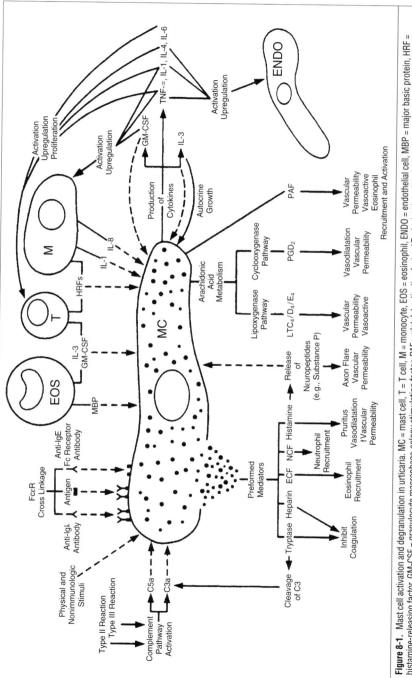

Figure 8-1. Mast cell activation and degranulation in urticaria. MC = mast cell, T = T cell, M = monocyte, EOS = eosinophil, ENDO = endothelial cell, HRF = histamine-releasing factor, GM-CSF = granulocyte macrophage-colony stimulating factor, PAF = platelet activating factor, IL = interleukin, LT = leukotriene, MBP = major basic protein, NCF = neutrophil chemotactic factor, ECF = eosinophil chemotactic factor, λ = antibody, black box = antigen, arrow = degranulation stimulus.

neutrophils and eosinophils, with scattered mononuclear cells initially and T lymphocytes sub-sequently. Clinically, the reactions are manifested as burning, pruritus, erythema, and induration that peak at 6–8 hours and resolve by 24–48 hours. Most urticarial lesions do not seem to have a late-phase component. However, it is seen when patients with autoimmune urticaria (see below) are injected with autologous sera containing autoantibodies to IgE receptor (FcεRI), sug-gesting that late-phase reactions may be involved in this form of urticaria.

17. **Describe contact urticaria (allergic or pseudoallergic).**
Contact urticaria refers to lesions that develop following skin contact with substances ranging from low-molecular-weight organic compounds to macromolecules. Nonimmunological contact urticaria (NICU) occurs without previous sensitization. Inducing substances include preserva-tives and fragrances in foods, cosmetics, and topical medicaments. Immunologic (allergic) con-tact urticaria is due to immediate-type hypersensitivity and involves IgE specific for the contact allergens. It may be associated with systemic and potentially life-threatening symptoms. Natural rubber latex is one of the most notable allergens.

18. **What is the role of foods in urticaria?**
Foods are a common cause of acute urticaria, which is often identified by the patients them-selves through association of the development of the lesions in proximity to ingestion of a par-ticular kind of foods on several occasions. Symptoms begin within minutes to several hours after ingestion. GI and respiratory symptoms may accompany or precede the urticarial reaction. IgE antibodies to food components are implicated. However, other mechanisms exist; for exam-ple, red wines may contain high concentrations of vasoactive amines, which can cause urticaria. The role of foods as a cause of chronic urticaria is controversial.

19. **What is known about NSAID sensitivity and urticaria?**
Urticaria may occur after a therapeutic dose of aspirin or other nonsteroidal anti-inflammatory drugs (NSAIDs), but the incidence is very small. NSAIDs can aggravate chronic urticaria in a substantial percentage of patients. The mechanisms of NSAID-sensitive urticaria are not fully understood but probably involve modulation of the arachidonic acid metabolic pathway, thus affecting mast cell responsiveness.

20. **What is familiar cold urticaria? Is it true urticaria?**
Familial cold urticaria is an autosomal-dominant systemic inflammatory disease that presents with recurrent attacks of a nonpruritic, nonurticarial, rash consisting of erythematous papules and plaques shortly after exposure to cold. The rash is associated with fever, chill, arthralgia, myalgia, fatigue, and swelling of the extremities and persists for 24–48 hours. The disease man-ifests in early childhood and persists throughout life. The genetic defect has been identified. Familial cold urticaria is a misnomer, since the skin lesions are not urticarial; thus, the condition has been renamed as familial cold autoinflammatory syndrome.

21. **Describe hereditary angioedema.**
Hereditary angioedema is a dominantly inherited disorder characterized by recurrent attacks of angioedema involving the skin, mucous membranes, and respiratory and gastrointestinal tracts. It is associated with a functional deficiency of the inhibitor of the first component of the comple-ment system, the C1 esterase inhibitor. About 85% of patients have decreased levels of the inhibitor; the remaining patients have a normal level of the inhibitor, but it is nonfunctional. The condition can be diagnosed by clinical presentation, positive family history, and a characteristic complement profile (normal C1, C3, decreased C4) during attacks.

22. **Define urticarial vasculitis.**
The urticarial lesions have pronounced central clearing and a purpuric component and may be painful, burning as well as pruritic. The individual lesions may last for greater than 24 hours and

result in residual hyperpigmentation after resolution. There may be associated systemic symptoms such as low-grade fever, arthralgia, and gastrointestinal, pulmonary or ocular complaints. Histopathologically, the lesions have the characteristics of leukocytoclastic vasculitis.

23. **What systemic diseases may be associated with urticarial vasculitis?**
    Urticarial vasculitis is idiopathic in many patients but can also occur in the context of autoimmune disorders, infections, drug reactions, or a paraneoplastic syndrome. Patients can be subgrouped into normocomplementemic or hypocomplementemic, according to serum complement levels. Normocomplementemic patients usually have minimal or no systemic involvement and often have a better prognosis. Hypocomplementemic patients tend to have underlying systemic diseases, such as systemic lupus erythematosus, Sjögren's syndrome, and cryoglobulinemia.

    Venzor J, Lee WL, Huston DP: Urticarial vasculitis. Clin Rev Allergy Immunol 23:201–216, 2002.

24. **What is autoimmune urticaria?**
    Autoimmune urticaria designates a subset of patients with chronic urtiaria who have autoantibodies with histamine-releasing activity. The existence of these autoantibodies was recognized initially by the observation that sera from affected patients induced an immediate urticarial response on injection into their own skin. It was then shown that the sera induced histamine release from basophils and mast cells. It is now well established the autoantibodies responsible for this activity are those recognizing FcεRI and, less commonly, IgE.

25. **Describe the role of anti-FcεRI antibodies in chronic urticaria.**
    Anti-FcεRI autoantibodies are found in a high percentage of patients with chronic urticaria. They can induce histamine release by cross-linking to the receptor. Anti-FcεRI autoantibodies with and without histamine-releasing activity have been found, and only sera containing the former induce positive skin responses. The clinical presentation of patients with and without these autoantibodies is similar. However, patients with histamine-releasing autoantibodies tend to have more severe urticaria compared to those with non-histamine-releasing autoantibodies.

26. **Are anti-FcεRI antibodies associated only with urticaria?**
    Anti-FcεRI antibodies are not detectable in patients with dermographism or cholinergic urticaria. However, they are also present in other autoimmune diseases, including pemphigus vulgaris, dermatomyositis, systemic lupus erythematosus, and bullous pemphigoid. Nevertheless, only antibodies from patients with chronic urticaria are able to induce histamine release from basophils.

27. **What is the association between chronic urticaria and thyroid autoimmunity?**
    An increasing number of reports suggest the association of thyroid autoimmunity with urticaria. A substantial percentage (5–25%, depending on the studies) of patients with chronic urticaria have antithyroid autoantibodies. Such patients may be clinically and biochemically euthyroid. Moreover, among patients with thyroid diseases, a significantly higher percentage of those with autoantibodies have chronic urticaria compared to those without autoantibodies.

    Heymann WR: Chronic urticaria and angioedema associated with thyroid autoimmunity. J Am Acad Dermatol 40:229–32, 1999.

28. **What other systemic diseases may present with urticaria?**
    - Serum sickness
    - Systemic lupus erythematosus
    - Hepatitis C virus infection with cryoglubulinemia
    - Sjögren's syndrome
    - Schnitzler's syndrome (IgM gammopathy)

29. **What is known about infection and chronic urticaria?**
Whether chronic infection causes chronic urticaria is controversial. No convincing evidence substantiates this link. Eliminating an infection in a patient with chronic urticaria may sometimes cause a decrease in severity of the condition but rarely results in resolution.

30. **Can malignancies cause urticaria?**
Urticarial vasculitis has been associated with visceral and hematologic malignancies, but the connection is extremely rare.

31. **Describe a general diagnostic approach for chronic urticaria.**
The history is the most important part of the work-up of chronic urticaria. There is no need for routine extensive laboratory tests, unless indicated by the history. The following tests are appropriate in the initial evaluation of chronic urticaria: erythrocyte sedimentation rate and white blood cell count, including the differential count. Blood eosinophilia should prompt examination for parasitic infestations. Otherwise, extensive searches for occult infections are unwarranted. Current information does not support a routine exhaustive evaluation for an occult neoplasm.
Kozel MM, Bossuyt PM, Mekkes JR, Bos JD: Laboratory tests and identified diagnoses in patients with physical and chronic urticaria and angioedema: A systematic review. J Am Acad Dermatol 48:409–16, 2003.

KEY POINTS: DIAGNOSIS OF URTICARIA

1. Laboratory tests should be performed only when indicated by history.

2. Urticarial vasculitis should be suspected when individual urticarial lesions last for more than 24 hours. A skin biopsy should be performed.

3. A search for thyroid autoantibodies is appropriate for all chronic urticaria not responding to antihistamines because of the high prevalence of thyroid autoimmunity in patients with chronic urticaria.

4. Autoimmune urticaria due to autoantibodies to the IgE receptor FcεRI is a common cause of chronic urticaria.

32. **What are the appropriate laboratory tests if a systemic cause for urticaria is suspected?**
A raised erythrocyte sedimentation rate may suggest a work-up of systemic diseases. If history and physical examination suggest a collagen vascular disease (particularly if urticarial vasculitis is present), appropriate tests include complement assay, cryoglobulin, antinuclear antibody (ANA), rheumatoid factor, serum electrophoresis, hepatitis panel, and quantitative immunoglobulin.

33. **How should one approach the identification of foods as cause of chronic urticaria?**
If foods or food additives are suspected by history, an elimination diet or a diet low in food dyes and preservatives can be tried. If there is substantial improvement, a double-blind, placebo-controlled challenge should be considered.

34. **When should one consider thyroid autoimmunity?**
A search for thyroid autoantibodies is appropriate for all patients with chronic urticaria not responding to antihistamines, especially women and patients with a family history of thyroid

diseases or other autoimmune disorders. The search should include testing for antibodies against thyroid peroxidase and thyroglobulin.

35. **Describe methods for diagnosing autoimmune urticaria.**
The diagnosis is not possible by clinical assessment alone. Anti-FcεRI autoantibodies in the sera can be detected in vivo by intradermal injection of autologous serum or in vitro by testing the histamine-releasing activity using basophils or skin mast cells. Both methods are nonspecific for anti-FcεRI autoantibodies and detect anti-IgE autoantibodies as well as other yet-to-be-identified histamine-releasing molecules. The autoantibodies can also be detected by nonfunctional assays, such as immunoblot analysis using purified recombinant alpha chain of FcεRI. These assays detect autoantibodies both with and without histamine-releasing activity.

36. **What is the role of skin biopsy in managing urticaria?**
Skin biopsy is not necessary for routine management of clinically typical urticaria that responds to antihistamines. However, histology may sometimes provide useful therapeutic guides. Lymphocyte-predominant urticaria can often be controlled by antihistamines, while neutrophil-predominant urticaria is often unresponsive to antihistamines alone but may respond to dapsone or colchicine. Skin biopsy is indicated in severe cases of chronic urticaria, particularly when urticarial vasculitis is considered.

KEY POINTS: ROLE OF SKIN BIOPSY

1. Skin biopsy is not necessary for routine management of clinically typical urticaria that responds to antihistamines.

2. Histology may sometimes provide useful therapeutic guides.

3. Skin biopsy is indicated in severe cases of chronic urticaria, particularly when urticarial vasculitis is considered.

37. **Describe the management of acute urticaria.**
The goal of the management of acute urticaria is to identify and then remove the trigger of the process and offer symptomatic relief. H_1 antihistamine is the mainstay of the treatment of acute urticaria.

38. **Describe the management of chronic urticaria.**
Patients should be informed that (1) although the diagnosis is clear, in most cases the cause may not be identifiable; (2) the condition is not contagious, serious, or a sign of cancer; (3) unless it is related to underlying systemic diseases, the condition will resolve eventually. The treatment is removal of triggers or aggravating factors, if identified, and the use of medications that provide symptomatic relief.

39. **What should patients with chronic urticaria be told about the use of aspirin?**
Avoidance of aspirin and other nonsteroidal anti-inflammatory drugs should usually be recommended. Patients taking low-dose aspirin for its antithrombotic properties can usually continue regular treatment.

40. **List current FDA-approved antihistamines.**
Antihistamines include those that inhibit H_1 receptors and H_2 receptors.

First-generation H$_1$ antihistamines include ethylenediamines (e.g., tripelennamine), ethanolamines (e.g., diphenhydramine), alklyamines (e.g., chlorpheniramine), phenothiazines (e.g., promethazine), piperazines (e.g., hydroxyzine), and piperidines (cyproheptadine).

Second-generation H$_1$ antihistamines include cetirizine, fexofenadine, loratadine, and desloratadine.

H$_2$ antihistamines include cimetidine, ranitidine, and amotidine.

The tricyclic antidepressant **doxepin** is an antagonist for both H$_1$ and H$_2$ receptors and has potent antihistaminic effects.

41. **How do antihistamines work?**

    H$_1$ antihistamines competitively inhibit the binding of histamine on H$_1$ receptors, which belong to the family of G protein-coupled receptors. They reduce itch, wheal, or both. The new-generation H$_1$ antihistamines also exert anti-inflammatory effects such as inhibition of cytokine release from basophils and mast cells. **H$_2$ antihistamines** appear to influence vasodilatation and vaso-permeability through binding to H$_2$ receptor.

42. **Describe the difference between first- and second-generation antihistamines.**

    Histamine functions as a neurotransmitter and is important in maintaining a state of arousal and awareness within the central nervous system (CNS). The first-generation antihistamines are lipophilic and can penetrate through the blood-brain barrier and thus cause sedation. The second-generation antihistamines have much reduced propensity to enter the CNS and therefore exert no or markedly reduced sedative effects.

    Slater JW, Zechnich AD, Haxby DG: Second-generation antihistamines: A comparative review. Drugs 57:31–47, 1999.

43. **Describe how antihistamines are used in managing urticaria.**

    The second-generation antihistamines should be considered as first-line symptomatic treat-ment. The use of the first-generation antihistamines as monotherapy for chronic urticaria is less desirable because of their sedative effect. Many cases of chronic urticaria can be controlled with a single H$_1$ antihistamine; however, some respond better to a combination of two H$_1$ antihista-mines. A combination of a nonsedating antihistamine in the morning and a sedating antihista-mine in the late evening may be useful, especially when sleep is disturbed by itching. In some patients suffering from anxiety and depression due to chronic urticaria, the use of doxepin in the evening may be beneficial.

44. **What is the role of H$_2$ antihistamines in treatment of urticaria?**

    H$_2$ blockers alone offer little in the management of urticaria. However, an H$_2$-antihistamine administered in conjunction with an H$_1$-antihistamine may be beneficial in some patients refrac-tory to treatment with H$_1$-antihistamines alone. The existing literature does not support the rou-tine use of combination treatment.

45. **Describe the treatment of physical urticaria.**

    Most cases of physical urticaria respond to H$_1$ antihistamines. Treatment of dermographism may require a combination of H$_1$ and H$_2$ antihistamines. Treatment of delayed pressure urticaria may be very difficult because classic antihistamines have a limited effect. High-dose cetirizine (30 mg/day) and NSAIDs have been reported to be effective. Many patients require use of sys-temic corticosteroids.

46. **Discuss the possible adverse effects of H$_1$ antihistamines.**

    Sedation occurs with the use of all first-generation H$_1$ antihistamines and is the most common side effect. Other adverse effects include dizziness, blurred vision, and paradoxical symptoms of CNS stimulation, such as nervousness, insomnia, and tremor. Anticholinergic effects, such as dryness of mucous membranes, urinary retention, and increased intraocular pressure, also may be seen.

47. **Can antihistamines be used during pregnancy?**
It is best to avoid all antihistamines during pregnancy, especially in the first trimester, although none has been shown to be teratogenic in humans. If an antihistamine must be prescribed during pregnancy, the consensus is that chlorpheniramine is among the safest.

48. **What is the role of systemic corticosteroids in urticaria?**
Corticosteroids do not inhibit cutaneous mast-cell degranulation directly, but they affect the function and cytokine production of various inflammatory cell populations.
Systemic corticosteroids should not be used as a regular therapy for chronic urticaria. They may be required for severe chronic urticaria not responding to full-dose antihistamines, delayed pressure urticaria, and urticarial vasculitis. It is prudent to perform biopsy before starting systemic corticosteroids and pulse therapy, and alternate-day therapy should be considered.

49. **List immunosuppressive therapies for treatment of chronic urticaria.**
Immunosuppressive therapy has been shown to be useful in treating chronic urticaria. Available agents include:
- Azathioprine
- Cyclophosphamide
- Cyclosporine
- Intravenous immunoglobulin
- Methotrexate
- Mycophenolate mofetil

50. **Name other treatment options for chronic urticaria.**
Numerous other therapies have been reported for antihistamine-unresponsive chronic urticaria. Examples include leukotriene inhibitors, calcium channel blockers, and mast cell inhibitors (cromolyn and ketotifen). Colchicine and dapsone are useful for the treatment of neutrophil-predominant urticaria. Psoralen ultraviolet-A range (PUVA) and plasmapheresis have been shown to be effective for the treatment of urticaria. Anabolic agents, such as danazol (a gonadotropin inhibitor) and stanozolol (an anabolic steroid), are useful in hereditary angioedema. Because the severity of urticaria may fluctuate and spontaneous remission may occur, it is recommended that the treatment be reevaluated every 3–6 months.

KEY POINTS: TREATMENT OF URTICARIA

1. Antihistamines are the first-line treatment of chronic urticria.

2. Urticarial vasculitis usually does not respond to antihistamines alone.

3. Corsticosteroids and other immunosuppressive therapies may be necessary for treatment of chronic urticaria.

4. Patients with chronic urticaria associated with thyroid autoimmunity should receive thyroid hormone replacement, whether they are hypothyroid or euthyroid, especially if they have been unresponsive to standard therapy.

51. **What therapies are available for urticarial vasculitis?**
Various therapeutic agents have been shown to be efficacious, although the response to treatment is variable. For urticarial vasculitis manifesting only as non-necrotizing skin lesions, the

initial treatment may include antihistamines, dapsone, colchicine, hydroxychloroquine, and indomethacin, but corticosteroids are often required. For cases with necrotizing skin lesions or visceral involvement, corticosteroids are regularly indicated. Cases of corticosteroid-resistant urticarial vasculitis may require treatment with other immunosuppressive agents, such as those listed in question 52.

52. **How should urticaria associated with thyroid autoimmunity be treated?**
Patients with chronic urticaria and thyroid autoimmunity benefit from treatment with thyroid hormone replacement therapy or antithyroid drugs. The best response is actually seen in euthyroid patients treated with levothyroxine. The current recommendation is that patients with chronic urticaria associated with thyroid autoimmunity should receive thyroid hormone replacement for at least 8 weeks, whether they are hypothyroid or euthyroid, especially if they have been unresponsive to standard therapy for chronic urticaria. The hormone should be discontinued when patients are in remission for 1–2 months and readministered if the urticaria recurs.

WEBSITE

American Academy of Allergy, Asthma and Immunology: www.aaaai.org

BIBLIOGRAPHY

1. Beltrani VS: An overview of chronic urticaria. Clin Rev Allergy Immunol 23:147–170, 2002.
2. Charlesworth EN: Chronic urticaria: Background, evaluation, and treatment. Curr Allergy Asthma Rep 1:342–347, 2001.
3. Grattan CEH, Sabroe RA, Greaves MW: Chronic urticaria. J Am Acad Dermatol 46:645–657, 2002.
4. Greaves M: Autoimmune urticaria. Clin Rev Allergy Immunol 23:171–83, 2002.
5. Heymann WR: Chronic urticaria and angioedema associated with thyroid autoimmunity. J Am Acad Dermatol 40:229–32, 1999.
6. Kozel MM, Bossuyt PM, Mekkes JR, Bos JD: Laboratory tests and identified diagnoses in patients with physical and chronic urticaria and angioedema: A systematic review. J Am Acad Dermatol 48:409–16, 2003.
7. Slater JW, Zechnich AD, Haxby DG: Second-generation antihistamines: A comparative review. Drugs 57:31–47, 1999.
8. Tharp MD: Chronic urticaria: Pathophysiology and treatment approaches. J Allergy Clin Immunol 98:S325–30, 1996.
9. Venzor J, Lee WL, Huston DP: Urticarial vasculitis. Clin Rev Allergy Immunol 23:201–16, 2002.
10. Zuberbier T. Greaves MW, Juhlin L, et al: Definition, classification, and routine diagnosis of urticaria: A consensus report. J Invest Dermatol Symp Proc 6:123–7, 2001.

CHAPTER 9

ATOPIC DERMATITIS

Rosemary L. Hallett, M.D.

1. **What is atopic dermatitis?**

   Atopic dermatitis is a chronic, relapsing inflammatory skin condition characterized by extreme pruritus, edema, exudation, crusting, and scaling. It has been termed "the itch that rashes" because there is no primary skin lesion. The rash is caused by scratching and excoriation in response to pruritus. Atopic dermatitis usually presents in childhood and usually has a chronic course. Irritation and rubbing lead to lichenification. All of the skin is prone to generalized dryness, even uninvolved areas.

2. **What diseases make up the allergic triad?**

   Asthma, allergic rhinitis, and atopic dermatitis (Fig. 9-1). Children with atopic dermatitis tend to experience allergic rhinitis and asthma subsequently. These three diseases affect 8–25% of the worldwide population. The incidence is higher in developed countries and urban areas, particularly western societies, but they may occur in any race or geographic location. Children with atopic dermatitis tend to have more severe asthma than asthmatic children without atopic dermatitis. The allergen sensitization through the skin may cause a more severe and persistent respiratory disease.

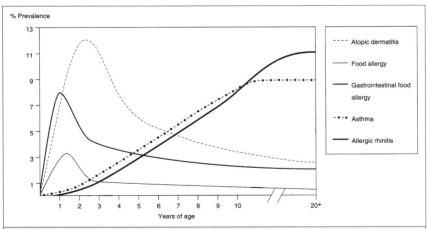

Figure 9-1. The atopic march. Several studies have suggested that treatment approaches to atopic dermatitis early in life may reduce progression to asthma and allergic rhinitis later in life. (From Beck LA: Atopic dermatitis. In Lichtenstein LM, Busse WW, Geha RS (eds): Current Therapy in Allergy, Immunology, and Rheumatology, 6th ed. St. Louis, Mosby, 2004, Fig. 1, p 89.)

3. **Is there a genetic basis for atopic dermatitis?**

   Almost 50% of patients with atopic dermatitis have a family history of atopy. Clinical studies have demonstrated a higher risk of atopy with a history on the maternal side. Other inheritance patterns may involve chromosome 5q31-33, which contains genes for interleukin (IL)-3, IL-4,

IL-5, IL-13, and granulocyte macrophage-colony stimulating factor (GM-CSF). Other chromoso-mal linkages have been reported, and there is a higher incidence among monozygotic twins.

4. **Has the incidence of atopic dermatitis changed?**
The incidence has increased, paralleling the increase in asthma and allergic rhinitis. Atopic der-matitis affects between 10% and17% of the total population; most patients are diagnosed before age 5 years.

5. **What are the specific anatomic distributions of atopic dermatitis? How do they vary with age?**
The infantile form is characterized by lesions on the face, trunk, neck, and extensor surfaces of the extremities. The anatomic distribution changes in older children and adults, in whom the lesions occur on the flexor surfaces, antecubital fossa, popliteal fossa, neck, hands, and feet. Adults may have more hand involvement associated with occupational work (e.g., hand washing or exposure to chemicals). Any area of the body can be involved in severe cases, although it is uncommon to see lesions in some flexor surfaces, such as the axillary, gluteal, or groin area. If such lesions are present, another diagnosis should be considered.

6. **At what age does atopic dermatitis start?**
It usually begins in infancy; 49–75% of patients present by 6 months of age, usually within the first 2–3 months of life. By 5 years, 80–90% of patients have the disease. Patients tend to grow out of atopic dermatitis, and the incidence drops to 10–15% by age 14. However, if an adolescent has moderate-to-severe atopic dermatitis, it is likely to persist into adulthood in more than 80% of patients. Characteristics indicating a poorer prognosis include severe childhood disease, a family history of atopic dermatitis, associated asthma or allergic rhinitis, onset before the age of 1 year, and female gender. Adult-onset disease should raise a higher index of suspicion of other diseases.

7. **What are the different stages of atopic dermatitis?**
Acute lesions are characterized by erythema and scaling. Tiny erythematous vesicles may rup-ture and weep. Subacute lesions develop mild scaling and lichenification. As the lesions become more chronic, scaling and lichenification are more prominent, with minimal skin erythema. Chronic lesions may be hyperpigmented or hypopigmented. On biopsy, intraepidermal vesicula-tion (spongiosis) is present, but this finding is not specific for the disease.

8. **How is the diagnosis of atopic dermatitis made?**
The diagnosis is clinical; there are no definitive lab tests. The main feature is pruritus. Other key findings include a chronic, relapsing course, personal or family history of atopy, early age of onset, and anatomic distribution associated with defined age groups. Other characteristics include accentuated lines or grooves below the margin of the lower eyelid (atopic pleat, Dennie's line, or Morgan's fold), periorbital darkening, palmer hyperlinearity, and keratosis pilaris (rough sandpaper texture from follicular accentuation to lateral aspects of the arms and thigh). Major and minor criteria have been suggested, with three major and three minor criteria indicative of the disease. The sensitivity and specificity of the criteria vary, and they are more often used as a guideline that summarizes the clinical findings and triggers.

9. **List the major criteria for diagnosis of atopic dermatitis.**
1. Pruritus
2. Typical distribution and morphology
   - Adults/older children: flexural surfaces
   - Infants: face and extensor surfaces
3. Chronic or relapsing dermatitis
4. Personal or family history of atopy

10. List the minor criteria for diagnosis of atopic dermatitis.
 1. **Clinical features:** facial pallor or erythema, hypopigmented patches, infraorbital darkening, infraorbital folds or wrinkles, cheilitis, recurrent conjunctivitis, anterior neck folds.
 2. **Triggers:** foods, emotional factors, environmental factors, skin irritants (e.g., wool, solvents, sweat).
 3. **Complications:** susceptibility to cutaneous viral and bacterial infections, impaired cell-mediated immunity, keratoconus, anterior subcapsular cataracts.
 4. **Other factors:** early age of onset, dry skin, hyperlinear palms, hand and foot dermatitis, keratosis pilaris, nipple eczema, white dermatographism, perifollicular accentuation, immediate skin test reactivity, raised serum IgE, ichthyosis.

KEY POINTS: CHARACTERISTICS OF ATOPIC DERMATITIS

1. Chronic, relapsing dermatitis

2. Pruritus

3. Characteristic distribution based on age

   - Adults/teenagers: flexural surfaces

   - Infants: face and extensor surfaces

4. Personal or family history of atopy

11. What other diagnoses need to be considered?
 - Other eczematous and dermatitis conditions (e.g., nummular eczema, dyshidrotic eczema, psoriasis, seborrheic dermatitis)
 - Allergic and irritant contact dermatitis (which can be seen with atopic dermatitis)
 - Stasis dermatitis
 - Systemic diseases
 - Immunodeficiency diseases
 - Malignancies
 - Infections
 - Scabies

12. Describe the typical features of nummular and dyshidrotic eczema.
 Nummular eczema is characterized by circular or oval, coin-like lesions. The most common locations are on the trunk or the extensor surfaces of the extremities, particularly on the pretibial areas or dorsum of the hands. **Dyshidrotic eczema** is located on the palmar and plantar sides of the palms, fingers and soles.

13. What are the typical features of seborrheic dermatitis?
 Seborrheic dermatitis describes greasy, pink-red scales usually seen on the scalp. In infancy, it often begins as "cradle cap." It also may involve sides of the nose, eyebrows, and eyelids. Sometimes in infancy it is difficult to distinguish seborrheic dermatitis from atopic dermatitis, particularly when the face is primarily involved. Seborrhea in infancy has a shorter course than atopic dermatitis and responds much more rapidly to treatment.

14. **Describe the characteristics of allergic contact dermatitis. What are the most common causes?**

    Allergic contact dermatitis first requires sensitization to an antigen, which takes approximately 1 week. On repeat exposure to the antigen, an eczematous reaction may become clinically apparent in 1–2 days. The lesions may be linear, arcuate, or well-demarcated patches in the configuration of contact with the offending agent. Lesions are usually not seen in the flexural areas. Common causes include neomycin, preservatives in topical ointments, poison ivy and related plants (oak and sumac), nickel, cosmetics, and latex.

15. **How is irritant contact dermatitis characterized?**

    Irritant dermatitis in a nonallergic reaction caused by various compounds; it is an extremely common form of eczema. It also has a sharply demarcated morphologic configuration in the area of the applied irritant. It is commonly seen in infancy in the perioral area (due to fruit juices) and diaper areas.

16. **What do allergic and irritant contact dermatitis have in common?**

    Both allergic and irritant contact dermatitis can have acute, subacute, and chronic forms. Patients with atopic dermatitis are prone to both allergic and irritant contact dermatitis. Patients with atopic dermatitis usually have more exposure to numerous creams and medications. Patients with active or inactive atopic dermatitis have a greater skin response to an irritant compared with healthy controls. The mechanism is unclear but may be secondary to an intrinsic hyperreactivity in inflammatory cells.

17. **What is stasis dermatitis? What other lesions may be mistaken for atopic dermatitis?**

    Stasis dermatitis develops on the lower extremities secondary to venous incompetence and chronic edema. Early findings may consist of mild erythema and scaling associated with pruritus with pigmented hemosiderin deposits. Psoriasis has scaly, silvery patches that may be mistaken for atopic dermatitis. The lesions are variably pruritic. Common areas for psoriasis are the elbows, knees, gluteal cleft, and scalp; lesions are usually symmetric. Ichthyosis vulgaris causes scales that are larger than those of atopic dermatitis. The pruritus is usually milder.

18. **Which systemic diseases may cause skin lesions resembling atopic dermatitis?**

    Langerhan cell histiocytosis (also known as histiocytosis X, Letterer-Siwe disease, Hand-Schüller-Christian disease, and diffuse reticuloendotheliosis), acrodermatitis enteropathica, and phenylketonuria (PKU) are systemic diseases occurring early in life. Newborns are routinely screened for PKU. Langerhan cell histiocytosis may present as failure to thrive; hemorrhagic manifestations are common in the eczematous eruptions. Acrodermatitis enteropathica is due to a deficiency of zinc absorption, resulting in dermatitis around the rectal, genitourinary, nasal, and oral areas.

19. **What immunodeficiency diseases may be associated with skin lesions resembling atopic dermatitis?**
    - Wiskott-Aldrich syndrome
    - X-linked agammaglobulinemia (Bruton's agammaglobulinemia)
    - Ataxia-telangiectasia
    - Hyper-IgE syndrome
    - Biotinidase deficiency

20. **What malignances need to be considered in the differential diagnosis?**

    Mycosis fungoides and Sézary syndrome are indolent non-Hodgkin's lymphomas of T-cell origin with primary involvement of the skin. Some patients may have initial patches that evolve into infiltrated plaques with a more generalized distribution. They also may present as generalized erythroderma with atrophic or lichenified skin. Patients are almost always intensely symptomatic from pruritus and scaling, and often have lymphadenopathy. Both malignancies need to be considered, particularly in adults and nonresponsive patients.

21. **What infectious agents may be confused with atopic dermatitis?**
Fungal infections with candida, herpes, *Staphylococcus aureus*, and scabies should be considered. Fungal infections often involve the intertriginous areas. Scabies lesions are located on the palms and soles with vesicles and commonly start with large papules on the upper back. The mite of scabies or its ova can be seen in scrapings from the vesicles. Herpes zoster or herpes simplex usually presents with painful vesicles. *S. aureus* can present as an impetigo or folliculitis.

22. **Describe the immunologic abnormalities behind atopic dermatitis.**
Atopic dermatitis is caused by an inflammatory process that is similar to the inflammatory cascade in the airways of asthmatics. Atopy is characterized by an increase in the TH2 type of T cells and the cytokines interleukin (IL)-4, IL-5, and IL-13. The result is an increase in IgE and eosinophilia. Other immunologic abnormalities include a decreased number of immunoregulatory T cells, increased costimulatory markers on antigen presenting cells (CD86), reduced cell-mediated immunity, and defective antibody-dependent cellular cytotoxicity. There is also a high incidence of elevated total IgE and IgE-mediated responses on skin testing to food and inhaled antigens and total IgE.

23. **Explain the differences in acute versus chronic inflammatory processes associated with atopic dermatitis.**
Acute lesions of atopic dermatitis have an increased numbers of cells expressing IL-4 and IL-13. IL-4 and IL-13 promote isotype switching to IgE, resulting in activation of mast cells, inhibition of TH2 cytokines, and upregulation of the low-affinity IgE receptor, FcεRII, (CD23) on monocytes and B cells. They also stimulate expression of RANTES cells (regulated on activation normally, T-cell expressed and secreted), eotaxin, and monocyte chemotactic protein (MCP)-1, leading to a local eosinophil infiltration. Acute lesions also demonstrate a reduced ability to produce interferon (IFN)-gamma. Chronic disease has increased IFN-gamma, IL-4, IL-5, IL-12, IL-13, and GM-CSF with an infiltration of eosinophils and macrophages. This pattern suggests a combined response of TH1 and TH2 cells. IL-5 is a potent chemotactic agent for the migration of eosinophils.

24. **What determines the location of allergic disease?**
The location of allergic disease is determined by the route of allergen sensitization, chemokine expression, and tissue compartmentalization of immune responses. T cells migrate to different tissues based in their homing receptors. T cells that infiltrate the skin express higher levels of a cell adhesion molecule, called cutaneous lymphocyte-associated (CLA) antigen, than T cells from asthmatics airways. CLA-positive T cells secrete IL-5 and IL-13, prolong eosinophil survival, and induce IgE synthesis. The chemokines RANTES, MCP-4 and eotaxin also are in higher concentrations in the skin of patients with atopic dermatitis and attract eosinophils and TH2 lymphocytes into the skin. Langerhan cells are important antigen-presenting cells in the skin and bear high-affinity IgE receptors (FcεRI) and allergen-specific IgE. They capture antigens, activate memory TH2 cells, and may migrate to the lymph nodes to stimulate naive T cells.

25. **What promotes the chronicity of atopic dermatitis on an immunologic basis?**
Eosinophils and monocytes have a prolonged survival in atopic skin, perhaps secondary to the expression of IL-5, which promotes eosinophil survival and function. Epidermal keratinocytes and infiltrating macrophages also cause an increase in GM-CSF, which maintains survival and function of monocytes, Langerhan cells, and eosinophils. Epidermal keratinocytes, when stimulated with IFN-gamma and tumor necrosis factor alpha (TNF-α), produce increased levels of

RANTES, which enhance the chemotaxis of eosinophils. Mechanical trauma also can induce the release of TNF-α and other cytokines.

26. **Explain the immunologic basis for the pruritus.**
The cause of pruritus is not completely understood, but proinflammatory mediators and cytokines are thought to play a role. Histamine injected into the skin demonstrates a lower itch threshold in atopic skin. Patients with atopic dermatitis have elevated histamine levels in all areas of skin, not just affected areas. Lichenified areas are characterized by an increase in mast cells, a potent histamine releaser. Substance P, a neuropeptide, induces mast-cell degranulation and increases releasability of histamine from basophils. Other mediators, such as leukotrienes, acetylcholine, proteases, and other neuropeptides, can induce pruritus. Nonantigenic mechanisms may also play a role in pruritus and inflammatory response. Patients with atopic dermatitis have a lower threshold of cutaneous hyperreactivity. Mechanical trauma to the keratinocytes results in a cytokine and proinflammatory cascade, possibly causing the pruritus.

27. **What cells are seen in the skin of patients with atopic dermatitis?**
Antigen-presenting cells in the skin, such as Langerhan cells and macrophages, have surface-bound IgE molecules and present antigens to promote an immune response. Acute lesions have activated memory T cells with CD3, CD4, and CD45RO, indicating prior sensitization. Mast cells are present in various stages of degranulation. Acute skin lesions have spongiosis, whereas chronic lesions have a minimal amount. A hyperplastic epidermis is present, and hyperkeratosis is prominent in areas of lichenification. Eosinophil proteins are found in the elastic fibers throughout the upper dermis. Eosinophil major basic protein, eosinophil cationic protein, and eosinophil-derived neurotoxin are elevated in atopic dermatitis sera and correlate with disease severity.

28. **What pathologic mechanisms other than immunologic abnormalities are associated with atopic dermatitis?**
A defective skin barrier decreases water content in the skin, resulting in reduced water-binding capacity and higher transepidermal water loss.

29. **What are the common triggers for a flare of atopic dermatitis?**
Irritants, allergens, soaps, detergents, fabric softeners, excessive bathing or hand washing, and physical environment. Infectious agents, emotional stressors, and abrasive or occlusive clothing also can trigger flares. In adolescent patients, these triggers may be reason to avoid certain occupations (excessive hand washing, certain exposures).

30. **What recommendations should be made about altering the physical environment?**
Extremes of heat and humidity should be avoided. A warm climate with moderate humidity is optimal for most patients. Exposure to sunlight and salt water is of benefit to many patients, but nonirritating sunblock should be used to avoid sunburn. In humid conditions, care should be taken to avoid sweat retention, which can lead to prickly heat rash or miliaria rubra and miliaria pustulosa. Clothing should be light and loose-fitting. Cotton is less irritating than polyester or wool.

31. **How do food allergies manifest in children with atopic dermatitis?**
Food allergies have a greater significance in childhood. The onset of dermatitis frequently coincides with the introduction of certain foods into the infant's diet. Common food allergies and possible triggers for atopic dermatitis in children include egg, milk, peanut, soy, and wheat. Overall, about 20–30% of children with eczema have food hypersensitivity to one or more of these food allergens. Patch testing may also play a role in identifying food allergy. Currently, there are no standardized tests or interpretations. Even continued ingestion of small amounts can provoke chronic inflammation. Children tend to outgrow food allergies, which are not com-

mon triggers for atopic dermatitis in adults. Arbitrary exclusion of numerous foods from the diets of infants without clear evidence that they are involved can lead to malnutrition, and the causative agent should be identified through double-blinded food challenges.

32. **What is the significance of food allergies in adults?**
Adults should be evaluated for food allergies if they have a relevant history. Routine skin testing and specific IgE assays for food have a high incidence of false-positive results. Immediate skin tests to specific allergens do not always indicate clinical sensitivity, and patients who outgrow atopic dermatitis frequently continue to have positive skin tests. This finding suggests that the relationship is not exclusively dependent on IgE-mediated mast-cell degranulation. If food is believed to be a possible cause in patients with serious atopic dermatitis, an elemental diet may be followed with reintroduction of foods one at a time and observation for flares.

33. **Describe the role of aeroallergens and household allergens in atopic dermatitis.**
Aeroallergens play more of a role as the atopic child grows older. Studies have shown worsening of symptoms with patch testing of aeroallergens. Inhalation of aeroallergens may exacerbate the skin disease. Sera from 95% of patients with atopic dermatitis had IgE to house dust mites compared with 42% of asthmatic patients. House dust mite–specific lymphocyte stimulation is greatly elevated in infants with atopic dermatitis. Recommendation of empiric avoidance of dust mite and animal dander may be warranted because avoidance improves symptoms.

34. **Immunotherapy improves symptoms of allergic rhinitis and asthma. Can it be used for atopic dermatitis?**
There is no role for immunotherapy in patients with atopic dermatitis. Anecdotally it has been associated with both aggravation and improvement of dermatitis. Immunotherapy may help other atopic diseases in the patient.

35. **What role do infectious agents play in flares of atopic dermatitis?**
Patients with atopic dermatitis have an increased tendency for development of bacterial and fungal skin infections. In general, dry skin creates small fissures that can serve as an entry to skin pathogens. However, compared with other dry skin conditions, such as psoriasis, there is still an increased susceptibility for infections. A deficiency in antimicrobial peptides was found in the skin of patients with atopic dermatitis compared to the skin of patients with psoriasis, leading to a susceptibility to *S. aureus*. *S. aureus* is colonized on the skin of 90% of patients with atopic dermatitis compared with only 5% of healthy people. Empirical treatment with oral antibiotics often results in improvement, even if no active infection is seen. Observation of pustules indicates that *S. aureus* may be present.
    Ong, PY, Ohtake, T, Brandt, C, et al: Endogenous antimicrobial peptides and skin infections in atopic dermatitis. N Engl J Med 347:1151–1160, 2002.

36. **How are bacterial skin infections treated?**
An antibiotic with good staphylococcal coverage, such as cephalexin or dicloxacillin should be administered for 3–4 weeks. Some patients may require longer treatment (6–12 weeks). Bactroban can be used for early topical treatment and also can be applied to the nares of staphylococcal carriers who experience frequent relapses when antibiotics are discontinued. However, other topical antibiotics are of little therapeutic value and can lead to sensitization to the agents, particularly neomycin.

37. **Describe the immunologic mechanism of a flare caused by *S. aureus*.**
S. aureus secretes toxins that act as superantigens. These superantigens activate T cells and macrophages. Cultures of *S. aureus* on the skin of atopic patients show that one-half of the organisms secrete enterotoxins A and B and toxic shock syndrome toxin-1 (TSST-1). The enterotoxins act as superantigens with marked activation of the cells, increased IgE synthesis,

and induced corticosteroids resistance. Most patients with atopic dermatitis make specific IgE antibodies directed against the staphylococcal toxins found on skin.

38. **What other infections can contribute to atopic dermatitis?**
   Malassezia furfur (Pityrosporum ovale) is a saprophytic yeast that can be part of normal skin flora. It is commonly present in seborrheic areas of the skin. Patients with atopic dermatitis may have IgE antibodies to *M. furfur*; such antibodies are more common in patients with head and neck dermatitis. Healthy controls or asthmatic patients rarely have IgE sensitization to *M. furfur*. Treatment involves antimycotic therapy. Other skin lesions include common warts and molluscum contagiosum, which probably result not from an immunologic mechanism but from decreased inherent resistance and increased autoinoculation.

39. **How does herpes simplex manifest in atopic dermatitis?**
   Herpes simplex may begin as a cold sore and become generalized. It may present as umbilicated vesicles or grouped erosions. Systemic dissemination associated with generalized vesicular and pustule lesions, fever, and constitutional symptoms has a 20% mortality rate.

40. **What can be recommended for prevention of atopic dermatitis?**
   Breast-feeding during the first 3 months has been associated with a lower incidence of atopic dermatitis in patients with a family history of atopic dermatitis. In children, food allergen sensitization can be reduced by delaying the introduction of solid foods until after 6 months of age. Breast-feeding mothers should avoid ingestion of high-risk foods in atopic-prone infants to reduce sensitization. Gut microflora may play a role in decreasing atopy. Lactobacilli administered to pregnant women and postnatally to the infant for 6 months lead to a decrease in atopic eczema, suggesting an immunomodulatory role. Other gut microflora may be protective, including enterococci and bifidobacetria, whereas more atopy has been seen with gut flora containing clostridia and *S. aureus*.
   Kalliom Ski, M, Salminen, S, Arvilommi, H, et al: Probiotics in primary prevention of atopic disease: A randomized placebo-controlled trial. Lancet 357:1076–1079, 2001.)

41. **Is atopic dermatitis associated with an autoimmune component?**
   Early studies showing sensitivity to human skin dander and an increase in cell proliferation with human skin extracts in patients with atopic dermatitis suggest that an autoallergen component may be involved. IgE to human intracellular proteins has been seen in patients with severe disease. These antibodies were not seen in patients with other autoimmune diseases, such as chronic urticaria and systemic lupus erythematosus, or normal controls.
   Valenta R: Autoallergy: a pathogenetic factor in atopic dermatitis? J Allergy Clin Immunol 105:432–437, 2000.

42. **Discuss the role of emotional stressors in atopic dermatitis.**
   Emotional stressors induce flares of atopic dermatitis. Patients should be advised to reduce stress at school and home and seek psychological counseling or behavior modification if appropriate.

43. **What ocular symptoms may be seen?**
   Atopic keratoconjunctivitis (AKC) is a severe, vision-threatening form of conjunctivitis that occurs in up to 25% of patients with atopic dermatitis. Corneal thinning, or keratoconus, has been reported in up to 15% of patients with AKC. In addition, anterior subcapsular cataracts are often associated with AKC, and the use of corticosteroids may cause worsening of posterior cataracts. Long-term eye rubbing may contribute to these findings.

44. **How is atopic dermatitis treated?**
   Standard treatment for atopic dermatitis is focused on topical anti-inflammatory preparations and lubrication of the skin. Advances in treatment have focused on nonsteroidal topical immunomodulators, which now play a larger role in the treatment of atopic dermatitis.

45. **What measures should be taken to protect the skin?**
Treatment should be aimed at controlling the itch-scratch cycle and hydrating the skin. The keys are avoidance of triggers and good skin care. The general principles of skin care include hydration and emollients. Hydration involves short baths (15–20 minutes) in tepid water. Patients should avoid excessively hot water and extended submersions. As little soap as possible should be used, and it should be nondrying (e.g., Cetaphil). Bubble baths can cause excessive irritation. Colloidal oatmeal or baking soda can be added to the bath for an antipruritic effect. Bath oils, however, are not effective because they coat the outer layer of the skin and may seal out the moisture in the hydrated skin. Patients should pat dry and avoid excessive toweling and rubbing. Nails should be trimmed short, and cotton gloves can be worn at night to decrease scratching during sleep.

46. **What emollients should be recommended?**
Lotions have a high water and low oil content and may contain alcohol. Creams (e.g., Eucerin in a tub) are thicker in consistency, have a low water content, and are preferred over lotions. Creams should be applied immediately after bathing to retain hydration. Ointments (e.g., petroleum jelly, Aquaphor, Petrolatum), which have zero water content, offer better protection against xerosis. Emollients are less expensive than corticosteroids, control the itch, and have no side effects. Emollients containing alcohol should be avoided. The cheaper alternatives, including petroleum jelly, mineral oil, and Crisco, can be just as effective. Another cheap but highly effective alternative is udder cream (Bag Balm). Care should be taken to avoid irritating ingredients such as methylsalicylate.

47. **What medication is recommended for treatment of atopic dermatitis?**
The backbone of topical medication for atopic dermatitis is corticosteroids. Topical immunomodulators have been approved in the past several years and also play an important role in treatment. The goal of therapy should be low-potency corticosteroids and emollients for maintenance therapy and mid- and high-potency corticosteroids for exacerbations. For facial involvement, topical immunomodulators (tacrolimus, pimecrolimus) may be considered as first-line treatments.

48. **How should topical steroids be prescribed?**
Hydrocortisone 1% (purchased over the counter) or 2.5% (available by prescription) is low-potency and useful for patients with mild disease. A medium-potency corticosteroid ointment (triamcinolone 0.1%) can be used for more severe disease. Higher-potency topical steroids can be used for a short period in some patients with acute flares and then reduced to a lower potency when lesions improve. Areas of lichenified skin may require stronger steroids in a thicker form for prolonged periods. Topical steroids should be applied twice daily and may be mixed with an emollient base. Ointments and creams have a thicker consistency and may increase the potency of a chemically equivalent steroid in a lotion. Occlusive bandages further increase the potency of the steroid. Systemic steroids may be used for severe flares, but dramatic rebound flares may be seen on discontinuation. Therefore, patients should have a good understanding of stepping up and down the medication. Short courses can be used in conjunction with an intensified topical program. Patients may also benefit from maintenance dosing (2–3 times per week) to keep flares in check.

49. **What are the side effects of topical steroids?**
Side effects include skin atrophy, telangiectasia, striae, and suppression of the hypothalamic-pituitary-adrenal axis. The ultra-high potency steroids have a more pronounced side-effect profile and must be prescribed judiciously. Patients must be educated about duration of usage and areas to avoid. High-potency corticosteroids should be avoided on the face, genitalia, and intertriginous areas and should be used only for a short period.

50. **Describe the role of the nonsteroidal topical immunomodulators tacrolimus and pimecrolimus.**
Tacrolimus (Protopic) and pimecrolimus (Elidel) are topical, nonsteroidal medications for atopic dermatitis. They act by decreasing the inflammatory cytokine transcription in activated T cells.

Tacrolimus ointment also reduces staphylococcal colonization of atopic dermatitis lesions. Systemic absorption is minimal, and the side effects of steroids are avoided. There is no increase in infections, and response to common antigens is not impaired. The main role of these agents is for facial involvement, including eyelids, and pediatric patients. The potency is roughly equivalent to a mid-potency steroid. Tacrolimus and pimecrolimus are much more expensive than topical steroids and should therefore be used appropriately.

51. **What are adverse effects of tacrolimus and pimecrolimus?**
Adverse affects include skin burning and pruritus upon application, which should decrease with repeated use. It is recommended to wear sunblock with these medications. Tacrolimus is available in 0.03% for ages over 2 years old and 0.1% for ages over 12 years old. Pimecrolimus 1% is approved for children over 2 years of age but has been used safely in infants as young as 3 months of age.

52. **Describe the role of antihistamines.**
Many patients experience relief of the pruritus with antihistamines, but it is unclear whether it is due to the antipruritic or sedative effect. Nighttime dosing can provide antihistamine effect without daytime sedation. The H_1 blockers hydroxyzine and cetirizine are particularly effective because they block some of the IgE-mediated, late-phase response. Hydroxyzine can be used in large doses (2 mg/kg/day or 75–100 mg) at bedtime. Daily use of cetirizine may reduce the use of additional H_1 antihistamines and may have a corticosteroid-sparing effect by decreasing the duration of high potency topical steroid use. Because topical antihistamines can be sensitizing, direct application to the skin is not recommended. A single dose of doxepin, a tricyclic antidepressant with antihistamine effects, can be effective. H_2 blockers may be a helpful adjunct for refractory pruritus.

KEY POINTS: TREATMENT FOR ATOPIC DERMATITIS

1. Hydration and topical emollients

2. Avoid excessive skin drying with soaps and hot water

3. Topical steroids

4. Topical immunomodulators (tacrolimus and pimecrolimus)

53. **What effect do dressings have on atopic dermatitis?**
Wet dressings are highly effective as an adjunct to therapy and for acute flares. Ointment is applied directly after bathing, followed by wet dressings with a dry cover. Wet pajamas can be applied over lotions if the extremities are involved, covered with a pair of dry pajamas or sweat suit. Socks and gloves can be used for the face and hands. This approach is best suited for overnight use.

54. **Describe the use of coal tar extracts for severe disease.**
Coal tar extracts may be applied during bathing if the above measures are not effective. Acute use can cause stinging and irritation and is not well tolerated because of the odor.

55. **Discuss the role of phototherapy.**
Phototherapy combined with PUVA (psoralens plus ultraviolet A radiation) or combinations of ultraviolet A (UVA) and ultraviolet B (UVB) help to control the disease. The combination of UVA

and UVB is better than either therapy alone. Disadvantages include an increased risk of skin cancer and the expense. The treating physician should have experience with both atopic dermatitis and phototherapy.

56. **How is cyclosporine used? What are its side effects?**
Oral cyclosporine (3–6 mg/kg/day) has been shown to be beneficial for severe atopic dermatitis unresponsive to topical corticosteroids, but its use is limited by side effects, including nausea, hypertrichosis, hypertension, paresthesias, and hepatic and renal toxicity. Blood pressure and renal function should be monitored. Cyclosporine typically is used for 6 weeks, and the disease may flare on discontinuation. Topical cyclosporine has not been shown to be effective. Oral tacrolimus (FK 506) has a similar side-effect profile and has also been used.

57. **What other drugs have been used?**
Azathioprine and methotrexate may be helpful. Interferon gamma may be helpful for refractory atopic dermatitis. Intravenous immunoglobulin dosed at 2 gm/kg showed clinical improvement, decreased steroid usage, and reduced skin-test reactivity to allergens. These modalities are expensive and require patient education. Leukotriene antagonists may have a role in treatment of atopic dermatitis. Chinese herbal medicines have been reported to be helpful, but the content has not been well characterized. Many formulations contain corticosteroids, and there has been an association with liver toxicity.

58. **What recommendations should be made for patients with atopic dermatitis in regard to smallpox vaccinations?**
Smallpox has become a concern as an agent of bioterrorism. Vaccinations have been offered to select groups; however, patients with atopic dermatitis (or a history of atopic dermatitis) should not receive the vaccine due to a concern of eczema vaccinatum. Patients whose household contacts have acute or chronic exfoliative skin conditions should also not receive the immunization. Eczema vaccinatum is a local or disseminated vesicopapular dermatitis, and in one study required prolonged hospitalization in 60% of patients. It can develop in patients with complete remission of the atopic dermatitis. Intravenous immunoglobulin may play a role in safely immunizing patients with eczema.

59. **List the indications for referral to a dermatologist or an allergist.**
- Severe or persistent disease
- Disease unresponsive to first-line therapy
- Erythroderma or extensive exfoliation
- Disease that requires more than one course of systemic corticosteroids or hospital admission
- Need to identify allergens and triggers
- Patients in need of intensive education
- Associated asthma or rhinitis
- Impaired quality of life
- Complications of the disease
- Uncertainty of diagnosis

60. **What is the prognosis of atopic dermatitis?**
Atopic dermatitis is a chronic, relapsing disease that can be extremely frustrating for families. It usually can be controlled with minimizing triggers and local treatments. Counseling of patients should include the fact that no immediate cure is available. Quality of life can be severely impaired due to disruption of school and family interactions and poor sleep due to intense pruritus. Parents of patients with atopic dermatitis and asthma believed that atopic dermatitis was more difficult to deal with. Education and support are vital. An atopic dermatitis action plan (similar to those used for asthma) may be useful. For additional information the patient can contact the National Eczema Association for Science and Education (800–818–7456; *www.nationaleczema.org*).

WEBSITE

National Eczema Association for Science and Education: www.nationaleczema.org

BIBLIOGRAPHY

1. Bjorksten B, Sepp E, Julge K, et al: Allergy development and the intestinal microflora during the first year of life. J Allergy Clin Immunol 18:516–520, 2001.

2. Boguniewicz, M, Fiedler, VC, Raimer, S, et al: Pediatric Tacrolimus Study Group. A randomized, vehicle-controlled trial of tacrolimus ointment for treatment of atopic dermatitis in children. J Allergy Clin Immunol 102:637–644, 1998.

3. Bratton DL, et al: GM-CSF inhibition of monocyte apoptosis contributes to the chronic monocyte activation in atopic dermatitis. J Clin Invest 95:211–218, 1995.

4. Bratton DL, May KR, Kailey JM, et al: Staphylococcal toxic shock syndrome toxin-1 inhibits monocyte apoptosis. J Allergy Clin Immunol 103; 895–900, 1999.

5. Bunikowski R, Mielke M, Skarabis H, et al: Prevalence and role of serum IgE antibodies to the *Staphylococcus aureus*-derived superantigens. J Allergy Clin Immunol 103:119–124, 1999.

6. Carucci JA, Washenik K, Weinstein A, et al: The leukotriene antagonist zafirlukast as a therapeutic agent for atopic dermatitis. Arch Dermatol 134:785–786, 1998.

7. Christophers E, Henseler T: Contrasting disease patterns in psoriasis and atopic dermatitis. Arch Dermatol Res 279 Suppl:S48–51, 1987.

8. Cookson WO, Young RP, Sanford AJ, et al: Maternal inheritance of atopic IgE responsiveness on chromosome 11q. Lancet 340:381–384, 1992.

9. Cookson WO, Ubhi B, Lawrence R, et al: Genetic linkage of childhood atopic dermatitis to psoriasis susceptibility loci. Nat Genet 27:372–373, 2001.

10. Cooper KD: Atopic dermatitis: recent trends in pathogenesis and therapy. J Invest Dermatol 1994; 102:128–137, 1994.

11. Cooper KD, Kazmierowski JA, Wuepper KD, Hanifin JM: Immunoregulation in atopic dermatitis: functional analysis of T-B cell interactions and the enumeration of Fc receptor-bearing T cells. J Invest Dermatol 80:139–345, 1983.

12. Diepgen TL: Early Treatment of the Atopic Child Study Group. Pediatr Allergy Immunol 13:278–286, 2002.

13. Eichenfield LF, Lucky AW, Boguniewicz M, et al: Safety and efficacy of pimecrolimus (ASM 981) cream 1% in the treatment of mild and moderate atopic dermatitis in children and adolescents. J Am Acad Dermatol 46:495–504, 2002.

14. Forrest S, Dunn K, Elliott K, et al: Identifying genes predisposing to atopic dermatitis. J Allergy Clin Immunol 104:1066–1070, 1999.

15. Gdalevich M, Mimouni D, David M, Mimouni M: Breast-feeding and the onset of atopic dermatitis in childhood: A systematic review and meta-analysis of prospective studies. J Am Acad Dermatol 45:520–527, 2001

16. Hanifin JM, Ling MR, Langley R, et al: Tacrolimus ointment for the treatment of atopic dermatitis in adult patients: part I, efficacy. J Am Acad Dermatol 44:S28–38, 2001.

17. Hanifin JM, Rajka G: Diagnostic features of atopic dermatitis. Acta Derm Venereol 92(suppl):44–47, 1980.

18. Hanifin JM, Schneider LC, Leung DY, et al: Recombinant interferon gamma therapy for atopic dermatitis. J Am Acad Dermatol 28:189–197, 1993.

19. Hopkins T, Clark RAF: The Eczemas. In Callen JP(ed): Current Practice of Dermatology. New York, McGraw, 1996, pp 68–75.

20. Joint Task Force on Practice Parameters, *Ann Allergy Asthma Immunol.* 79:197–211, 1997.

21. Jolles S, Hughes J, Rustin M, et al: Intracellular interleukin-4 profiles during high-dose intravenous immunoglobulin treatment of therapy-resistant atopic dermatitis. J Am Acad Dermatol 40:121–123, 1999.

22. Jones SM, Sampson HA: The role of allergens in atopic dermatitis. Clin Rev Allergy 11:471–490, 1993.

23. Kalliomaki M, Salminen, S, Arvilommi, H, et al: Probiotics in primary prevention of atopic disease: a randomized placebo-controlled trial. Lancet 357:1076–1079, 2001.

24. Keane FM: Analysis of Chinese herbal creams prescribed for dermatological conditions: BMJ 318:563–564, 1999.

25. Klein PA, Clark RA: An evidence-based review of the efficacy of antihistamines in relieving pruritus in atopic dermatitis. Arch Dermatol; 135:1522–1525, 1999.

26. Koro OF, Furutani K, Hide M, et al: Chemical mediators in atopic dermatitis: Involvement of leukotriene B4 released by a type I allergic reaction in the pathogenesis of atopic dermatitis. J Allergy Clin Immunol 103:663–670, 1999.

27. Kuster W, Peterson M, Christophers E, et al: A family study of atopic dermatitis: Clinical and genetic characteristics of 188 patients and 2,151 family members. Arch Dermatol Res 282:98–102, 1990.

28. Lane JM, Ruben FL, Neff JM, Millar JD: Complications of small pox vaccination, 1968. National surveillance in the United States. N Engl J Med 281:1201–1208, 1969.

29. Larsen FS, Holm NV, Henningsen K: Atopic dermatitis. A genetic-epidemiologic study in a population-based twin sample. J Am Acad Dermatol 15:487–494, 1986.

30. Lee YA, Wahn U, Kehrt R, et al: A major susceptibility locus for atopic dermatitis maps to chromosome 3q21. Nat Genet 26:470–473, 2000.

31. Leroy BP, Boden G, Sachapelle JM, et al: A novel therapy for atopic dermatitis with allergen-antibody complexes: a double-blind, placebo controlled study. J Am Acad Dermatol 28:232–239, 1993.

32. Leung DYM: Atopic dermatitis: New insights and opportunities for therapeutic intervention. J Allergy Clin Immunol 105: 860–876, 2000.

33. Mazer BD, et al: An open-label study of high-dose intravenous immunoglobulin in severe childhood asthma. J Allergy Clin Immunol 87:976–983, 1991.

34. Meingassner JG, Grassberger M, Fahrngruber H, et al: A novel anti-inflammatory drug, SDC ASM 981, for the topical and oral treatment of skin diseases: in vivo pharmacology. Br J Dermatol 137:568–576, 1997.

35. Morale J, et al: CTACK, a skin-associated chemokine that preferentially attracts skin-homing memory to T cell. Proc Natl Acad Sci USA 96: 14470–14475, 1999.

36. Nickel RB, Beck LA, Stellato C, et al: Chemokines and allergic disease. J Allergy Clin Immunol 104:723–742, 1999.

37. Ong, PY, Ohtake, T, Brandt, C, et al: Endogenous antimicrobial peptides and skin infections in atopic dermatitis. N Engl J Med 347:1151–1160, 2002.

38. Picker LJ, Martin RJ, Trumble A, et al: Differential expression of lymphocyte homing receptors by human receptors by human memory/effector T cells in pulmonary versus cutaneous immune effector sites. Eur J Immunol 24:1269–1277, 1994.

39. Pincelli CF, et al: Neuropeptides in skin from patients with atopic dermatitis: An immunohistochemical study. Br J Dermatol 122: 745–750, 1990.

40. Reinhold U, Kukel S, Brzoska J, et al: Systemic interferon gamma treatment in severe atopic dermatitis. J Am Acad Dermatol 29:58–63, 1993.

41. Reitamo S: Tacrolimus: A new topical immunomodulatory therapy for atopic dermatitis. J Allergy Clin Immunol 107:445–448, 2001.

42. Reitamo S, Rustin M, Ruzicka T, et al: Efficacy and safety of tacrolimus ointment compared with that of hydrocortisone butyrate ointment in adult patients with atopic dermatitis. J Allergy Clin Immunol 109:547–555, 2002.

43. Reitamo S, Van Leent EJ, Ho V, et al: Efficacy and safety of tacrolimus ointment compared with that of hydrocortisone acetate ointment in children with atopic dermatitis. J Allergy Clin Immunol 109:539–546, 2002.

44. Reitamo S, Wollenberg A, Schopf E, et al: Safety and efficacy of 1 year of tacrolimus ointment monotherapy in adults with atopic dermatitis. The European Tacrolimus Ointment Study Group. Arch Dermatol 136:999–1006, 2000.

45. Remitz A, Kyllonen H, Granlund H: Tacromlimus ointment reduces staphylococcal colonization of atopic dermatitis lesions. J Allergy Clin Immunol107: 196, 2001.

46. Rikkers SM, Holland GN, Drayton GE, et al: Topical tacrolimus treatment of atopic eyelid disease. Am J Ophthalmol 135:297–302, 2003.

47. Ruiz RG, Kemeny DM, Price JF: Higher risk of infantile atopic dermatitis from maternal atopy than from paternal atopy. Clin Exp Allergy 22:762–766, 1992.

48. Ruzicka T, Bieber T, Schopf E, et al: A short-term trial of tacrolimus ointment for atopic dermatitis. European Tacrolimus Multicenter Atopic Dermatitis Study Group. N Engl J Med 337:816–821, 1997.

49. Sharp JC, Fletcher WB: Experience of anti-vaccinia immunoglobulin in the United Kingdom. Lancet 1:655, 1973.

50. Shaw JC: Atopic dermatitis. Up-to-Date, Version 11.2, 2003.

51. Sheehan MP, Atherton DJ: A controlled trial of traditional Chinese medicinal plants in widespread non-exudative atopic eczema. Br J Dermatol 126:179–184, 1992.

52. Shimizu EA, Abe R, Ohkawara A, et al: Increase production of macrophage migration inhibitory factor by PBMCs of atopic dermatitis. J Allergy Clin Immunol 104:659–664, 1999.

53. Sicherer SH, Sampson H: Food hypersensitivity and atopic dermatitis: Pathophysiology, epidemiology, diagnosis and management. J Allergy Clin Immunol 104:114–122, 1999.

54. Sly RM: Allergic Disorders: Atopic Dermatitis. In Behrman RE, Kliegman RM, Jenson HB (eds): Nelson Textbooks of Pediatrics, 16th ed. Philadelphia, W.B. Saunders Company, 2000, pgs 681–684.

55. Taha RA, Leung DYM, Ghaffar O: In vivo expression receptor mRNA in atopic dermatitis. J Allergy Clin Immunol 102:245–550, 1998.

56. Trepka MJ, Heinrich, J, Wichmann, HE: The epidemiology of atopic diseases in Germany: an east-west comparison. Rev Environ Health 11:119–131, 1996.

57. Valenta R: Autoallergy: a pathogenetic factor in atopic dermatitis? J Allergy Clin Immunol 105:432–437, 2000.

58. Van Leent EJM, et al: Effectiveness of the ascomycin macrolactam ADZ ASM 981 in the topical treatment of atopic dermatitis. Arch Dermatol 134:805–809, 1998.

59. Wollenberg A, Kraft S, Oppel T, Bieber T: Atopic dermatitis: pathogenetic mechanisms. Clin Exp Dermatol 25:530–534, 2000.

60. Wollenberg A, Sharma S, von Bubnoff D, et al: Topical tacrolimus (FK506) leads to profound phenotypic and functional alterations of epidermal antigen-presenting dendritic cells in atopic dermatitis. J Allergy Clin Immunol 107:519–525, 2001.

61. Yawakar N, et al: Enhanced expression of eotaxins and CCR3 in atopic dermatitis. J Invest Dermatol 113:43–48, 1999.

CHAPTER 10

OCULAR ALLERGIES

Mark Zlotlow, M.D.

1. **Which diseases are included in the study of ocular allergies?**
   The terms *ocular allergy* and *allergic conjunctivitis* are often used interchangeably. There are several types of ocular allergic disease.
   - Allergic conjunctivitis
   - Allergic keratoconjunctivitis
   - Vernal conjunctivitis
   - Giant papillary conjunctivitis
   - Contact allergy

2. **Why are these diseases important?**
   The importance of these diseases, especially allergic conjunctivitis, lies in their frequency. Both allergic keratoconjunctivitis and vernal conjunctivitis can produce corneal lesions and visual impairment. In general, however, these disorders do not permanently impair vision.

3. **What other ocular disorders are relevant to the allergist?**
   Dry eyes syndrome and blepharitis are important because of their frequency, but they are not allergic diseases. The differential diagnosis of red eyes and conjunctival inflammation is also important. For the allergist a major question is treatment versus referral to an ophthalmologist.

4. **What makes the conjunctiva an active immunologic organ?**
   Because the conjunctiva forms a barrier to exogenous substances, it is expected to have a sophisticated immunologic repertoire. Under normal circumstances, various cells active in phagocytosis and in the processing and elimination of antigen are present. These cells include lymphocytes, neutrophils, and plasma cells. Specific structures are involved in some of these functions. The papillae of the palbebral conjunctiva contain collections of nonspecific inflammatory cells and tissue elements. Follicles can be found in the normal conjunctiva, especially in the lower fornix. These follicles are filled with lymphocytes, predominantly CD8+, in various stages of development. Both CD4+ and CD8+ lymphocytes are found in the substantia propria. Mononuclear cells in the epithelium also include Langerhans cells.
   Friedlaender MH: Ocular Allergy. In Middleton E, Reed CE et al (eds): Allergy: Principles and Practice, 4th ed. St. Louis, Mosby, 1993 p 1651.
   Bielory L: Allergic and immunologic disorders of the eye. In Middleton E, Ellis E et al (eds): Allergy: Principles and Practice, 5th ed. St. Louis: Mosby, 1998, p 1148.

5. **What types of mast cells are found in the conjunctiva?**
   Two types of mast cells are found in the conjunctiva: MC_t and MC_{tc}. The former contains only tryptase in its granules. It predominates at mucosal surfaces and increases markedly in aeroallergen sensitivity. Its function depends on the presence of T lymphocytes. MC_{tc} contains both tryptase and chymase in its granules. It is T cell independent and found in fibrotic processes. In normal conjunctiva, the mast cells are predominantly of the MC_{tc} subtype.
   Irani A: Ocular mast cells and mediators. Allergy Clin North Am 17:1–13, 1997.

6. **How do you examine the conjunctiva?**
To examine the bulbar conjunctiva, gently retract the opposite lid and then ask the patient to look up or down as appropriate. The lower palpebral conjunctiva can be everted for examination by placing a finger by the lid margins and drawing downward. The upper palpebral conjunctiva is examined by everting the lid. While the patient is looking down, the upper lid is grasped at its base with a cotton swab. It is then pulled out and up. To return the lid to its normal position, ask the patient to look up.

7. **How do you do a conjunctival scraping for eosinophils? Why is it useful?**
The lower conjunctival sac is anesthetized with a topical anesthetic eye drop. After a sufficient interval, the inner surface of the lower lid is gently scraped with a platinum spatula several times. The material is spread on a glass slide and stained with an appropriate stain such as Hansel stain. The slides are examined for the presence of eosinophils or eosinophil granules.
Nonallergic people do not have eosinophils. Therefore, the presence of eosinophils or granules strongly supports a diagnosis of allergic conjunctivitis. The rate of positive scrapings is variable, depending on the patient population and the chronicity of the disease.
Bielory L, Frielander M, Fujishima H: Allergic conjunctivitis. Allergy Clin North Am 17:19–31, 1997.

KEY POINTS: KEY IMMUNOLOGY OF THE CONJUNCTIVA

1. Because the conjunctiva forms a barrier to exogenous substances, it has a sophisticated immunologic repertoire.

2. Under normal circumstances, various cells (lymphocytes, neutrophils, and plasma cells) are active in phagocytosis and in the processing and elimination of antigens.

3. The papillae of the palpebral conjunctiva contain collections of nonspecific inflammatory cells and tissue elements.

4. Follicles in the normal conjunctiva, especially in the lower fornix, are filled with lymphocytes, predominantly CD8+, in various stages of development.

5. Both CD4+ and CD8+ lymphocytes are found in the substantia propria.

6. Mononuclear cells in the epithelium also include Langerhans cells.

ALLERGIC CONJUNCTIVITIS

8. **List the symptoms of allergic conjunctivitis.**
   - Itching, both ocular and periocular
   - Redness
   - Tearing
   - Burning
   - Stinging
   - Watery discharge
   - Photophobia

9. **Which of these symptoms is most characteristic of AC?**
Itching of the eye is the most characteristic and often the predominant symptom. In contact dermatitis it is itching of the lid. Itching occurs in other disorders, such as dry eyes, but it is not usually the predominant symptom.

Bielory L, Frielander M, Fujishima H: Allergic conjunctivitis. Allergy Clin North Am 17:19–31, 1997.

10. **List the signs of AC.**
    - Redness: usually mild to moderate in severity. Severe redness suggests another diagnosis.
    - Swelling (chemosis): usually subtle and visualized with a slit lamp. Occasionally it is marked and disproportionate to the redness.
    - Milky appearance of the palpebral conjunctiva. Because of edema, the blood vessels are obscured, giving the milky appearance. A velvety, beefy red appearance suggests a bacterial cause.
    - A white exudate can occur in the acute stage. It can become stringy in the chronic stage.
    - Lid edema and ecchymoses (allergic shiners) are frequent. Allergic shiners have been attributed to impaired venous return from the skin and subcutaneous tissue. However, proof of this attribution is lacking.
    - Since AC usually occurs with allergic rhinitis, symptoms and signs of allergic rhinitis are present.

11. **What are the differences between seasonal and perennial AC?**
    Both disorders share the same pathophysiology. The differences are primarily in the length of symptoms and the aeroallergens provoking symptoms. **Seasonal AC** occurs much more frequently, usually with allergic rhinitis. The symptoms are caused by seasonal aeroallergens, usually specific pollens. In 78% of patients specific IgE is increased. In 96% of affected patients, specific tear fluid IgE is also elevated. The length of the season correlates with the pollinating seasons of the specific aeroallergens.

    Perennial AC occurs less frequently. Dust mites, animal dander, and feather sensitivity are the usual causative aeroallergens. Although, as the name implies, the symptoms are perennial, seasonal exacerbations may occur. High rates of both specific serum and tear fluid IgE to the causative agent are also found.

    Bielory L, Frielander M, Fujishima H: Allergic conjunctivitis. Allergy Clin North Am 17:19–31, 1997.

12. **What is the conjunctival provocation test?**
    An offending pollen is instilled into the conjunctival sac. In sensitive people the typical symptoms and signs of AC are produced. Reactions are scored through a system that includes such objective and subjective factors as conjunctival erythema, chemosis, tearing, and pruritus.

    Irani A: Ocular mast cells and mediators. Allergy Clin North Am 17:1–13, 1997.

13. **Why is conjunctival provocation useful?**
    It is one of the original methods of establishing specific sensitivity and is particularly useful in the evaluation of antiallergic medication, immunotherapy and the pathophysiology of the disorder. As a diagnostic test, it may reveal specific eye sensitivities that do not provoke nasal symptoms. In one study, conjunctival provocation correlated with RAST in 71% of the cases. Of the 29% of the uncorrelated cases, the provocation test was positive but the RAST negative in 6% of cases. As a diagnostic test, it is more useful in patients who only have a small number of sensitivities.

    Bielory L: Allergic and immunologic disorders of the eye. In Middleton E, Ellis E et al (eds): Allergy: Principles and Practice, 5th ed. St. Louis: Mosby, 1998, p 1148.

14. **Describe a standardized technique for performing a provocation test.**
    In the standardized technique the contralateral eye is the control. At the initial visit the threshold of sensitivity is determined. If a drug is being studied, the test is bilateral. Incremental allergen doses are administered every 10 minutes until a positive test is achieved. Factors such as erythema, chemosis, tearing, and pruritus are evaluated according to a predetermined scoring system. After approximately 3 to 7 days the threshold dose is again administered to ensure the reproducibility of the effect.

Approximately 1 week later, the test drug is administered in one eye and the placebo control in the other. Ten minutes later the threshold dose is administered to both eyes. Symptoms and signs are evaluated at 3 and 10 minutes later. Rechallenge is performed 2–4 hours later to assess the duration of the drug effect.

Abelson MB, Smith LS: Levocabastine: Evaluation in the histamine and compound 40/80 models of ocular allergy in humans. Ophthalmology 95:1494–1497,1988.

15. **In conjunctival challenges, there are early-phase and late-phase reactions. Other than time of onset, how do these reactions differ?**
    In both reactions, mast cells are central to the process. Administration of grass pollen extract to a sensitized person results in marked symptoms within 20 minutes. They subside in 40 minutes. During this time there is a marked increase in tryptase, histamine, and TAME-esterase from mast cell degranulation. Tumor necrosis factor alpha (TNF-α) is also released within minutes.

    At 6 hours there is a second reaction with another peak of histamine and an increase in eosinophilic cationic protein. There is no increase in tryptase and few basophils. At this point the cellular infiltrate contains mast cells, neutrophils, eosinophils, and macrophages. There are few CD4+ and CD8+ T cells. The adhesion molecules, E-selectin and ICAM-1, are increased. This scenario explains the increase in both eosinophils and granulocytes in the late-phase reaction.

    McGill JL, Holgate ST, Church MK, et al: Allergic eye disease mechanisms. Br J Ophthamol 82:1203–1214,1998.

16. **What subtypes of mast cells are increased in AC?**
    MC$_t$ mast cells are modestly increased in both the epithelium and the subepithelium in both seasonal and perennial AC. Many proinflammatory mediators are increased in AC. They include histamine, leukotriene, prostaglandin (PGD$_2$), tryptase, carboxypeptidase A, cathepsin G, platelet activating factor, and other chemoattractants.

    McGill JL, Holgate ST, Church MK, et al: Allergic eye disease mechanisms. Br J Ophthamol 82:1203–1214,1998.

17. **What cytokines are released in AC and vernal keratoconjunctivitis?**
    See Table 10-1.

TABLE 10-1. CYTOKINES RELEASED IN AC AND VERNAL KERATOCONJUNCTIVITIS			
Cytokine	Tear	Tissue	Serum
IL-1β	↑VKC	↓VKC	↑VKC
IL-2	↑SAC-PAC		
IL-4	↑SAC-PAC	↑SAC	
IL-5	↑SAC-PAC	↑SAC	
IL-6	↑VKC	↑SAC–VKC	
IL-8		↑SAC	
IL-10	↓SAC-PAC		
TNF-α	↑SAC	↑SAC	↑VKC
IFN-γ	↓SAC-PAC		

IL = interleukin, TNF-α = tumor necrosis factor alpha, IFN-γ = interferon gamma.
From Bonini S, Lambiase A, Sacchetti M, Bonini S: Cytokines in ocular allergy. Int Ophthamol Clin 43:95–103, 2003.

18. What are the functions of the soluble factors that are released?
    See Table 10-2.

TABLE 10-2.	FUNCTIONS OF SOLUBLE FACTORS
Factor	**Function**
Interleukin-4	1. Switches B cells to IgE production from IgM production
	2. Promotes T helper cell growth and differentiation
Interleukin-5	1. Promotes growth and differentiation of eosinophils
	2. Chemoattractant and priming agent for eosinophils
Interleukin-6	1. Augments T and B-Cell function
	2. Potentiates IL-4 synthesis of B-cells
Stem cell factor	1. Regulates mast cell growth and differentiation
	2. Enhances IgE dependent mast cell mediator release
	3. Cytokine generation and release
	4. Chemoattractant for mast cells
TNFα	1. Primary agent for mediator secreting cells
	2. Upregulation of adhesion molecules

19. Eosinophils are characteristically found in large numbers in AC. What factors do they release that contribute to the pathology?
    - Major basic protein
    - Eosinophil cationic protein
    - Eosinophil-derived neurotoxin

20. What are classes of drugs are available for treatment? What are their advantages and disadvantages?
    See Table 10-3.

21. What do over-the-counter antihistamine-decongestant combinations have in common?
    All have an antihistamine, usually pheniramine or antelzoline. The decongestant is naphazoline. The concentrations differ only slightly among the various brands.

22. Why this combination of antihistamine and a decongestant?
    In several clinical studies, the combination proved to be more effective than either agent singly or placebo. These studies employed conjunctival challenge with allergen. Itching and redness were the clinical symptoms evaluated.

23. Are the available topical antihistamine preparations effective?
    Levocabastine was specifically developed as an H_1-receptor antagonist for ocular use. In animal studies, it has been a potent and specific agent with little affinity for H_2, serotonin, and muscarinc receptor sites. In human clinical studies, it had an onset of action within 15 minutes and duration of approximately 16 hours.
    Emedastine is also a highly selective and potent antihistamine. In several environmental allergy clinical studies it was superior in efficacy to levocabastine. In a conjunctival challenge test, it proved superior to nedocromil in controlling itching and redness. It was similar in efficacy to ketotifen fumarate 0.025% in controlling itching.

TABLE 10-3.   ADVANTAGES AND DISADVANTAGES OF DRUGS USED TO TREAT ALLERGIC CONJUNCTIVITIS

Drug Class	Advantages	Disadvantages
Oral antihistamines	Ease of administration Particularly useful with coexisting allergic rhinitis Some are available over counter or as generics; thus less expensive	Often need to be supplemented with topical agents May have systemic side effects May increase dry eyes
Topical antihistamine-decongestants (e.g., Opcon-A or Naphcon-A)	Available over-the-counter Few side effects May be considered first-line treatment in mild cases	Overuse results in conjunctivitis medicamentosa, increase in conjunctival injection, and rebound hyperemia that may persist after discontinuing drops Usually effective only in mild cases
Topical antihistamines (e.g., levocabastine, azelastine, emedastine)	Proven potency as topical antihistamine in laboratory and clinical studies	Requires prescription
Topical antihistamine and mast cell stabilizer (e.g., olopatadine, ketotifen)	Dual mode of action Usually requires only twice-dailiy dosage	Requires prescription
Mast cell stabilizer (e.g., cromolyn, lodaxamide)	Inhibits both early- and late-phase reactions Safe	Effect not present until used 2–5 days; maximum benefit in 15 days Needs to be used regularly 4–6 times/day; this regimen decreases compliance
NSAID-like agents (e.g., ketorolac)	Specifically indicated to relieve itching Analgesic properties	Safety in aspirin-allergic patients not yet demonstrated
Topical corticosteroids	Effective for short-term use	Raise intraocular pressure Risks of incurring infection of cornea and conjunctiva Risks of cataract formation

Azelastine is the third topically active selective antihistamine with efficacy in the treatment of AC.

Siret DJ: Oral and topical antihistamines: Pharmacologic properties and therapeutic potential in ocular allergic disease. J Am Optometr Assoc 69(2):77–87,1998.

Orfeo V, Vardaro A, Lena P, et al: Comparison of emedastine 0.05% or nedocromil sodium 2% eye drops and placebo in controlling local reactions in subjects with allergic conjunctivitis. Eur J Ophthalmol 12(4):262–266, 2002.

D'Arienzo PA, Leonardi A, Bensch G: Randomized, double-masked, placebo-controlled comparison of the efficacy of emedastine difumarate 0.05% ophthalmic solution and ketotifen fumarate 0.025% ophthalmic solution in the human conjunctival allergen challenge model. Clin Ther 24(3):409–416, 2002.

Verin P, Easty DL, et al: Clinical evaluation of twice-daily emedastine 0.05% eyedrops (Emadine eye drops) versus levocabastine 0.05% eyedrops in patients with allergic conjunctivitis. Am J Opthalmol 131:691–698, 2001.

Secchi A, Leonardi A, et al: An efficacy and tolerance comparison of emedastine difumarate 0.05% and levocabastine hydrochloride 0.05%: Reducing chemosis and eyelid swelling in subjects with seasonal allergic conjunctivitis. Acta Ophthal Scand Suppl 230:48–51, 2000.

Secchi A, Ciprandi G; et al: Safety and efficacy comparison of emedastine 0.05% solution compared to levocabastine 0.05% ophthalmic suspension in pediatric subjects with allergic conjunctivitis. Acta Ophthal Scand Suppl 230:42–47, 2000.

24. **Discuss the role of oral antihistamines.**

All oral antihistamines have some efficacy in AC, since it is frequently associated with allergic rhinitis. Thus the oral preparations may be useful monotherapy for both disorders. They may reduce the need for topical therapy to an as-needed basis. The newer nonsedating antihistamines have not been proved to be any more efficacious for AC. They also share the anticholinergic side effects of the older preparations. Dryness of the mucosal membranes, both conjunctival and oropharyngeal, may occur. The conjunctival dryness may precipitate symptoms of dry eye syndrome.

Oral decongestants, which are frequently used in combination with antihistamines, can produce mydriasis. In a predisposed person, it may precipitate an attack of acute closed-angle glaucoma.

25. **How useful are mast cell–stabilizing drugs?**

These agents appear to stabilize mast cell membranes and thereby inhibit the release of mediators of inflammation. In studies, **Iodaxamide** prevented the release of histamine, leukotrienes, and SRS-A. It also inhibits eosinophil chemotaxis. All mast cell–stabilizing drugs have negligible systemic absorption. Side effects are topical only. They include burning or stinging, hyperemia, tearing, itching, and dry eyes. They all require several days of usage to begin working and are maximally effective only after several weeks of regular use. Thus, therapy for seasonal AC needs to be commenced several weeks before the onset of the season for maximal efficacy.

Cromolyn sodium 4% is the oldest drug of this class. It has been widely used for AC and has been mildly effective for this purpose. It requires frequent use (4 times/day) for maximal effect.

Lodaxamide is a more potent mast cell stabilizer than cromolyn. It has greater activity in vernal conjunctivitis, atopic keratoconjunctivitis, and giant papillary conjunctivitis.

Nedocromil 2% solution is another mast cell stabilizer with proven efficacy in AC. In one double-blind, placebo-controlled allergen challenge test, it was equally effective with levocabastine after 2 weeks. It reduced the concentration of histamine and PGD_2 in the tears and the percentage of 3H4-positive mast cells. In contrast, levocabastine had antihistamine properties but also reduced the expression of ICAM-1 on conjunctival blood vessels.

Pemirolast 0.1%, like cromolyn, requires dosing 4 times/day.

Abelson MB, McGarr PJ, Richard KP: Anti-allergic therapies. Textbook of Ocular Pharmacology, 1997, pp 609–633.

Ahluwalia P; Anderson D; et al: Nedocromil sodium reduces the symptoms of conjunctival allergin challenge by different mechanisms. J Allergy Clin Immunol 108:449–454, 2001.

26. **Why is ketorolac, a nonsteroidal anti-inflammatory drug, effective for AC?**

Ketorolac tromethamine (Acular) 0.5% has been effective in relieving the itching in AC. It is a highly potent NSAID that inhibits prostaglandin synthetase. It has been shown to reduce prostaglandin E_2 in tears. Both PGE_2 and PGI_2 have been demonstrated to induce pruritus. In seasonal environmental studies, it was superior to placebo in reducing symptoms of inflammation, itching, swollen eyes, burning, and stinging. Some burning on administration is the most common side effect. Safety in aspirin-sensitive people has not been established.

27. **Summarize the efficacy of drugs with combined antihistamine and mast cell-stabilizing properties.**

Comparative trials to date indicate that mast cell-stabilizing/antihistamine drugs are probably the most effective treatment for allergic conjunctivitis with the exception of corticosteroids. In the United States they are definitely not the least expensive.

28. **How does ketotifen fumarate compare with cromolyn?**

Ketotifen, the parent compound of ketotifen fumarate 0.025%, has been available for many years for treatment of asthma and allergic rhinitis. In a controlled allergen challenge study, a single dose of ketotifen proved superior to a 2-week course of cromolyn administered 4 times/day. Dosing of Ketotifen is 2–3 times/day.

Greiner JV, Michaelson C, McWhirter CL, Shams NB: Single dose of ketotifen fumarate .025% versus 2 weeks of cromolyn sodium 4% for allergic conjunctivitis. Adv Ther 19(4):185–193, 2002.

29. **How does olopatadine compare with other specific treatments?**

Olopatadine (Patanol) is a highly selective and potent H_1 blocker. It is also a potent inhibitor of mast cell degranulation. It has the advantage of dosing 2–3 times/day. The duration of action is 8 hours. Olopatadine has been compared to a number of other drugs in AC. In a comparison with ketorolac in an allergen challenge study, it proved to be more effective in reducing both hyperemia and ocular itching. In another study it was more effective and comfortable than nedocromil sodium 2%, a pure mast cell stabilizer. It proved superior to azelastine hydrochloride 0.05%, a selective antihistamine, in controlling itching. In a controlled challenge study, after a 2-week course of olopatadine, lopredenol, a topical steroid, or placebo, olopatadine was superior in inhibiting itching and redness. It also relieved itching better and was better tolerated than ketotifen in another controlled challenge study.

Butrus S, Greiner JV, Discepola M, Feingold J: Comparison of the clinical efficacy and comfort of olopatadine hydrochloride 0.1% ophthalmic solution and nedocromil sodium 2% ophthalmic solution in the human conjunctival allergen challenge model. Clin Ther 22:1462–1472, 2000.

Spangler DL, Bensch G, Berdy GJ: Evaluation of the efficacy of olopatadine hydrochloride 0.1% ophthalmic solution and azelastine 0.05% ophthalmic solution in the conjunctival allergen challenge model. Clin Ther 23:1272–1280, 2001.

Berdy GJ, Stoppel JO, Epstein AB: Comparison of the clinical efficacy and tolerability of olopatadine hydrochloride 0.1% ophthalmic solution and lotepredenol etabonate 0.2% suspension in the conjunctival allergen challenge model. Clin Ther 24:918–929, 2002.

Berdy GJ, Spangler DL, et al: A comparison of the relative efficacy and clinical performance of olopatadine hydrochloride 0.1% ophthalmic solution and ketotifen fumarate 0.025% ophthalmic solution in the conjunctival antigen challenge model. Clin Ther 22:826–833, 2000.

30. **What are the benefits of topical corticosteroids?**

Corticosteroids, as potent anti-inflammatory drugs, are very effective in relieving the symptoms of allergic conjunctivitis. Their efficacy as a group generally exceeds the other classes of drugs previously discussed.

A newer preparation, lotepredenol etabonate, may offer an improved safety profile for AC. Lotepredenol is a modification of prednisolone that is rapidly hydrolyzed in the anterior chamber to an inactive metabolite. In one study it did not raise intraocular pressure by 10 mmHg or more after a 6-week course of 4 times/day dosing.

Of the older preparations, fluormethalone (FML) and medrysone (HMS) are favored for the treatment of AC. Although less potent than other preparations, they also have less risk of side effects. FML is mildly hydrophobic and concentrates in the epithelial layer of the cornea before passing through to the hydrophobic layers of the stroma. It is inactivated in the anterior chamber. HMS, available in a 1.0% suspension, also has a weak effect on the cornea.

Dell SJ, Lowry GM, et al: A randomized, double-masked, placebo-controlled study of lotepredenol etabonate in patients with season allergic conjunctivitis. JACI 102:251–255, 1998.

31. **What are the risks of topical corticosteroids?**
Subcapsular cataracts. Both topical and systemic preparations are associated with the development of subcapsular cataracts. Although the pathogenesis of this complication is not fully understood, both total dosage and duration of treatment are associated with its development. Discontinuation of the drug does not alter the opacity.

Increased ocular pressure. Increased ocular pressure has been demonstrated with the use of both systemic and topical preparations. The effect is reversible with the discontinuation of the drug. However, the increase in pressure can cause optic nerve damage and visual field changes similar to open-angle glaucoma. The ability to produce this effect varies amongst the various preparations. Genetic differences, age, and coexistent diabetes are also contributing factors.

Immune suppression. Steroids suppress the activation and migration of leukocytes. Both conjunctivitis and keratitis, bacterial and viral, can occur. Vision-threatening infections such as fungal keratitis, fungal endophthalmitis, and toxoplasmic chorioretinitis are potential risks of treatment.

Systemic effects. Systemic absorption can also occur. For example, decreased serum cortisol levels were found after 6 weeks of treatment with topical 0.1% dexamethasone sodium phosphate.

Other complications may include acute anterior uveitis with associated mydriasis, ptosis, and loss of accommodation. Refractive changes, blurring vision, increased corneal thickening, and pseudotumor cerebri also have been reported.

Abelson MB, McGarr PJ, Richard KP: Anti-allergic therapies. Textbook of Ocular Pharmacology, 1997, pp 609–633.

32. **Summarize the risk-benefit ratio of corticosteroids in the treatment of AC.**
The efficacy of corticosteroids for AC is more than matched by the potential for serious complications. They should be used only for a short period and only if other agents have failed. Given the required caution, monitoring by an ophthalmologist is certainly a wise choice. Prescribing this class of medicine without examination and with at-will refills is definitely unwise.

KEY POINTS: ALLERGIC CONJUNCTIVITIS

1. Itching, both ocular and periocular, is the most prominent symptom.

2. Mild-to-moderate redness is the most prominent sign.

3. Conjunctival provocation tests are useful both in determining specific sensitivities and in evaluating the efficacy of medication.

4. Mast cell–stabilizing/antihistamine drugs are probably the most effective treatment currently available with the exception of corticosteroids.

5. Corticosteroid eye drops with their potential for significant side effects should be used with great caution and for short periods of time. Monitoring treatment by an ophthalmologist is certainly a wise choice.

VERNAL KERATOCONJUNCTIVITIS

33. **What are the symptoms of vernal keratoconjunctivitis (VKC)?**
The most common symptom is itching of the eye, which often is quite intense. A thick, ropy discharge is present. The discharge consists of mucus, eosinophils, epithelial cells, and neutrophils. Photophobia (often intense), burning, and a foreign body sensation are other symptoms.

34. **What are the signs of VKC?**
The principal findings are giant papillae on the superior tarsal and sometimes limbal conjunctiva. These papillae give the surface a cobblestone appearance. A stringy mucus coats the cobblestones. The limbal form of the disease is characterized by translucent globular deposits at the limbus in the form of an arc or even a complete circle. Within these deposits Horner-Trantas dots can be found. These chalky white infiltrates are composed of clumps of degenerating epithelial cells, eosinophils, and neutrophils. Horner-Trantas dots are virtually pathognomonic of the disease. More severe cases may be associated with a diffuse epithelial keratitis. A shield ulcer may be present in rare case; it is a well-defined, centrally located epithelial defect of the cornea.

35. **Discuss the epidemiology of VKC.**
Worldwide VKC is said to account for 0.1–0.5% of all ocular disorders. It is particularly prevalent in hot, dry environments. It is primarily a disease of childhood with a majority of patients being between 5 and 25 years. Until puberty there is a male predominance of approximately 2:1 to 3:1. By age 20, the distribution between the sexes is even. There may be recurrent episodes over a 2- to 10-year period before resolution. In more temperate climates, VKC has a seasonal predilection for spring and summer. There is usually a family and personal history of atopy. There is also a high frequency of positive skin tests to relevant inhalant allergens, particularly pollens. However immunotherapy has not been particularly effective for VKC.
Lee Y, Raizman M: Vernal conjunctivitis. Allergy Clin North Am 17:33–51, 1997.

36. **Summarize the role of mast cells in the pathogenesis of VKC.**
Mast cells play an important role in VKC. The predominant cell, MC_{tc} is found in high numbers in both epithelial and subepithelial levels of the conjunctiva. There is also an increase in MC_t cells. Approximately 80% of the mast cells are degranulated. Histamine levels are 10-fold higher than normal—due in part to a decrease in histaminase levels.
Abelson MB, McGarr PJ, Richard KP: Anti-allergic therapies. Textbook of Ocular Pharmacology, 1997, pp 609–633.

37. **Discuss the role of eosinophils in the pathogenesis of VKC.**
Eosinophils are found in increased numbers within the epithelial and subepithelial layers. Only in VKC may more than two eosinophils per high-powered field be found on light microscopy. Since many of the eosinophils are degranulated, there is a marked increase in major basic protein. This protein has been recovered on the mucoid plaque overlying the shield ulcer and from elution from the ulcer itself. It is thought to be integral to the formation of the ulcer. Eosinophil cationic protein has also found to be elevated in the tears. In VKC 70% of the eosinophils express estrogen and progesterone receptors. This finding may in part explain the predominance of the disorder in prepubertal children and the decline in incidence with age. Besides eosinophils, high levels of the CC chemokines, eotaxin-1 and eotaxin-2 are found are found in the tears of patients. They are correlated with both the eosinophil count and disease severity.
Lee Y, Raizman M: Vernal conjunctivitis. Allergy Clin North Am 17:33–51, 1997.
Bonini S, Sacchetti M, Lambiasi A, Bonini S: Cytokines in ocular allergy. Int Ophthalmol Clin 43:27–31, 2003.

38. **How are lymphocytes affected in VKC?**
The lymphocyte population shows an increase in CD4+ T cells but not CD8+ T cells. The T cells are predominantly of the TH-2 phenotype and appear to be produced locally. With cytokine profiles showing the TH-2 phenotype, there is a suggestion that VKC results from a maturation shift

of CD4+ T cells to a pattern stimulating a mast cell and eosinophil response. In approximately 30–50% of nonatopic patients with VKC there was specific IgE in tears, suggesting local production.

Bielory L: Allergic and immunologic disorders of the eye. In Middleton E, Ellis E et al (eds): Allergy Principles and Practice, 5th ed. St.Louis, Mosby, 1998, p 1153.

39. **Discuss nonpharmacologic treatments for VKC.**
Cool compresses and ice packs are often helpful, perhaps due to a vasoconstricting effect. Sleeping in an air-conditioned room may provide increased comfort. Artificial tears used frequently may dilute mediators and act as a barrier. Rubbing the eyes should be discouraged because the trauma may increase mediator release.

For some patients, patching the eye provides relief from photophobia. Both patches and goggles may reduce allergen exposure. General allergen control measures such as dust mite controls and avoiding the outdoors on windy days and during peak pollination times offer some benefit. Although immunotherapy is not specifically effective for VKC, it may be useful in patients with coexisting allergic rhinoconjunctivitis.

40. **What pharmacologic treatments are available?**
The drugs used for allergic conjunctivitis are useful for VKC:
- Both systemic and topical antihistamines may reduce itching.
- Cromolyn and lodaxamide have specific indications for VKC. Lodaxamide has been shown to prevent keratitis and shield ulcers. It may also reverse some corneal changes. In one controlled study it proved superior to cromolyn in providing relief from both the symptoms and signs of VKC.
- Ketorolac has not been specifically approved for use in VKC. However, 1% suprofen, an NSAID indicated for inhibition of intraoperative miosis, has demonstrated activity for VKC.
- Olopatadine and ketotifen are not specifically indicated for VKC. Their modes of action as mast cell stabilizers and antihistamines make some benefit a logical inference.
- Topical cyclosporine has been used in severe cases. However, it must be dissolved in an alcohol-oil base because it is lipophilic. The vehicle itself causes significant tearing, erythema, and irritation.
- Topical corticosteroids should be reserved for severe cases and used only for short-term treatment, particularly in view of the self-limited nature of VKC and the numerous side effects of corticosteroids.

Tuft SJ, Kemeny DM, Dart JK, Buckley RJ: Clinical features of atopic keratoconjunctivitis. Ophthalmology 98:150–158, 1991.

41. **Are any surgical treatments available?**
Cryotherapy of the tarsal conjunctiva often provides temporary relief. Conjunctival autografts have been performed with limited benefit. Superficial keratectomy of plaques may aid re-epithelization. Excimer laser phototherapeutic keratectomy has been used to treat central corneal lesions. It may prove useful for superficial corneal scars. Corneal shield ulcers may also respond to soft contact lenses, patching and tarsorrhaphy.

KEY POINTS: VERNAL KERATOCONJUNCTIVITIS

1. Like AC, itching is the most common symptom. However, it is usually accompanied by a ropey discharge.

2. The principal sign is giant papillae on the superior tarsal conjunctiva that have a cobblestone appearance.

3. VKC is a worldwide disorder. It is usually a disease of childhood between the ages of 5 and 25. Until puberty there is a male predominance.

4. The drugs used for AC are useful for VKC.

ATOPIC KERATOCONJUNCTIVITIS

42. **Discuss the epidemiology of atopic keratoconjunctivitis (AKC).**
AKC is strongly associated with atopic dermatitis. However, some patients who have other atopic diseases, such as asthma, have AKC without skin involvement. The disorder starts in late adolescence and early adulthood. Spontaneous resolution is rare. There is a male predominance.

43. **What are the symptoms of AKC?**
The principal symptoms, as with VKC, are tearing, itching, and photophobia. The involvement is bilateral. A stringy mucous discharge may be present.

44. **Summarize the physical findings in AKC.**
One study of 37 patients with AKC reported significant lid involvement. Eczematous changes of the skin of the lids occurred in 81%. Clinical blepharitis and meibomitis were found in almost 90%. *Staphylococcus aureus* was frequently recovered with the blepharitis. About half of the patients had maceration of the inner and outer canthi. Punctal ectropion, ptosis, and loss of lashes were also seen in about 50% of the patients. All of the patients had papillae greater than 0.9 mm in diameter on both the upper and lower lids. In 10 of 37 patients the papillae were greater than 1.0 mm in the upper eyelid. Reticular scarring was found in 28 of 37. Symblepharon was found in 10 of 37.

Multiple corneal lesions are also seen in AKC. Punctate erosions were found in all patients. Neovascularization was found in 65% of the patients. Shield ulcers and sheets of mucus adherent to the ulcers were found in about half of the patients. Keratoconus occurred in about one-third. Cataracts can develop in severe chronic forms of the disease, especially in young patients. These cataracts are frequently bilateral and may progress quickly to complete opacification. Because the cataract is frequently a posterior capsular one, identical to that produced by corticosteroids, it is difficult to determine whether the cause is the disease or the treatment.

Zhan H, Smith L, Calder V, et al: Clinical and immunological features of atopic keratoconjunctivitis. Int Ophthamol Clin 43:59–71, 2003.

Tuft SJ, Kemeny DM, Dart JK, Buckley RJ: Clinical features of atopic keratoconjunctivitis. Ophthamology 98:150–158, 1991.

45. **How can AKC be differentiated from allergic conjunctivitis and vernal keratoconjunctivitis since many of the symptoms are the same?**
Allergic conjunctivitis usually occurs with allergic rhinitis. Usually lid changes do not occur with allergic conjunctivitis but are frequent in AKC. Lesions of atopic dermatitis usually occur on other skin surfaces.

VKC is usually a disease of prepubertal children, whereas AKC begins in young adults. Lid and blepharal involvement does not occur with VKC but is characteristic of AKC. The palpebral involvement of VKC is large papillae on the upper lid. In AKC both lower and upper palpebral conjunctiva are involved.

46. **Discuss the immunologic findings in AKC.**
As with atopic dermatitis, levels of IgE are elevated in serum and (with less frequency) in tear fluid. Although positive RAST and skin tests are frequent, they are not always of clinical significance as exacerbants of the disease.

Mast cells of the MC_{tc} subtype are increased. This subtype appears to be T cell independent and is characteristic of fibrotic processes. Eosinophils are also present in increased numbers.

As in VKC the number of CD4+ but not CD8+ T cells is increased. Most of the CD4+ cells are memory cells. In VKC and giant papillary conjunctivitis, about 50% of the cells coexpressed CD45RO and CD4RA. This coexpression was not found in AKC, which suggests that the T cells found in the conjunctiva in AKC may be recruited from circulating memory T cells. In VKC and GPC, the T cells are produced locally.

McGill JL, Holgate ST, Church MK, et al: Allergic eye disease mechanisms. Br J Ophthamol 82:1203–1214, 1998.

47.   What are the available treatments?

The blepharitis may be controlled by the usual measures of hot compresses and lid scrubs. Occasionally antibiotics may be necessary for patients. With specific allergic sensitivities, avoidance measures are indicated. Mast cell–stabilizing agents administered regularly are a mainstay of therapy. Ocular itching may be controlled with oral antihistamines or topical nonsteroidal antiinflammatory drugs. The topical nonsteroidals exert their effect by inhibiting prostoglandin production.Thus far there is little evidence for a role for combined topical mast cell stabilizing-antihistamine agents.

Topical steroids in bursts are often required to reduce both conjunctival and eyelid inflammation as well as keratitis. Topical cyclosporine has provided some relief in steroid-dependent cases. Systemic cyclosporine has been used in some severe cases.

Some of the complications may require surgical intervention. Lid surgery may be necessary for correction of ectropion or entropion. The development of cataracts often leads to surgical removal and replacement with a posterior chamber intraocular lens. Although keratoconus can frequently be managed with contact lenses, it may require corneal transplantation.

McGill JL, Holgate ST, Church MK, et al: Allergic eye disease mechanisms. Br J Ophthamol 82:1203–1214, 1998.

KEY POINTS: ATOPIC KERATOCONJUNCTIVITIS

1. AKC is strongly associated with atopic dermatitis.

2. Eczematous changes of the skin of the eyelids, blepharitis, and meibomitis are the most frequent signs.

3. The symptoms are similar to AC and VKC. However, AC usually occurs with allergic rhinitis. Both AC and VKC generally have no eyelid or blepheral involvement. In VKC, the palpebral involvement is generally in the upper lid. In AKC, both upper and lower lids are involved

GIANT PAPILLARY CONJUNCTIVITIS

48.   What is giant papillary conjunctivitis (GPC)?

GPC is named for the large papillae that are found on the upper tarsal surface. These papillae resemble the findings in VKC. GPC is associated most frequently with the wearing of soft contact lenses. No one particular soft lens has a higher incidence. It has also been reported with the following entities: rigid contact lenses, ocular prosthesis, exposed sutures in ocular surgery, limbal dermoid tumors, and cyanoacrylate tissue adhesive.

49.   What are the symptoms of GPC?

There is a decreased tolerance to the wearing of lenses. Irritation, redness, burning, and itching occur with this intolerance. Mucus production also occurs.

50.   What are the signs of GPC?

During the early stages of the disease, signs include increased awareness of the lens, mild itching, and mucus in the inner canthus upon arising. There may be a mucus coating of the lens which blurs vision. Papillae may be found on the upper tarsal conjunctiva.

With increased disease progression, symptoms, lens coating, and mucus production increase. The papillae increase in both size and number. There is marked injection of the conjunctiva with loss of the normal vascular pattern.

In the most advanced cases, there is a complete intolerance to lens wear. The mucus production is much increased, and the lids can be stuck together in the morning. The upper tarsal surface is thickened, and the vasculature is totally obscured. The papillae are large and may have flattened apices.

Donshik PC, Ehlers WH: Giant papillary conjunctivitis. Allergy Clin North Am 17:53–73, 1997.

51. Why mention GPC in a book on allergy?

There is significant usage of contact lenses, particularly soft contact lenses, in the general population. Symptoms of the early stages of GPC may be attributed by either the patient or referring physician to allergic conjunctivitis. Given the frequency of allergic conjunctivitis, it becomes important to differentiate between the two disorders. In the more advanced stages, the symptoms and the appearance of giant papillae mimic vernal keratoconjunctivitis.

Donshik PC, Ehlers WH: Giant papillary conjunctivitis. Allergy Clin North Am 17:53–73, 1997.

52. Discuss the histopathologic changes associated with GPC.

In GPC, mast cells, eosinophils, and basophils are found in both the epithelium and substantia propria. The concentration of inflammatory cells per mm^3 is similar to normal tissue. However, because of an increase in the total mass of tissue, the number of cells is increased. The histologic appearance is very similar to VKC. However, the histamine levels are about 25% less. In both GPC and VKC, mast cells are found in both the epithelium and substantia propria. In both normal controls and normal contact lens wearers, mast cells are found only in the substantia propria. In GPC, the mast cells are of the MC_{tc} subtype, whereas in VKC, the mast cells are of the MC_t subtype. Levels of immunoglobulins and complement are increased in the tear fluid. The level of neutrophil chemotactic factor is 15 times normal levels.

Secchi A, Leonardi A, et al: An efficacy and tolerance comparison of emedastine difumarate 0.05% and levocabastine hydrochloride 0.05%: Reducing chemosis and eyelid swelling in subjects with seasonal allergic conjunctivitis. Acta Ophthal Scand Suppl (230):48–51, 2000.

53. Summarize the pathophysiology of GPC.

There is still debate on this matter. It may be a primarily immunologic disorder. However, it seems that mechanical trauma or irritation initiates the immunologic changes that are found.

54. How is GPC treated?

The most obvious treatment, discontinuing contact lens wear, does not meet with the universal approval of patients. The lens itself can be made less irritating by reducing the coating. Improved cleaning, decreased time wearing the lenses, or a change in design or material may be sufficient. The use of a daily use disposable lens may improve or solve the problem.

The use of mast cell stabilizers and NSAIDs topically has been reported to be of some benefit. While topical steroids are effective, long-term use involves substantial risk of side effects.

KERATOCONJUNCTIVITIS SICCA AND DRY EYE SYNDROME

55. What is the difference between dry eye syndrome (DES) and keratoconjunctivitis sicca (KCS)?

DES is a constellation of symptoms and signs caused by a decrease in the quantity or abnormal quality of the tear film layer. KCS is a specific disorder caused by a quantitative or qualitative abnormality of lacrimal gland secretions.

56. What are the components of the tear film layer?

The tear film consists of three layers. The **outer layer of lipids** is secreted by the meibomian glands. These glands secrete a phospholipid that stabilizes the tear film layer and reduces the rate of evaporative loss. This layer is 1.0 μm thick.

The main and accessory lacrimal glands secrete the **middle aqueous layer**, which is 7.0 μm thick. It contains the water-soluble components of the tear film, such as immunoglobulins, lysozyme, and complement.

The **inner mucin layer** is derived from the goblet cells of the conjunctiva. It causes the hydrophilic aqueous layer to adhere to the hydrophobic corneal epithelium. This process helps make the tear film a smooth even layer over the entire conjunctiva. The tears are spread by blinking.

57. What are the symptoms of DES?

The most common complaint is a foreign body sensation, described by many as a feeling of sand in the eye. Tearing, pain, photophobia, and redness also occur. There may be a decrease in vision from an irregular tear film on the cornea. A reduction of the aqueous component may lead to eyelid crusting in the morning. Dry windy weather can exacerbate these symptoms.

Several conditions, including AC, GPC, and blepharitis, can mimic these symptoms. Patients with borderline dryness may develop the symptoms only when wearing contact lenses. This possibility is increased with the use of extended-wear soft lenses that have a higher water content, which is drawn from the tear layer.

58. What are the signs of DES?

A slit-lamp examination with minimal manipulation can show a continuous tear meniscus. In normal people it is 0.3 to 0.5 mm in height. It is decreased in DES. Redundant conjunctiva, injection of the conjunctiva and mild chemosis may be seen. In severe cases the epithelium may be keratinized. A stringy mucus may form in the inferior fornix.

Constad WH, Bhagat N: Keratitis sicca and dry eye syndrome. Allergy Clin North Am 17:89–102, 1997.

59. What are the common objective tests of the tear film?

Staining the tear film with fluorescein stain demonstrates any denuded areas of epithelium. It also demonstrates the tear meniscus.

Tear film break-up time quantitatively measures a mucus deficiency in the tear layer. After instillation of fluorescein, the patient is asked to blink and then keep the eye open at least 5–10 seconds. The time from the blink to the appearance of a dry spot is the tear breakup time. Any time less than 10 seconds indicates a mucin deficiency or meibomian gland dysfunction.

Rose bengal staining can also be used to evaluate the ocular surface. The Schirmer test quantitatively measures tear secretions by the lacrimal gland. The Jones test evaluates the patency of the nasolacrimal apparatus. Both of these latter tests are used for objective evaluation of dry eyes.

60. How is DES treated?

The initial treatment is the frequent use of tear substitutes. Most patients use them on as-needed basis. However, with the occurrence of symptoms there is a degree of damage to the ocular surface. Therefore, regular treatment, 4 times/day for several days to weeks, allows healing. Then reduction of dosage to as low as 2 times/day may be sufficient. Dry, windy weather necessitates more frequent treatment. The hypotonic, nonviscous solutions last up to 2 hours. The more viscous solutions, which generally have cellulose as a base, last longer but may cause some blurring of vision by creating a non-uniform tear layer. Ointments are useful for bedtime use and as adjuncts for severe dryness.

Surgical treatment involves ancicular occlusion, which decreases tear drainage. The occlusion may be done with temporary or permanent plugs. Cautery, diathermy, or argon laser can be used to create permanent occclusions.

61. What connective tissue diseases cause KCS?

- Sjögren's disease
- Rheumatoid arthritis
- Sarcoidosis
- Amyloidosis
- Systemic lupus erythematosus

CONTACT DERMATITIS OF THE EYE AND EYELID

62. **Why is contact dermatitis of the eye important?**
Contact dermatitis is the most common eruption of the eyelid. The eyelid, with its thin soft skin, is particularly vulnerable to delayed sensitivity reactions. With its location and cosmetic implications, affected people frequently seek medical attention.

63. **What are the most common contactants?**
Cosmetics applied to the hair, face, and fingernails are the most frequent sensitizers. Often they cause no problems at the site of application, but for reasons mentioned previously affect the eyelid. Irritant reactions may also occur from cosmetics applied around the eye. Although tolerance may develop to an irritant, an irritant contact dermatitis can develop. Clinically it cannot be differentiated from an allergic contact dermatitis.

64. **What are the common sensitizers?**
Water-based mascara contains emulsifiers that can be irritating. However, for some people it is the waterproof mascara itself that is not tolerated. A cake-type mascara or eyeliner can be a suitable alternative.

Products for eye and periorbital use contain antimicrobial preservatives to prevent contamination. Parabens, which are esters of parahydroxybenzoic acid, are the most commonly used. Although they may cause reactions when placed in the eye, they are usually tolerated topically on the lid. Quarternum 15 and imidazolidnyl urea are preservatives that generate formaldehyde. They may be antigenic in their own right or cause irritation from the formaldehyde they release. Other preservatives that are sensitizers include potassium sorbate, diisopropanolamine, and ditertiarybutly hydroquinone.

Some nail polish contains a toluene-sulfonamide formaldehyde resin that is a sensitizer when dry. Rubbing the eyes with the hands places the sensitizer on the lid. Paradoxically the nail beds and paronychial areas are not involved. Dubbed "ectopic dermatitis," it is a phenomenon that extends to hair products. The hypoallergenic nail polishes substitute a polyester resin.

Eyeliners, eyeshadows and artificial lashes may also be sources of sensitizers for the lid and conjunctiva. Eyelash liners and tweezers that contain nickel can also be sensitizers.

Bielory L: Contact dermatitis of the eye. Allergy Clin North Am 17:131–138,1997.

65. **What are the causes of contact dermatitis of the conjunctiva?**
"Conjunctivitis medicamentosa" typically arises from the repeated use of a topical ocular medication. After an initial improvement of the problem, a red eye returns. This return prompts the use of multiple medications with no relief. Often the treatment is the cessation of all topical medications for several days. The patient returns for relevant scrapings and cultures to diagnose the original problem.

The conjunctival response to this entity is marked by pronounced vasodilatation, chemosis, and a watery discharge. In severe cases there may even be keratitis. The skin of the lids becomes edematous, erythematous, and even ulcerated.

Topical anesthetics and glaucoma medications have been causative agents. However, preservatives are by far the most common cause. Benzalkonium and thimersol are the most commonly used preservatives and thus the most common culprits. All multiple dose preparations require some preservatives. In liquid preparations, chlorbutanol, a rare sensitizer, can be an alternative. In lubricants, sodium perborate, which generates hydrogen peroxide, can be an alternative preservative.

66. **How can these reactions be diagnosed?**
For lid involvement, patch testing is used. Interpretation is difficult because of frequent false-positive irritant reactions. Moreover, in the case of eye cosmetics the typical vesicular eruption often does not occur in the positive test. A use test is another means of determining sensitivity. The suspected material is applied to another area (e.g., forearm) 2 or 3 times/day for about 5 days. A positive test is generally clinically significant. However, false-negative tests are frequent.

KEY POINTS: CONTACT DERMATITIS OF THE EYE AND EYELID

1. Contact dermatitis is the most common eruption of the eyelid.

2. The most common sensitizers are cosmetics applied to the hair, face, and fingernails.

3. Contact dermatitis of the conjunctiva can arise from the repeated use of a topical eye medication.

4. Preservatives in eye medications are the most frequent cause.

INFECTIOUS CAUSES OF CONJUNCTIVITIS

67. **What do all infectious cases of conjunctivitis have in common?**
    All of the diseases mentioned below are associated with both irritation and discharge, and in all cases pupils and intraocular pressure are normal.

68. **List the symptoms of bacterial conjunctivitis.**
    - Redness
    - Irritation
    - Foreign body sensation
    - Copious mucopurulent discharge
    - Lids stuck together in the morning
    - Recent respiratory tract infection or blepharitis

69. **List the objective findings of bacterial conjunctivitis.**
    - Papillary reaction of palbebral conjunctiva
    - Mild-to-pronounced hyperemia of conjunctiva
    - Mild edema of the lids
    - Matted lashes
    - After fluorescein staining, punctate stain on inferior one-third of corneal conjunctiva

70. **Which organisms are commonly associated with bacterial conjunctivitis?**
    1. *Neisseria gonorrhoeae* and *N. meningitidis* can cause a hyperacute reaction characterized by a marked mucopurulent discharge, eyelid edema, and chemosis. Infection can cause ulceration, scarring, and even perforation leading to blindness. Inoculation from infected genitalia is the usual mode of transmission (Fig. 10-1).
    2. *Streptococcus* and *Haemophilus* species are most commonly seen in children and institutional settings. These organisms can cause petechial hemorrhages.
    3. *Staphylococcus* species are the most common cause of conjunctivitis in adults. Although usually an acute problem, the existence of chronic blepharitis can lead to chronic conjunctivitis (see Fig. 10-1).

71. **What are the symptoms of chlamydial conjunctivitis?**
    - Foreign body sensation
    - Lacrimation
    - Redness
    - Photophobia
    - Lid swelling
    - Mucopurulent discharge

KEY POINTS: INFECTIOUS CAUSES OF CONJUNCTIVITIS

1. *Neisseria gonorrhoeae* and *N. meningitidis* can cause a hyperacute reaction characterized by a marked mucopurulent discharge, eyelid edema, and chemosis.

2. *Streptococcus* and *Haemophilus* species are most commonly seen in children and institutional settings.

3. *Staphylococcus* species are the most common cause of conjunctivitis in adults.

4. Chlamydial infection is generally found in young adults and usually transmitted from infected genitalia.

5. Viral causes include adenovirus, herpes simplex, and varicella-zoster.

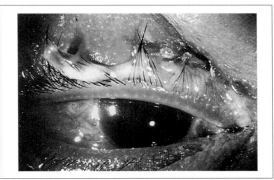

Figure 10-1. Gonococcal conjunctivitis with marked conjunctival injection and copious mucopurulent discharge on the eyelid margin. (From Kim T, Rodman RC, Cohen EJ: Corneal infections. In Vander JE, Gault JA (eds): Ophthalmology Secrets, 2nd ed. Philadelphia, Hanley & Belfus, p 86.)

72. **What is the incubation period of chlamydial conjunctivitis? How does the infection last?**
Incubation period is 2–10 days. Untreated infections can last for months.

73. **List the objective findings of chlamydial conjunctivitis.**
    - Palpebral conjunctiva with initial papillary hypertrophy
    - Chronic follicular response
    - Painless preauricular adenopathy may be present
    - Concomitant otitis media may be present
    - Corneal involvement may occur with epithelial keratitis, subepithelial opacities, phlyctencular lesions, or micropannus

74. **Summarize the epidemiology of chlamydial conjunctivitis.**
It is generally found in young adults and usually transmitted from infected genitalia.

75. **List the symptoms of viral conjunctivitis.**
    - Clear watery discharge
    - Soreness or pain
    - Foreign body sensation
    - Photophobia
    - Glare
    - Slight blurring of vision

76. List the objective findings of viral conjunctivitis.
    - Follicles, more prominent in the lower lid
    - Tender preauricular lymph nodes
    - Both epithelial and subepithelial keratitis may occur
    - Subepithelial opacities may occur

77. Which four clinical syndromes may be caused by adenovirus?
    1. **Epidemic keratoconjunctivitis** has an incubation period of 2–14 days and a self-limited course of 2–14 days. Diagnostic signs include tender preauricular nodes, diffuse subepithelial infiltrates, formation of a membrane on the upper or lower conjunctiva and petechial hemorrhage. Malaise, slight fever, and headache may precede the onset of symptoms.
    2. **Pharyngoconjunctival fever** is more common in children. Antecedent symptoms of sore throat and fever may precede the illness. Malaise, myalgia, headache, and gastrointestinal disturbance may accompany the eye disease. Because the virus is shed for up to 30 days in feces, a recent history of swimming in a pool or contact with a previously infected person may be obtained.
    3. **Nonspecific acute sporadic conjunctivitis**
    4. **Chronic papillary conjunctivitis**

78. Describe conjunctivitis due to herpes simplex virus.
    The key differentiating sign in herpes simplex conjunctivitis is small vesicles around the lid, particularly the lid margins. Other signs include follicular conjunctivitis, preauricular or submandibular lymphadenopathy, lid edema, and superficial punctate keratitis, which may occur 1–2 weeks after the conjunctivitis. The causative organism, HSV-1, can remain latent in the trigeminal ganglion and cause recurrent ocular infection in up to 25% of the cases.

79. Describe conjunctivitis due to varicella-zoster virus.
    Patients have other features of either varicella or zoster infection. Mild-to-severe ocular complications may occur in over 50% with the involvement of the trigeminal nerve.
    Jackson BW: Differentiating conjunctivitis of diverse origins. Surv Ophthalmol 38:91–104, 1993.
    Sendrowski DP: Acute conjunctival inflammation. In Bezan D, LaRussa F, Nishimoto J, et al (eds): Differential Diagnosis in Primary Eye Care. New York, Butterworth-Heineman, 1999, pp 107–113.

OTHER CAUSES OF AN ACUTE RED EYE

80. What are the symptoms and signs of acute angle glaucoma?
    The symptoms of acute glaucoma, which usually occurs in older female patients, stem from the sudden rise in intraocular pressure. They include blurred vision, ocular pain, frontal headache, colored haloes, nausea and emesis. The prominent findings are fixed and dilated pupil and a dull corneal reflex from the edematous cornea. *Acute angle glaucoma is an ocular emergency and requires immediate care by an ophthalmologist.*

KEY POINTS: NONALLERGIC, NONINFECTIOUS CAUSES OF ACUTE RED EYE

1. Acute angle glaucoma
2. Ruptured globe
3. Episcleritis
4. Idiopathic anterior uveitis
5. Iritis
6. Subconjunctival hemorrhage

81. **Discuss the symptoms and signs of a ruptured globe.**
Patients usually have a history of penetrating trauma to the globe. A sharp pain is present. Ocular complaints can vary. The most important diagnostic findings are hypotony, shallow anterior chamber, and a sluggish pupillary response to light. Subconjunctival hemorrhages and periocular abrasions may be seen. *Ruptured globe is an ocular emergency and requires urgent consultation with an ophthalmologist.*

82. **Discuss the symptoms and signs of episcleritis. With which systemic disorders is it associated?**
Patients are usually adults between the ages of 20–50 with a female predominance. The presenting symptoms are rapid onset of pain and irritation in one or both eyes. There may be tenderness over the area of redness. There is no circumlimbal injection or visual disturbance. The cornea and anterior chamber are normal. The symptoms usually progress over 3–5 days and resolve in 10 days. It is found in the following systemic diseases: systemic lupus erythematosus, polyarteritis, Lyme disease, rheumatoid arthritis, Crohn's disease, hepatitis B infection, gout, or syphillis.

83. **What are the symptoms and signs of idiopathic anterior uveitis?**
There is sudden onset of pain, redness of the eye and photophobia without a history of trauma. The disease is usually unilateral occurring in adults between the ages of 20–50. The affected pupil is miotic. The vasculature of the limbal area is engorged and reddened. Ptosis may occur secondary to blepharospasm.

84. **Discuss the symptoms and signs of iritis. With which systemic disorders is it associated?**
Symptoms include pain, photophobia, and circumlimbal injection. The pupil is miotic, and the intraocular pressure is decreased. The anterior chamber is abnormal. This disorder is usually found with the following systemic diseases: ankylosing spondylitis, Reiter's syndrome, ulcerative colitis, sarcoidosis, or Behçet's disease

85. **Explain the cause of subconjunctival hemorrhage.**
This common but benign problem presents suddenly without symptoms such as pain, discharge, or visual disturbance. The pupils, anterior chamber, and cornea are all normal. There is no history of discharge. Although usually idiopathic, it can occur with hypertension and bleeding disorders.
Sendrowski DP: Acute red eye. In Bezan D, LaRussa F, Nishimoto J, et al (eds): Differential Diagnosis in Primary Eye Care. New York, Butterworth-Heineman, 1999, pp.97–105.

WEBSITES

1. American College of Allergy, Asthma and Immunology: www.acaai.org

2. National Library of Medicine: www.nlm.nih.gov

BIBLIOGRAPHY

1. Abelson MB, McGarr PJ, Richard KP: Anti-allergic therapies. In Textbook of Ocular Pharmacology, 1997, pp 609–633.

2. Abelson MB, Smith LS: Levocabastine: Evaluation in the histamine and compound 40/80 models of ocular allergy in humans. Ophthalmology 95:1494–1497, 1988.

3. Ahluwalia P, Anderson D, et al: Nedocromil sodium reduces the symptoms of conjunctival allergin challenge by different mechanisms. J Allergy Clin Immunol 108:449–454, 2001.

4. Berdy GJ, Spangler DL, et al: A comparison of the relative efficacy and clinical performance of olopatadine hydrochloride 0.1% ophthalmic solution and ketotifen fumarate 0.025% ophthalmic solution in the conjunctival antigen challenge model. Clin Ther 22:826–833, 2000.

5. Berdy GJ, Stoppel JO, Epstein AB: Comparison of the clinical efficacy and tolerability of olopatadine hydrochloride 0.1% ophthalmic solution and lotepredenol etabonate 0.2% suspension in the conjunctival allergen challenge model. Clin Ther 24:918–929, 2002.

6. Bielory L: Contact dermatitis of the eye. Allergy Clin North Am 17:131–138,1997. Jackson BW: Differentiating conjunctivitis of diverse origins. Surv Ophthalmol 38:91–104,1993.

7. Bielory L: Allergic and immunologic disorders of the eye. In Middleton E, Ellis E et al (eds): Allergy Principles and Practice, 5th ed. St. Louis, Mosby, 1998, p 1153.

8. Bielory L, Frielander M, Fujishima H: Allergic conjunctivitis. Allergy Clin North Am 17:19–31, 1997.

9. Bonini S, Lambiase A, Sacchetti M, Bonini S: Cytokines in ocular allergy. Int Ophthalmol Clin 43:95–103,2003.

10. Bonini S, Sacchetti M, Lambiasi A; Bonini S: Cytokines in ocular allergy. Int Ophthamol Clin 43:27–31, 2003.

11. Butrus S, Greiner JV, Discepola M, Feingold J: Comparison of the clinical efficacy and comfort of olopatadine hydrochloride 0.1% ophthalmic solution and nedocromil sodium 2% ophthalmic solution in the human conjunctival allergen challenge model. Clin Ther 22:1462–1472, 2000.

12. Constad WH, Bhagat N: Keratitis sicca and dry eye syndrome. Allergy Clin North Am 17:89–102, 1997.

13. D'Arienzo PA, Leonardi A, Bensch G: Randomized, double-masked, placebo-controlled comparison of the efficacy of emedastine difumarate 0.05% ophthalmic solution and ketotifen fumarate 0.025% ophthalmic solution in the human conjunctival allergen challenge model. Clin Ther 24:409–416, 2002.

14. Dell SJ, Lowry GM, et al: A Randomized, double-masked, placebo-controlled study of lotepredenol etabonate in patients with season allergic conjunctivitis. J Allergy Clin Immunol 102:251–255, 1998.

15. Donshik PC, Ehlers WH: Giant papillary conjunctivitis. Allergy Clin North Am 17:53–73, 1997.

16. Friedlaender, MH: Ocular allergy. In Middleton E, Reed CE et al. (eds): Allergy: Principles and Practice, 4th ed. St. Louis, Mosby, 1993, p 1651.

17. Greiner JV, Michaelson C, McWhirter CL, Shams NB: Single dose of ketotifen fumarate .025% versus 2 weeks of cromolyn sodium 4% for allergic conjunctivitis. Adv Ther 19(4):185–193, 2002.

18. Irani A: Ocular mast cells and mediators. Allergy Clin North Am 17:1–13, 1997.

19. Lee Y, Raizman M: Vernal conjunctivitis. Allergy Clin North Am 17:33–51, 1997.

20. Leonardi A, Briggs RM, Bloch KJ, et al: Correlation between conjunctival provocation test (CPT) and systemic allergometric tests in allergic conjunctivitis. Eye 4:760–764, 1990.

21. McGill JL, Holgate ST, Church MK, et al: Allergic eye disease mechanisms. Br J Ophthalmol 82:1203–1214, 1998.

22. Orfeo V, Vardaro A, Lena P, et al: Comparison of emedastine 0.05% or nedocromil sodium 2% eye drops and placebo in controlling local reactions in subjects with allergic conjunctivitis. Eur J Ophthalmol 12(4):262–266, 2002.

23. Richard C, Triquand C, Bloch-Michel T: Comparison of topical 0.05% levocabastin and 0.1% lodaxamide in patients with allergic conjunctivitis. Eur J Ophthalmol. 8(4):207–216,1998.

24. Secchi A, Ciprandi G; et al: Safety and efficacy comparison of emedastine 0.05% solution compared to levocabastine 0.05% ophthalmic suspension in pediatric subjects with allergic conjunctivitis. Acta Ophthal Scand Suppl 230:42–47, 2000.

25. Secchi A, Leonardi A, et al: An efficacy and tolerance comparison of emedastine difumarate 0.05% and levocabastine hydrochloride 0.05%: reducing chemosis and eyelid swelling in subjects with seasonal allergic conjunctivitis. Acta Ophthal Scand Suppl (230):48–51, 2000.

26. Sendrowski DP: Acute conjunctival inflammation. In Bezan D, LaRussa F, Nishimoto J, et al (eds): Differential Diagnosis in Primary Eye Care. New York, Butterworth-Heineman, 1999, pp 107–113.

27. Sendrowski DP: Acute red eye. In Bezan D, LaRussa F, Nishimoto J, et al (eds): Differential Diagnosis in Primary Eye Care. New York, Butterworth-Heineman, 1999, pp 97–105.

28. Siret DJ: Oral and topical antihistamines: Pharmacologic properties and therapeutic potential in ocular allergic disease. J Am Optometr Assoc 69(2):77–87,1998.

29. Spangler DL, Bensch G, Berdy GJ: Evaluation of the efficacy of olopatadine hydrochloride 0.1% ophthalmic solution and azelastine 0.05% ophthalmic solution in the conjunctival allergen challenge model. Clin Ther 23:1272–1280, 2001.

30. Tuft SJ, Kemeny DM, Dart JK, Buckley RJ: Clinical features of atopic keratoconjunctivitis. Ophthamology 98:150–158, 1991.

31. Verin P, Easty DL, et al: Clinical evaluation of twice-daily emedastine 0.05% eyedrops (Emadine eye drops) versus levocabastine 0.05% eyedrops in patients with allergic conjunctivitis. Am J Opthalmol 131:691–698, 2001.

32. Zhan H, Smith L, Calder V, et al: Clinical and immunological features of atopic keratoconjunctivitis. Int Ophthamol Clin 43:59–71, 2003.

CHAPTER 11

ANAPHYLAXIS

Arif M. Seyal, M.D.

1. **Define anaphylaxis.**

   Anaphylaxis is a potentially life-threatening clinical syndrome characterized by the sudden onset of generalized, often unanticipated symptoms, affecting multiple organ systems in the body. Clinical features in anaphylaxis are induced by the mediators released by IgE-receptor cross-linking on mast cells and basophils previously sensitized by antigen.

2. **How does anaphylaxis differ from anaphylactoid reaction?**

   Anaphylactoid reaction is a systemic reaction that is clinically similar to anaphylaxis but is not caused by IgE-mediated immune response. Anaphylaxis and anaphylactoid reactions are usually immediate in nature and occur within 30 minutes after exposure to the causative agent, but in some cases onset may be delayed an hour or longer.

   Ring J, Behrendt H: Anaphylaxis and anaphylactoid reactions: Classification and pathophysiology. Clin Rev Allergy Immunol 17:469–496, 1999.

3. **What factors influence the incidence of anaphylaxis?**

   Factors that may influence the incidence of anaphylaxis include history of underlying atopy, route of administration of antigen/causative agent, and the patient's age and gender.

4. **Explain the influence of underlying atopy.**

   Approximately 50% of people who experience exercise-induced anaphylaxis have an underlying history of atopy. There also appears to be a higher incidence of anaphylaxis due to food, radio-contrast material, and latex in atopic patients.

5. **How does route of administration of the antigen influence the incidence of anaphylaxis?**

   The incidence of anaphylactic reactions is higher after parental administration of antibiotics and biologic agents. Oral administration of antibiotics appears to be considerably safer.

6. **Explain the role of age and gender.**

   Anaphylactic reactions are more common in adults than in children. Women appear to be affected twice as often by food-associated, exercised-induced anaphylaxis. Approximately 60% of the cases of anaphylaxis tend to occur in people younger than 30 years. The higher incidence of systemic allergic reactions due to Hymenoptera sting in males may be secondary to increased exposure.

7. **Summarize the role of histamine receptors in the pathogenesis of anaphylaxis and anaphylactoid reaction.**

   Most of the clinical features of anaphylaxis can be produced by intravenous infusion of the small doses of histamine, which, by acting through both H_1 and H_2 receptor subtypes, can cause vasodilation, increased mucus gland secretions, and hypotension (Table 11-1).

   Felix SB, Baumann G, Helmus S, Sattelberger U: Role of histamine in the cardiac anaphylaxis: Characterization of histaminergic H_1 and H_2 receptor effects. Basic Res Cardiol 5:531–539, 1988.

TABLE 11-1.   GRANULE-ASSOCIATED PREFORMED MEDIATORS OF ANAPHYLAXIS

Mediators	Pathophysiologic Effect	Clinical Effect
Histamine		
H$_1$ receptor-mediated effects	Increased capillary permeability	Flushing
	Vasodilation	Pruritus
	Contraction of smooth muscles (bronchial and intestinal)	Urticaria, angioedema
		Hypotension
	Coronary vasoconstriction	Wheezing
	Increased rate of depolarization of sinoatrial node	Abdominal cramps
		Tachycardia and myocardial ischemia
	Irritation of nerve endings	
	Neuropeptide release	Increased mucous gland secretions
	Increased mucous gland secretions	
H$_2$ receptor-mediated effects	Peripheral vasodilation	Hypotension
	Coronary artery vasodilation	Tachycardia
	Positive inotropic and positive chronotropic effects on cardiac smooth muscles	Atrial and ventricular arrhythmias
		Increased goblet cells and bronchial gland secretions.
	Decreased fibrillation	
	Increased glandular secretions	
H$_3$ receptor-mediated effects	Cardiovascular effects have been implicated in canine model of anaphylaxis	Potential implication for anaphylaxis in humans is not known.
Enzymes		
Tryptase	Neutral protease; activates complement C3	Plasma half-life = 2 hours
		Useful marker of mast cell activation
		Clinical effects unknown
Chymase	May act as angiotensin-converting enzyme	May play a role in response to hypotension
Chemotactic factors		
Eosinophilic and neutrophilic chemotactic factors (ECFA, NCFA)	Chemotactic factors for inflammatory cells (eosinophilic and neutrophilis)	Important for the late-phase reaction
Heparin	Anticoagulant, complement inhibitor	Probable anti-inflammatory effect

8. **Which effects are mediated by H$_1$ receptors?**
Increased vascular permeability, smooth muscle contraction, and enhanced bronchial mucus production. H$_1$ receptors also cause the stimulation of sensory nerves endings, leading to the release of neuropeptides. Cardiac effects include increased rate of depolarization of the sinoatrial node and coronary vasospasm.

9. **Which effects are mediated by H$_2$ receptors?**
Coronary artery vasodilation as well as inotropic and chronotropic effects on cardiac muscles. H$_2$ receptors also increase mucus secretion from goblet cells and bronchial glands.

10. **Name other biochemical mediators and chemotactic substances that are released systemically by the degranulation of mast cells and basophils during the anaphylactic reaction.**
Other mediators released in this process include tryptase, chymase, chemotactic factors, and heparin (see Table 11-1).

11. **What are the most common clinical features of anaphylaxis in order of relative frequency?**
Clinical features of anaphylaxis are frequently sudden in onset and may range from mild to very severe or occasionally fatal. Table 11-2 lists the clinical features of anaphylaxis according to relative frequency.

TABLE 11–2. RELATIVE FREQUENCY OF CLINICAL FEATURES OF ANAPHYLAXIS	
Clinical Features	**Percent of Patients**
Pruritus, urticaria, and angioedema	> 90
Dyspnea and wheezing	47–60
Dizziness, near syncope, syncope, and hypotension	30–33
Flushing of skin	> 28
Nausea, vomiting, and abdominal cramps	25–30
Laryngeal edema, tongue swelling, choking, and dysphonia	24
Rhinitis and nasal congestion	16
Substernal chest discomfort	6
Headache	> 5
Pruritus without rash	4
Seizure	1.5–2

12. **Discuss the pathophysiologic effects and clinical manifestation related to the newly synthesized mediators released by the mast cells and basophils.**
Newly generated lipid-derived mediators, such as leukotrienes, prostaglandins, and platelet activating factors, play a significant role in pro- or anti-inflammatory activity in anaphylaxis (Table 11-3).

13. **Explain the mechanism of radiocontrast material (RCM)-associated anaphylaxis.**
The exact mechanism of anaphylactoid reaction to RCM is unknown. IgE does not appear to be involved in this reaction. Possible mechanisms of RCM-induced anaphylactoid reaction include

TABLE 11-3.	NEWLY GENERATED MEDIATORS OF MAST CELLS AND BASOPHILS THAT PLAY A ROLE IN ANAPHYLAXIS AND ANAPHYLACTOID REACTIONS	
	Pathophysiologic Effect	**Clinical Manifestation**
Arachidonic acid metabolites lipoxygenase pathway		
Leukotrienes	Contraction of airway smooth	Wheezing
■ LTC4	muscles	Hypotension
■ LTD4	Increased vascular permeability	Possible late-phase reaction
■ LTB4	Chemotactic activity	
Cyclooxygenase pathway		
■ Prostaglandins	Bronchoconstriction	Hypotension
(PG D2 and PG F2)	Peripheral vasodilation	Wheezing
■ Thromboxane A_2	Coronary artery vasoconstriction	Myocardial ischemia
Platelet-activating factor (PAF)		
	Bronchoconstriction	Wheezing
	Vasodilation	Hypotension
	Increased vascular permeability	Cardiac arrhythmias
	Increased myocardial	Pump failure, probably in
	contractility	late-phase reaction

direct release of mediators from mast cells and basophils, complement activation, inhibition of cholinesterase, recruitment of inflammatory mediators, and indirect release of the prostacycline by vascular endothelial cells.

14. **What is the value of skin testing in the diagnosis of RCM-associated anaphylaxis?**
Skin testing has no value in the diagnosis of RCM-associated anaphylaxis.

15. **How can you reduce the risk of recurrent anaphylactoid reaction to hyperosmolar (HOS) radiocontrast material?**
The risk of recurrent anaphylactoid reaction to high-osmolality contrast material can be reduced to < 1% by use of low-osmolality contrast material and a pretreatment regimen.

16. **What foods are most commonly implicated in fatal anaphylactic reactions?**
Although any food can cause a fatal anaphylactic reaction, certain foods have been implicated more frequently than others including peanuts, tree nuts (walnuts, cashews, hazelnuts, pistachios, Brazil nuts), fish, shellfish (shrimps, crabs, oysters, lobster), certain fruits (kiwi), and seeds (psyllium, cottonseed, and sesame seed).

17. **What is exercise-induced anaphylaxis?**
Exercise-induced anaphylaxis (EIA) is a form of physical allergy that usually occurs after prolonged exercise and is manifested by the symptoms of generalized warmth, pruritus, urticaria, angioedema, nausea, vomiting, abdominal cramps, diarrhea, dyspnea, and vascular collapse.
    Sheffer AL, Austen KF: Exercise-induced anaphylaxis. J Allergy Clin Immunol 66: 106–111, 1980.

18. **What is cholinergic urticaria?**
    Cholinergic urticaria is also a form of physical allergy and is characterized by the small punctate (1–4 mm), intensely pruritic wheals (microhives) with surrounding erythema. It can be triggered by raising core body temperature or even by sweating induced by stress. Some patients may also experience systemic symptoms.

19. **How is EIA differentiated from cholinergic urticaria?**
    Passive heat challenge appears to be valuable diagnostic test in the differentiation of cholinergic urticaria from EIA.

20. **What is the role of antihistamine and systemic corticosteroids in prevention of EIA?**
    Prophylactic treatment of EIA with H_1 and H_2 antihistamine and corticosteroids has not proved effective.

21. **What is the possible mechanism of anaphylaxis induced by aspirin and other nonsteroidal anti-inflammatory drugs (NSAIDs)?**
    The mechanism by which nonsteroidal anti-inflammatory drugs lead to the development of an anaphylactic/anaphylactoid reaction is not well defined. It is likely that inhibition of cyclooxygenase by aspirin and other NSIADs may result in a shift of arachidonic acid metabolism from the cyclooxygenase to lipoxygenase pathway, thus leading to increased peptidoleukotriene production. Increased levels of peptidoleukotriene may result in the symptoms of hypotension, bronchoconstriction, increased mucus production, urticaria, and angioedema.
    Stevenson DD: Diagnosis, prevention, and treatment of adverse reactions to aspirin and nonsteroidal anti-inflammatory drugs. J Allergy Clin Immunol 74:617–622, 1984.

22. **How is the diagnosis of NSAID-induced anaphylaxis confirmed?**
    There is no reliable skin test or in vitro study to confirm the diagnosis. The aspirin/NSAID challenge can be performed in an intensive care setting.

23. **List the three basic mechanisms of anaphylaxis/anaphylactoid reactions.**
    - IgE-mediated
    - Non-IgE-mediated
    - Unknown

24. **Which reactions are mediated by IgE mechanisms?**
    - Foods: fish, shellfish, crustaceans, egg, milk, peanut, fruits (e.g., kiwi, banana), and seeds (cottonseed, sesame, and psyllium) are the most common foods implicated.
    - Animal and human proteins: stinging insects (Hymenoptera, fire ants), biting insects (kissing bug or triatoma), anti-lymphocyte globulin (ALG), avian-based vaccine (measles, mumps, influenza, and yellow fever), murine-derived monoclonal antibodies, human seminal plasma.
    - Hormones: insulin, corticotropin (ACTH).
    - Enzymes: streptokinase, chymopapain.
    - Aeroallergens: skin test or immunotherapy for pollens, house dust mite, molds, and other allergens.
    - Others: latex (gloves and other medical devices), protamine.
    - Haptens (IgE-mediated reactions against the protein hapten conjugate).
    - Antibiotics: penicillin, cephalosporins, sulfonamides, and streptomycin.
    - Disinfectants: ethylene oxide.
    - Smooth muscle relaxants, such as succinylcholine.
    Marshal CP, Pearson FC, Sagona MA, et al: Reaction during hemodialysis caused by allergy to ethylene oxide gas sterilization. J Allergy Clin Immunol 75:285–290, 1985.

25. **Which reactions are mediated by non-IgE mechanisms?**
    - Complement activation and generation of anaphylotoxins (C3a, C4a, C5a): human plasma and blood products, gamma globulin.
    - Direct activation of mast cells or basophil mediators release: opiates, tubucurare, dextran, radiocontrast materials, fluorescein dye for angiography, and some chemotherapeutic agents.
    - Modulators of arachidonic acid metabolism: nonsteroidal anti-inflammatory drugs (e.g., aspirin, ibuprofen, indomethacin).

26. **Which reactions are mediated by an unknown mechanism?**
    - Sulfites: food additives
    - Steroids: progesterone and hydrocortisone
    - Physical triggers: EIA, food-dependent EIA, systemic cold-induced urticaria, and systemic heat-induced urticaria
    - Systemic mastocytosis
    - Idiopathic anaphylaxis

27. **What are the shock organs in anaphylaxis?**
    The clinical course of anaphylaxis is determined by organ system involvement. It is based on the immune response and the location of the smooth muscles affected by the release of the chemical mediators. In humans, the major organs affected by the anaphylaxis are heart and lung, with common and potentially fatal clinical reactions of cardiovascular compromise, respiratory failure, and laryngeal edema.

28. **What common clinical conditions may mimic anaphylaxis/anaphylactoid reaction?**
    1. Shock
       - Hemorrhagic (massive gastrointestinal blood loss)
       - Cardiogenic (acute myocardial infarction)
       - Septic
    2. Vasovagal reaction
    3. Carcinoid syndrome
    4. Systemic mastocytosis
    5. Pheochromocytoma
    6. Hereditary angioedema
    7. Nonorganic causes
       - Panic disorder
       - Vocal cord dysfunction
       - Globus hystericus

29. **How can you differentiate a vasovagal reaction from true anaphylaxis or anaphylactoid response?**
    Vasovagal reactions may occur after an injection, and the usual clinical manifestations include dizziness, diaphoresis, pallor, weakness, sweating, nausea, hypotension, and bradycardia. Patients lack pruritus, urticaria, angioedema, tachycardia, and bronchospasm.

30. **What is the most appropriate treatment of vasovagal reaction?**
    An administration of atropine sulfate, 0.3–1 mg intramuscularly or intravenously, usually reverses a vasovagal reaction.

31. **Define carcinoid syndrome.**
    Carcinoid syndrome is usually associated with flushing, abdominal cramps, diarrhea, and occasionally broncospasm. This condition is caused by the release of vasoactive substances such as serotonin, bradykinin, and histamine by a slow-growing tumor usually located in the bronchi, stomach, pancreas, or small intestine.

KEY POINTS: VASOVAGAL REACTION

1. Vasovagal reaction, which is manifested by dizziness, pallor, diaphoresis, nausea, hypotension, and bradycardia, should be differentiated from anaphylaxis.

2. Patients with vasovagal reaction lack skin manifestations (urticaria and angioedema), tachycardia, and bronchospasm.

3. Administration of atropine sulfate, 0.3–1 mg intramuscularly or intravenously, usually reverses a vasovagal reaction.

32. **How is carcinoid syndrome diagnosed?**
Affected patients have elevated plasma level of 5-hydroxyindole acetic acid (5HIAA). An elevated level of 5HIAA in 24-hour urine collection is strongly suggestive of the diagnosis.

33. **What is the effect of epinephrine on carcinoid flush?**
Epinephrine is contraindicated because it may provoke carcinoid flush.

34. **Define systemic mastocytosis.**
Systemic mastocytosis is a clinical syndrome caused by the accumulation of mast cells in multiple organs, including skin, bone marrow, liver, and gastrointestinal tract. Clinical features of flushing, pruritus, and anaphylactic response may be associated with urticaria pigmentosa and may develop spontaneously or after taking NSAIDs, opiates, or alcohol. Other common features are osteoporosis, bone demineralization, and anemia due to bone marrow involvement.
Horan RF, Austen KF: Systemic mastocytosis: Retrospective review of a decade of clinical experience at the Brigham and Women's Hospital. J Invest Dermatol 96:5S–14S, 1991.

35. **How can you distinguish systemic mastocytosis from anaphylaxis/anaphylactoid reaction?**
In systemic mastocytosis baseline α-protryptase level is markedly elevated (> 20 mg/mL). This elevation presumably reflects the total mast cell burden and can be used to assess the response to treatment directed at lowering total mast cell load. In systemic anaphylaxis, serum β-tryptase level is > 5 ng/mL.

36. **Explain the significance of anemia and thrombocytopenia in systemic mastocytosis.**
Extensive bone marrow infiltration by mast cells in systemic mastocytosis is associated with hematologic abnormalities such as anemia, thrombocytopenia, eosinophilia, and lymphopenia. Anemia (especially hemoglobin < 11 gm/dL), thrombocytopenia, decreased bone marrow fat cells (< 20%), constitutional symptoms, and liver function abnormalities are associated with poor prognosis.

37. **What is the importance of serum tryptase as a diagnostic marker of anaphylaxis?**
Tryptase is neutral protease concentrated selectively in the secretory granules of the human mast cells and may be an important marker for mast cell activation in anaphylaxis. During anaphylaxis, tryptase is released into the blood after degranulation of the mast cells; therefore, plasma tryptase levels may correlate well with the severity of anaphylaxis. Since β tryptase is stored in the mast-cell secretory granules, its release is considered more specific for the mast cell activation during anaphylaxis than that of α protryptase, which is not stored in the granules and is constantly released from the mast cells in small amounts.

38. **What is the diagnostic value of a normal plasma histamine level 4 hours after insect sting–induced anaphylaxis?**

Plasma histamine levels peak at 10–15 minutes after insect-induced anaphylaxis and return to baseline within 30 minutes. In addition, during the blood clotting and specimen handling, basophils can release a significant amount of histamine and thus may make it difficult to interpret an elevated level of histamine that may have occurred in vivo or in vitro. Therefore, a normal or elevated plasma histamine level 4 hours after the anaphylactic reaction has no clinical significance.

39. **What is food-associated EIA?**

Anaphylactic reaction occurs when exercise is performed within 2–4 hours after ingestion of a specific food. The patient can ingest the same food without any apparent reaction and can exercise without any reaction as long as the specific food has not been ingested in the past several hours. Skin test to the specific food is usually positive.

Horan RF, Sheffer AL: Food-dependent, exercise-induced anaphylaxis. Immunol Allergy Clin North Am 11:757, 1991.

40. **Define idiopathic anaphylaxis.**

Idiopathic anaphylaxis (IA) is a diagnosis of exclusion. IA can be diagnosed after a meticulous history, review of emergency department records and the patient's diary, and laboratory studies have excluded any underlying causative factor.

41. **What are the possible mechanisms of IA?**

There is no known mechanism of idiopathic anaphylaxis (IA). The following possibilities have been considered:

- IA is a mast-cell activation syndrome that is precipitated by the inappropriate release of histamine-releasing factors (HRFs) from T lymphocytes.
- Autoantibodies against the IgE receptors may play a role. They may cross-link IgE on the mast cells and lead to the activation and release of mediators from the mast cells.

Patterson R, Clayton DE, et al: Fatal and near fatal idiopathic anaphylaxis. Allergy Proc 16(3);103–108, 1995.

42. **Define frequent IA.**

Frequent IA is defined as greater than 6 episodes of anaphylactic reactions per year or as 2 or more episodes in 2 months.

43. **What general principle guides the treatment of patients with frequent episodes of IA?**

The treatment regimen should be implemented on an individual basis in accordance with the severity and frequency of the IA episodes.

44. **What instructions should patients with frequent IA be given for self-treatment?**

Patients with IA should be instructed in self-administration of intramuscular epinephrine. They should also be instructed to self-administer 60 mg of prednisone and an antihistamine (hydroxyzine, 25 mg, or diphenhydramine, 50 mg) orally. Patients should then proceed to the emergency department.

45. **Describe the approach to treatment after the acute episode has resolved.**

After the acute episode of anaphylaxis has resolved, patients should be treated with 60 mg of prednisone daily for 1 week, followed by slow tapering (not more than 10 mg/month). An antihistamine (hydroxyzine, 25–50 mg 3 times/day) and an oral sympathomimetic (e.g., albuterol, 2 mg 3 times/day) are also added. IA appears to respond well to systemic glucocorticoids.

46. **What treatment regimen should be used once the patient is stable?**
Once the patient is stable, prednisone can be converted to alternate-day dosing. Patients with frequent episodes of IA may require long-term oral steroids to control the recurrent symptoms. Some patients with corticosteroid-dependent IA may be treated with oral cromolyn or ketotifen. This approach may allow further reduction in the dosage of oral corticosteroids. Ultimate prognosis is generally good, and most patients are eventualy able to discontinue the systemic corticosteroids.

47. **A 38-year-old woman with hypertension who is being treated with atenolol is stung by a honeybee and develops symptoms of anaphylaxis within 15 minutes. On arrival in the emergency department, her blood pressure is 90/54 mmHg. She has generalized urticaria, wheezing, and chest tightness. After repeated injections of epinephrine, her blood pressure is still 92/50 mmHg, and her heart rate is 82 beats/min. She continues to have wheezing and chest tightness. What should you do next?**
Patients treated with beta bockers generally respond poorly to epinephrine. In such patients hypotension should be treated with vigorous intravascular volume repletion. Atropine may be administered 0.2–0.5 mg subcutaneously every 10 minutes to the maximum of 2 mg. Atropine is helpful in reversing bradycardia. Glucagon exerts its inotropic and chronoprotic effect on heart muscles independently of beta receptors and can be given intravenously as a bolus of 1–5 mg given over 5 minutes followed by continuous infusion at the rate of 5–15 µg/min. Because glucagon can induce nausea and vomiting, all aspiration precautions should be observed. Occasionally, intravenous dopamine or isoproterenol is needed to treat protracted hypotension. Persistent bronchospasm may be treated with nebulized albuterol.

48. **Describe the late phase of systemic anaphylactic reaction. What is its clinical significance?**
Most anaphylactic reactions begin within 30 minutes after exposure to the causative agent. In most patients, the anaphylactic reaction is uniphasic and does not reoccur after complete resolution of the early phase. In some patients, however, a second episode of symptoms is seen approximately 6–8 hours (sometimes up to 12 hours) later without any repeat exposure to the offending agent. It is estimated that approximately 7–20% of patients have biphasic anaphylactic reaction.

Douglas DM, Sukenick E, Andrade WP, Brown JS: Biphasic anaphylaxis: An inpatient and outpatient study. J Allergy Cin Immunol 93(6):977–985, 1994.

49. **Explain the mechanism of the late-phase reaction.**
The exact mechanism of the late-phase systemic anaphylactic reaction is unclear. It is possible that this response is initiated by the release of newly formed mast cell mediators (especially chemoattractants such as eosiniphilic chemotactic factor and neutrophil chemotactic factor) and further release of cytokines, but so far no correlation between the symptoms of late anaphylaxis and mediator release has been found.

50. **Discuss the role of glucocorticoids in prevention of late-phase systemic anaphylactic reaction.**
Glucocorticoids and other medications (antihistamine and epinephrine) used in the treatment of anaphylaxis have not been shown to prevent late-phase anaphylactic response. Glucocorticoids are, however, generally administered to blunt or attenuate the late-phase systemic anaphylactic response because they have proved to be efficacious in other clinical situations associated with late-phase reaction.

51. **How long after the successful treatment of acute anaphylaxis should a patient be kept under observation in a medical facility?**
In general, no clinical features allow identification of patients likely to experience biphasic anaphylactic reaction. Several investigators have observed that patients with biphasic anaphylaxis

KEY POINTS: ANAPHYLAXIS

1. Generalized urticaria and angioedema are the most common manifestations of anaphylaxis.

2. Idiopathic anaphylaxis is one of the most common causes of anaphylaxis.

3. Foods implicated in cases of fatal anaphylaxis include peanuts, tree nuts, fish, and shellfish (shrimp, crab, oyster, and lobster).

4. Intramuscular injection of epinephrine into the lateral thigh is the preferred route and site of administration during the treatment of moderate-to-severe anaphylaxis.

required significantly more epinephrine to ameliorate the initial symptoms compared with uniphasic symptoms. It is important, therefore, to observe closely all patients with severe anaphylaxis, especially when they require significantly higher dose of epinephrine, for at least 12 hours after resolution of initial symptoms. Patients with mild reactions may be observed at home and instructed to return immediately at the slightest hint of recurrent symptoms. It is necessary to communicate with patients within 24 hours after the initial phase. Instruction in self-administration of epinephrine is also recommended.

52. **What are the common clinical characteristics of human seminal plasma hypersensitivity anaphylaxis?**
Common clinical features of human seminal fluid allergy vary from localized vulvar and vaginal burning, with itching and swelling, to generalized pruritus, urticarial eruptions, asthma, hypotension, and shock. Most affected women are between 20 and 30 years of age with an underlying history of atopy. Systemic reactions to human seminal plasma are mediated by the production of the IgE antibodies.

53. **Which tests are used to diagnose human seminal plasma hypersensitivity anaphylaxis?**
Diagnosis can be confirmed by percutaneous skin testing. Skin testing, however, is not a reliable marker for the diagnosis of localized allergic reactions to seminal fluid. On the basis of available data, in vitro tests (ELISA or RAST) of serum-specific IgE appear to be less sensitive than skin testing. Finally the diagnosis of human seminal plasma allergy (local and systemic) can be established by complete prevention of symptoms with the use of condoms.

54. **Describe the treatment of human seminal plasma hypersensitivity anaphylaxis.**
Treatment of human seminal plasma allergy includes the use of condoms. For patients with latex allergy, latex-free condoms should be substituted. In addition to systemic antihistamines, pretreatment with intravaginal cromolyn sodium may be used in mild cases. Patients with a history of systemic anaphylactic reaction may be considered for parenteral or intravaginal immunotherapy. Successful pregnancies have been achieved after intravaginal desensitization.
    Park JW, Ko SH, Kim CW: Seminal plasma anaphylaxis: Successful pregnancy after intravaginal desensitization and immunodetection of allergens. Allergy 54:990–993, 1999.

55. **What is progesterone-induced anaphylaxis?**
Unexplained anaphylaxis usually occurs in young females during pregnancy or menstruation. Such patients usually undergo remission during lactation. Episodes of anaphylaxis can also be

provoked by administration of progesterone and luteinizing hormone-releasing hormone (LHRH). Anaphylaxis, however, cannot be provoked by administration of estrogen.

Burstein M, Rubinow A, Shalit M: Cyclic anaphylaxis associated with menstruation. Ann Allergy 66:36–38, 1991.

56. **How is progesterone-induced anaphylaxis treated?**
Treatment includes administration of LHRH analog. Sometimes bilateral oophorectomy is necessary.

57. **What are the cardiovascular effects of the histamine released by mast cells and basophils?**
Histamine causes a reduction in systemic vascular resistance and thus leads to a fall in systolic, diastolic, and mean aortic pressure and an increase in the heart rate. This effect is mediated through both the H_1 and H_2 receptors. In addition to the peripheral vasodilatation, H_2 receptors cause an increase in heart rate and cardiac muscle contractility as well as coronary vasodilatation. H_1 receptors mediate chronotropic effects and coronary vasoconstriction. Histamine administration after H_2 receptor blockade alone with cimetidine may intensify coronary vasoconstriction.

58. **Describe the cardiovascular effects of the platelet-activating factor (PAF) released by mast cells and basophils.**
PAF causes cardiac arrhythmias and myocardial pump failure. PAF may be responsible for the late or protracted phase of anaphylaxis. Arachidonic acid metabolites, peptid-leukotrienes (LTC4, LTD4, and LTE4), are powerful coronary vasoconstrictors in guinea pigs, rats, and monkeys. In humans, peptid-leukotrienes can induce transient hypotension, increased heart rate, and coronary artery vasoconstriction.

Felix SB, Bauman G, Hashemi T, et al: Characterization of cardiovascular events mediated by the platelet activating factor during systemic anaphylaxis. J Cardiovasc Pharmacol 6:987–997, 1990.

59. **What agents may contribute to the release of vasoactive mediators from mast cells?**
The antigens and various other agents such as protamine, general anesthetics, and intravenous contrast media can be involved in the anaphylactoid reaction and can directly activate cardiac mast cells, thus leading to the release of vasoactive mediators. Clinically anaphylaxis has been associated with myocardial ischemia and infarction, ST-T wave abnormalities on the EKG, atrial and ventricular arrhythmias, and conduction abnormalities.

60. **Why is the detection of anaphylaxis during general anesthesia usually delayed?**
Detection of anaphylaxis during general anesthesia may be delayed due to patient's inability to verbalize initial symptoms. Clinical features of urticaria and erythema can be masked by the drapes used during the surgical procedure. Furthermore, anesthetics can directly produce hemodynamic instability without causing anaphylactic or anaphylactoid response.

Moscicki RA, Sockin SM, Corsello BF, et al: Anaphylaxis during induction of general anesthesia: Subsequent evaluation and management. J Allergy Clin Immunol 86:325–332, 1990.

61. **What symptoms and signs aid in the detection of anaphylaxis during general anesthesia?**
Often the early observable clinical features of anaphylaxis during general anesthesia include sudden onset of hypotension, bronchospasm, and sudden oxygen desaturation or increased airway pressure. Elevated serum beta tryptase is helpful in diagnosis of anaphylactic reaction.

62. **List the probable causes of anaphylaxis during general anesthesia.**
Because many drugs are administered over a very short time in the perioperative period, it may difficult to determine a causative agent. However, the following commonly used drugs have been implicated:
   - Thiopental
   - Muscle relaxants (e.g., succinylcholine)
   - Opioids
   - Intravenous antibiotics
   - Hypertonic intravenous solutions (e.g., mannitol)
   - Blood products
   - Intravenous radiocontrast material (RCM)
   - Latex
   - Ethylene oxide (used for gas sterilization of medical and surgical equipment)
   - Topical antibiotics (Bacitracin)

63. **How common is thiopental-induced anaphylaxis? Are other intravenous hypnotics equally implicated?**
The incidence of anaphylaxis secondary to thiopental is 1:400–1:30,000. Other intravenous hypnotics, such as ketamine and etomidate, are rarely the cause of systemic allergic reaction.

64. **By what mechanism do muscle relaxants produce anaphylaxis?**
Muscle relaxants may produce dose-dependent, non-IgE-mediated release of mediators. In some cases there is evidence for the IgE-mediated mechanism.

65. **By what mechanism do opioids produce anaphylaxis?**
Systemic reactions to the opioids are due to direct (non-IgE-mediated) mediator release.

66. **Can bone cement cause anaphylaxis?**
Bone cement (methylmethacrylate) has been known to cause hypotension, hypoxia, and noncardiogenic pulmonary edema. The mechanism is unknown.

67. **What is the incidence of serious systemic anaphylactic reaction due to allergen immunotherapy?**
In the United States the incidence of fatal reactions due to immunotherapy have been reported to be 1 fatality per 2 million injections. Frequency of severe systemic reactions ranges from < 1% in patients receiving conventional immunotherapy to ≥ 36% in patients treated with rush immunotherapy.

68. **List the potential risk factors for fatal or near-fatal anaphylactic reactions due to the allergen immunotherapy.**
   - Poorly controlled asthma
   - High pretreatment sensitivity to aeroallergens
   - Compromised pulmonary functions
   - Concurrent use of beta-adrenergic blocking agents

69. **What is the pretreatment recommendation for prevention of anaphylactoid reaction to RCM?**
In patients with a history of anaphylactoid reactions to RCM, pretreatment with oral glucocorticoids, H_1 and H_2 antihistamines, and ephedrine has been recommended for prevention of recurrent reaction. Use of radiocontrast material with low osmolality is also highly recommended. If possible, beta-adrenergic blocking agents and ACE inhibitors should be discontinued before the procedure.

70. **Outline a specific regimen for use of each of these agents.**
    - Prednisone, 50 mg, is given orally 13 hours, 7 hours, and 1 hour before RCM administration.
    - Diphenhydramine, 50 mg, is given orally or intramuscularly 1 hour before the procedure.
    - Ephedrine, 25 mg (when not contraindicated), is given orally 1 hour before administration of RCM.

    Modification of this regimen includes additional use of H_2 antihistamine, a lower dose of corticosteroids, and exclusion of ephedrine.

71. **What approach is recommended in emergency situations?**
    In emergency situations, 200 mg of hydrocortisone every 4 hours and 50 mg of diphenhydramine intramuscularly 1 hour before the procedure has proved successful.

72. **Should a patient with history of topical sensitivity to iodine be given pretreatment before undergoing a procedure requiring RCM?**
    Patients with topical sensitivity to iodine are not at increased risk for the RCM reaction. Therefore, no pretreatment is needed.

73. **What is the role of monoclonal anti-IgE therapy in the treatment of peanut-induced anaphylaxis?**
    Recent studies suggest that, when treated with monoclonal anti-IgE therapy, patients with a history of peanut-induced anaphylaxis experience at least partial protection from accidental peanut ingestion.

74. **Describe the possible mechanism of action.**
    Humanized anti-IgE is a monoclonal antibody against IgE that binds with high affinity to epitope in the CH3 domain of IgE, thus preventing IgE from binding to the high-affinity IgE receptors on mast cells and basophils. In addition, it also downregulates the expression of FcεRI on human basophils and may inhibit allergen-specific activation of T cell through interference with the processing of antigen-presenting cells mediated by the FcεRII or FcεRI.

75. **Specify the three keys to successful management of an episode of acute anaphylaxis/anaphylactoid reaction in the emergency department.**
    Early recognition, prompt treatment, and close observation are the keys to the successful management of anaphylaxis. Because anaphylactic reactions may vary from mild localized urticaria and pruritus to severe hypotension, airway obstruction, and cardiovascular collapse, initial treatment should be determined by the clinical features on presentation and by a high index of suspicion. After treatment, the strategy can be modified as necessary.

76. **What immediate interventions are recommended in the emergency department?**
    1. Quickly assess the patient, including airways, vital signs, and level of consciousness.
    2. Establish and maintain oropharyngeal airway and administer oxygen (5–6 L/min).
    3. Promptly administer aqueous epinephrine, the most important drug for the treatment of anaphylaxis. The adult dosage is 0.3–0.5 mL (of 1:1000 aqueous solution); for children, give 0.01 mL/kg body weight intramuscularly. This dosage can be repeated every 5 minutes as necessary. In life-threatening anaphylaxis, epinephrine can be administered intravenously in 1:10,000 or higher dilution at slow rate.

77. **What specific measure is recommended for anaphylaxis due to injection?**
    Place the tourniquet above the injection site and infiltrate the site with 0.10–0.20 mL of epinephrine (1:1000) to slow further absorption of injected medication.

78. **What are the recommendations for diphenhydramine and ranitidine?**
Diphenhydramine, 25–50 mg given intravenously, is recommended for adults; for children, give 1–2 mg/kg body weight. In mild cases the drug may be given orally.
   Ranitidine, 50 mg in adults and 12.5–50 mg (1 mg/kg) in children, is administered intravenously in 5% dextrose solution. Alternatively, cimetidine (4 mg/kg) may be administered in adults.

79. **Summarize the role of systemic glucocorticosteroids.**
Systemic glucocorticosteroids, such as methylprednisolone (1–2 mg/kg per 24 hours) should be given intravenously. Mild cases can be treated with oral prednisone. Corticosteroids are usually not helpful acutely but may prevent protracted reactions and/or relapses.

80. **How are bronchospasm, hypotension, and reflex bradycardia treated?**
   - **Bronchospasm** may be treated with nebulized albuterol.
   - **Hypotension** is treated with intravenous fluids and vasopressors. Dopamine is the vasopressor of choice.
   - **Reflex bradycardia** is treated with atropine.

81. **What special issues apply to patients receiving beta-adrenergic blockers?**
Patient receiving beta-adrenergic blockers may not respond to epinephrine. In addition to intravenous fluids, they may be treated with 1 mg of glucagon, administered intravenously slowly, followed by continuous infusion at the rate of 1–5 mg/hour.

82. **What is the best route for administration of epinephrine during the treatment of anaphylaxis?**
Intramuscular administration is the route of choice for the treatment of an acute anaphylactic reaction. Recently published reports suggest that absorption of epinephrine is complete and more rapid in children who receive epinephrine intramuscularly in the thigh with an autoinjector. Comparative studies in adults also show that higher peak plasma levels are achieved when epinephrine is injected intramuscularly into the lateral thigh rather than either intramuscularly or subcutaneously in the deltoid region of the arm.
   Simons FER, Gu X, Simons KJ: Epinephrine absorption in adults: Intramuscular versus subcutaneous injection. J Allergy Clin Immunol 108:871–873, 2001.

WEBSITES

1. Food Allergy and Anaphylaxis Network: www.foodallergy.org
2. National Library of Medicine: www.nlm.nih.gov

BIBLIOGRAPHY

1. Burstein M, Rubinow A, Shalit M: Cyclic anaphylaxis associated with menstruation. Ann Allergy 66:36–38, 1991.
2. Douglas DM, Sukenick E, Andrade WP, Brown JS: Biphasic anaphylaxis: An inpatient and outpatient study. J Allergy Cin Immunol 93(6):977–985, 1994.
3. Felix SB, Bauman G, Hashemi T, et al: Characterization of cardiovascular events mediated by the platelet activating factor during systemic anaphylaxis. J Cardiovasc Pharmacol 6:987–997, 1990.

4. Felix SB, Baumann G, Helmus S, Sattelberger U: Role of histamine in the cardiac anaphylaxis: Characterization of histaminergic H_1 and H_2 receptor effects. Basic Res Cardiol 5:531–539, 1988.

5. Fisher MM: Clinical observation on the pathophysiology and treatment of anaphylactic cardiovascular collapse. Anesth Intens Care 14:14–21, 1986.

6. Hogan AD, Schwartz LB: Markers of mast cell degranulation. Methods 13:43–52, 1997

7. Horan RF, Austen KF: Systemic mastocytosis: Retrospective review of a decade of clinical experience at the Bringham and Women's Hospital. J Invest Dermatol 96:5S–14S, 1991.

8. Horan RF, Sheffer AL: Food-dependent, exercise-induced anaphylaxis. Immunol Allergy Clin North Am 11:757, 1991.

9. Kemp SF, Lockey RF: Anaphylaxis: A review of causes and mechanisms. J Allergy Clin Immunol 110:341–348, 2002.

10. Kemp SF, Lockey RF, Wolf BL, Lieberman P: Anaphylaxis: A review of 266 cases. Arch Intern Med 155:1749–1751, 1995.

11. Leung DY, Sampson HA, Yunginger JW, et al: Effect of anti-IgE therapy in patients with peanut allergy. N Engl J Med 348:986–993, 2003.

12. Marshal CP, Pearson FC, Sagona MA, et al: Reaction during hemodialysis caused by allergy to ethylene oxide gas sterlization. J Allergy Clin Immunol 75:285–290, 1985.

13. Moraes PS, Taketomi EA: Allergic vulvovaginitis. Ann Allergy Asthma Immunol 85:253–265, 2000.

14. Moscicki RA, Sockin SM, Corsello BF, et al: Anaphylaxis during induction of general anesthesia: Subsequent evaluation and management. J Allergy Clin Immunol 86:325–332, 1990.

15. Nicklas RA, et al: Editors' diagnosis and management of anaphylaxis. J Allergy Clin Immunol 101(6 Part 2), 1998.

16. Park JW, Ko SH, Kim CW: Seminal plasma anaphylaxis: Successful pregnancy after intravaginal desensitization and immunodetection of allergens. Allergy 54:990–993, 1999.

17. Patterson R, Clayton DE, et al: Fatal and near fatal idiopathic anaphylaxis. Allergy Proc 16(3):103–108, 1995.

18. Ring J, Behrendt H: Anaphylaxis and anaphylactoid reactions: Classification and pathophysiology. Clin Rev Allergy Immunol 17:469–496, 1999.

19. Sampson HA: Anaphylaxis and emergency treatment. Pediatrics 111:1601–1608, 2003.

20. Sampson HA: Fatal food-induced anaphylaxis. Allergy 53 (Suppl 46):125–130, 1998.

21. Schwartz LB: Tryptase: A clinical indicator of mast cell-dependent events. Allergy Proc 15(3):119–123, 1994.

22. Sheffer AL, Austen KF: Exercise-induced anaphylaxis. J Allergy Clin Immunol 66:106–111, 1980.

23. Simons FER, Roberts JR, GU X, Simons KJ: Epinephrine absorption in children with history of anaphylaxis. J Alergy Clin Immunol 101:33–38, 1998.

24. Simons FER, Gu X, Simons KJ: Epinephrine absorption in adults: Intramuscular versus subcutaneous injection. J Allergy Clin Immunol 108:871–873, 2001.

25. Simpson JK, Metcalfe DD: Mastocytosis and disorders of mast cell proliferation. Clin Rev Allergy Immunol 22:175–188, 2002.

26. Slater JE, Kaliner M: Effects of sex hormones on the histamine release in the recurrent idiopathic anaphylaxis. J Allergy Clin Immunol 80:285–290, 1987.

27. Stark BJ, Sullivan TJ: Biphasic and protracted anaphylaxis. J Allergy Clin Immunol 78:76, 1986.

28. Stevenson DD: Diagnosis, prevention, and treatment of adverse reactions to aspirin and nonsteroidal anti-inflammatory drugs. J Allergy Clin Immunol 74:617–622, 1984.

29. Wasserman SL: The heart in anaphylaxis. J Allergy Clin Immunol 77:663–666, 1986.

30. Yocum MW, Butterfield JH, Klien JS, et al: Epidemiology of anaphylaxis in Olmsted County: A population-based study. J Allergy Clin Immunol 104:452–456, 1999.

CHAPTER 12

AUTOIMMUNE DISEASE

Gurtej S. Cheema, M.D.

1. **Define autoimmunity.**

The human immune system is composed of several different types of cells and molecules with specific functions aimed at defending the body against infection. Only the cells that are able to distinguish between self and non-self antigens are allowed to get into the peripheral circulation. The process by which the autoreactive cells are eliminated or neutralized is known as tolerance. Any breakdown of this procedure can result in the immune system misdirecting its response against the body itself. These aberrant responses of the immune system are referred to as autoimmunity.

Marrack P, Kappler J, Kotzin BL: Autoimmune disease: Why and where it occurs. Nature Med 7:899–905, 2001.

2. **Is all autoreactivity pathologic?**

No. In fact, a low level of autoimmunity is actually considered to be crucial to normal immune function. Autoimmunity can be demonstrated by the presence of autoantibodies or T lympho- cytes reactive to the host antigen.

3. **Name the most important components of the immune system.**

The most obvious and visible part of the immune system is the skin. It, along with the mucosal tissue, houses the highly specialized cells known as the dendritic cells. They act as antigen- presenting cells. The thymus (in infants), spleen, lymphatics, complement components, and white blood cells (both T and the B lymphocytes) comprise the immune system.

4. **Name the different types of T lymphocytes.**

T cells are responsible for providing specific cellular immunity. There are several different phe- notypic subpopulations of T-cells with a diverse set of functions. These include:
1. CD4-positive
   - T helper 1 (Th1)
   - T helper 2 (Th2)
2. CD8-positive or cytotoxic T cells
3. Natural killer cells (NK cells)

5. **Describe the functions of Th1 cells.**

After stimulation with specific antigen on the surface of antigen-presenting cells (APCs) in com- plex with the components of major histocompatibility class II (MHC II), Th1 cells acquire their specificity and exert functions of helper T cells. They help B cells in antibody production, activa- tion of macrophages, and production of proinflammatory cytokines interleukin (IL)-2 and interferon (IFN)-gamma.

6. **What is the function of Th2 cells?**

After stimulation Th2 cells produce anti-inflammatory cytokines such as IL-4, IL-5, and IL-10 and participate in the anti-inflammatory and suppressor functions of T cells.

7. **What is the function of CD8-positive T cells?**
   CD8 membrane antigen-positive cells also acquire their specificity in contact with APCs, but in association with the components of MHC class I. They exert predominantly functions of cyto-toxic T-cells (CTLs), killing specific foreign cells.

8. **How do NK cells function?**
   NK cells also kill foreign cells, but their actions are quite nonspecific.

9. **Summarize the process by which T cells are activated.**
   T cells are activated by a highly complex series of events that is initiated as a result of the cross-linking of the antigen receptor on the cell surface. After a string of interactions, a number of different biochemical pathways downstream are activated, leading to cellular proliferation and differentiation. Different T cells along with NK cells, B cells, macrophages, and dendritic cells, are responsible for providing immune surveillance and maintaining immunologic homeostasis in the human body.

10. **Discuss the role of B cells in the immune system.**
    B cells are responsible for providing *humoral* immunity, so called because B cells generate soluble proteins, the immunoglobulins, found in the *humors* (blood). All B cells have one or another type of immunoglobulin molecule on their surface. Each immunoglobulin molecule has the ability to recognize a specific epitope. Circulating immunoglobulins are also referred to as antibodies.

11. **What is an epitope?**
    An epitope is a unique three-dimensional configuration consisting of different amino acids on the antigen surface that give it a specific identity.
    Dighiero G, Rose NR: Critical self-epitopes are key to the understanding of self-tolerance and autoimmunity. Immunol Today 20: 423–428, 1999.

12. **Explain the process of clonal selection.**
    B cells capable of detecting the appropriate antigen with the help of their surface immunoglobu-lin are eventually activated. They then proliferate, resulting in a large population of cells that secrete immunoglobulin targeting the specific antigen. Activated B-cell clone differentiates into plasma cells and memory cells.

13. **What are the differences between plasma cells and memory cells?**
    Plasma cells are B cells that produce a specific antibody that is then able to bind the stimulatory antigen. They are able to generate up to 2000 antibody molecules in a second. However, their life span is limited to 5–7 days.
    Memory cells are B cells that are maintained in the circulation for as long as decades. They are responsible for a rapid secondary response to an antigenic stimulus that they are able to recognize.

14. **Describe the process of central B-cell tolerance to self-antigens.**
    Immature B cells are the earliest cell type in the lineage to express antigen-specific B cell receptors (BCRs). Selection against autoreactive B cells begins at this stage of development and takes place in the bone marrow. A functional BCR binds extracellular molecules and initiates antigen-specific cytoplasmic signaling. If the B cell does not bind with the antigen, BCR signaling remains at a basal level, and the cell enters the transitional stage for release into the peripheral circulation. If the immature B cell encounters extracellular antigen capable of cross-linking its BCR, it experiences an increase in BCR-mediated signaling, accompanied by developmental arrest.

15. **What are the consequences of B-cell developmental arrest?**
    Developmental arrest indicates that the B cell has responded to an autoantigen and will be blocked from further development. In addition, the B cell initiates the receptor editing process to produce BCR with new antigen-binding specificities. If it cannot alter its BCR effectively, the

immature B cell is deleted by apoptosis to prevent development into an autoreactive mature B cell. Some autoreactive B cell clones escape deletion and enter the peripheral circulation in an anergic state. These cells are not responsive to antigen stimulation but potentially can be activated with pathogen-derived ligands that mimic the autoantigen.

Marrack P, Kappler J, Kotzin BL: Autoimmune disease: Why and where it occurs. Nature Med 7:899–905, 2001.

16. **Describe the process of inducing peripheral B-cell tolerance.**
B cells, like the T cells, continue to undergo surveillance peripherally to purge self-reactive cells in order to maintain tolerance. After leaving the bone marrow, the relatively immature B cells migrate to the outer T-cell zone of the spleen. Most of the negative selection of B cells takes place in the splenic environment. These cells are cleared by a process that (1) induces anergy; (2) prevents migration of these cells into B-cell follicles; and (3) accelerates apoptosis. The lifespan of self-reactive B cells in the spleen is only about 1–3 days. However, some self-reactive anergic B cells can still bind to high-avidity antigens, thereby contributing to the immune response against foreign antigens. These cells then can be recruited to the immune repertoire.

Mackay IR: Tolerance and autoimmunity. BMJ 321:93–96, 2000.

17. **What conditions are required for activation of naive B cells by T lymphocyte-dependent antigens?**
Most protein antigens require the presence of T cells to recognize the immune system. In order for naive B lymphocytes to proliferate, differentiate, and mount an antibody response against T lymphocyte–dependent antigens, the B cells need to interact with the CD4-positive T lymphocytes.

18. **Describe the two steps in activation of B lymphocytes.**
The **first step** is the binding of surface immunoglobulin molecule on the B cell, which also functions as the B-cell receptor (BCR), with the epitope of the T cell-dependent antigen.

The **second step** involves the binding of complement component C3b to the complement receptor on the B-cell surface. These events activate the naïve B-lymphocytes, which results in increased expression of MHC II costimulatory molecules, such as B7 and CD40, and receptors for T lymphocyte–derived cytokines on its cell surface.

19. **What happens after the antigen is engulfed by the B lymphocytes?**
After being engulfed by the B lymphocytes, the antigen is degraded into peptides by the lysosomes. Just as in the case of macrophages and dendritic cells, these peptides are then expressed in conjunction with the MHC II molecules on the surface of the B lymphocyte. These B lymphocytes can interact with the different subclasses of T lymphocytes, especially Th2 cells. This interaction occurs via the binding of costimulatory molecules, such as CD28 and CD40L, on the Th2 cell with the B7 and CD40 molecules on the B lymphocyte, respectively. This interaction stimulates the Th2 lymphocyte to secrete cytokines (e.g., IL-2, IL-4, IL-5, IL-6).

Marrack P, Kappler J, Kotzin BL: Autoimmune disease: Why and where it occurs. Nature Med 7:899–905, 2001.

20. **List the functions of the cytokines.**
The cytokines act simultaneously to fulfill the following functions:
- Help in proliferation of B cells
- Stimulate B cells to produce antibodies
- Promote differentiation of B lymphocytes into plasma cells
- Help antibody-producing cells to switch class of antibody being produced

21. **Discuss T lymphocyte–independent stimulation of B lymphocytes.**
Carbohydrates and lipid molecules activate the B lymphocytes in a process that is independent of T lymphocytes. Good examples of these antigens are the bacterial lipopolysaccharides from

the cell wall of gram-negative bacteria. These capsular polysaccharides are remarkable for multiple and repeating subunits.

22. **What are the two types of T lymphocyte–independent antigens?**
    Type 1 antigens are derived from the outer membranes of gram-negative cell wall and bacterial nucleic acid and stimulate the B lymphocyte via the specific toll-like receptors rather than the B cell receptors.

    Type 2 antigens, like the capsular polysaccharides, have multiple repeating subunits and stimulate the B lymphocytes by cross-linking several B-cell receptors together.

23. **Describe the process of inducing central tolerance in the T cells.**
    The central T-cell tolerance is the deletion of self-reactive T cells in the thymus. Immature T cells migrate from the bone marrow to the thymus, where they complete the assembly of their antigen-specific T cell receptor (TCR). The developing T cells are exposed to peptides derived from endogenous proteins (self-antigens) bound to major-histocompatibility-complex (MHC) molecule on the surface of the thymic epithelial cells and the dendritic cells derived from the bone marrow. Since the process occurs in the thymus, it is known as central tolerance. It therefore requires presence of self-antigens in the thymus.
    Mackay IR: Tolerance and autoimmunity. BMJ 321:93–96, 2000.

24. **What are the three possible outcomes of the above interactions?**
    1. Spontaneous apoptosis occurs if the TCR-MHC-peptide bond is absent or too weak.
    2. Negative selection may occur—i.e., a process leading to active deletion of the T cells with high-affinity bonding between the TCR-MHC-peptide culminating in cell death. This process removes T-cell clones that react too strongly with host molecules and pose a risk of autoimmunity.
    3. The remaining T cells, which have receptors with an intermediate affinity for TCR-MHC-peptide complexes, continue to develop into more specialized T-cell subsets.

25. **Why is peripheral T-cell tolerance also necessary?**
    Because not all self-antigens occur in the thymus, a peripheral mechanism that participates in T-cell tolerance is also necessary. Regulation of T-cell function continues to occur even after the T cell has left the thymus. This process is important to prevent breakdown of tolerance if the T cells encounter any self-antigen to which it was not exposed in the thymus (Fig. 12-1).

Generation of T Cells in Bone Marrow and Thymus

↓

Central Tolerance

(antiself lymphocytes deleted by negative selection)

↓

Leakage of antiself lymphocytes to periphery controlled by

↓

Peripheral Tolerance

↓

If tolerance fails due to wrong environment or wrong genes

↓

Autoimmune disease

Figure 12-1. Mechanisms of central and peripheral tolerance.

26. **List the three mechanisms by which peripheral T-cell tolerance prevents development of autoimmunity.**
Ignorance, deletion, and regulation.

27. **Explain the mechanism of ignorance.**
Usually potentially autoreactive T cells simply ignore their antigens, maintaining self-tolerance. This process may be mediated by several mechanisms, some of which are lack of sufficient antigen load, anatomic separation of the T cell from the antigen (e.g., blood-brain barrier), and absence of costimulatory molecules.

28. **Explain the mechanism of deletion.**
Peripheral deletion of self-reactive T cells may result from depletion of growth factors or activation of Fas molecule by its ligand. Stimulation of T cells in the absence of costimulatory molecules may also lead to cell death.

29. **Explain the mechanism of regulation.**
Anergic T cells are T cells that do not produce IL-2 on encountering their antigen. As a result, they cannot be activated adequately. These cells produce IL-10 instead, a potent suppressor of T-cell activation. Cytotoxic T-lymphocyte-associated protein 4 (CTLA-4) molecule on the surface of T cells binds to CD80 and CD86 molecules on B cells with a much greater affinity than to CD28 and results in inhibition of the T cells. Other T cells, like the CD4+ subtype, may suppress activated T cells. This process may have a protective role in the prevention of autoimmunity.
Mackay IR: Tolerance and autoimmunity. BMJ 321:93–96, 2000.

30. **Define autoimmune disease.**
Disease caused by breakdown of self-tolerance and subsequent immune response against self or autologous antigens, resulting in tissue injury, is called autoimmune disease. There are many theories to explain the development of autoimmune disease, and probably many mechanisms underlie the process. Autoimmune diseases can be caused by abnormal secretion of antibodies by activated B cells that bind to antigens in particular cells or by antigen-antibody complexes that form in the circulation and are then deposited in the blood vessel walls. Occasionally, T-lymphocytes may cause tissue injury either by directly killing target cells or by a delayed type of hypersensitivity reaction.
Marrack P, Kappler J, Kotzin BL: Autoimmune disease: Why and where it occurs. Nature Med 7:899–905, 2001.

31. **How common are autoimmune diseases?**
Autoimmune diseases affect approximately 3–5% of the population.

32. **List factors that predispose to the development of autoimmunity.**
  - Genetic factors
  - Person's age
  - Environmental factors such as infectious agents

33. **How are autoimmune diseases classified?**
Autoimmune diseases are generally classified on the basis of the organ or tissue involved (Table 12-1). These diseases may fall in an organ-specific category in which the immune response is directed against antigen(s) associated with the damaged target organ or a non–organ-specific category in which the antibody is directed against an antigen not associated with the target organ. The antigen involved in most autoimmune diseases is evident from the name of the disease. This classification, although clinically useful, does not does not necessarily correspond to difference in causation.

TABLE 12-1.	CLASSIFICATION OF AUTOIMMUNE DISEASES ON THE BASIS OF ORGAN INVOLVEMENT
Organ Involved	**Autoimmune Diseases**
Nervous system	Multiple sclerosis, myasthenia gravis, autoimmune neuropathies such as Guillain-Barré, autoimmune uveitis
Blood	Autoimmune hemolytic anemia, pernicious anemia, autoimmune thrombocytopenia
Skin	Psoriasis, dermatitis herpetiformis, pemphigus vulgaris, vitiligo
Gastrointestinal system	Crohn's disease, ulcerative colitis, primary biliary cirrhosis, autoimmune hepatitis
Endocrine	Type 1 or immune-mediated diabetes mellitus, Graves' disease, Hashimoto's thyroiditis, autoimmune oophoritis and orchitis, autoimmune disease of adrenal gland

A more useful division distinguishes between diseases associated with a general alteration in the selection, regulation, or death of T cells or B cells and diseases in which an aberrant response to a particular antigen, self or nonself, causes autoimmunity (Table 12-2).

34. **List the most common systemic autoimmune diseases.**
    - Rheumatoid arthritis
    - Systemic lupus erythematosus
    - Scleroderma
    - Polymyositis
    - Dermatomyositis
    - Sjögren's syndrome
    - Spondyloarthropathies (e.g., ankylosing spondylitis, Reiter's syndrome, psoriatic arthritis)
    - Vasculitides (e.g., polyarteritis nodosa, Wegener's granulomatosis, microscopic polyangiitis, giant-cell arteritis)
    - Insulin-resistant diabetes
    - Atopic allergy
    - Antiphospholipid syndrome

35. **What are cytokines?**
    Cytokines are a unique family of growth factors. Secreted primarily from leukocytes, cytokines stimulate the humoral and cellular immune responses as well as the activation of phagocytic cells. Cytokines that are secreted from lymphocytes are termed **lymphokines,** whereas those secreted by monocytes or macrophages are termed **monokines.** Many of the lymphokines are also known as interleukins (ILs), since they are not only secreted by leukocytes but also able to affect the cellular responses of leukocytes. Specifically, interleukins are growth factors targeted to cells of hematopoietic origin.

36. **Describe briefly the normal functions of cytokines.**
    Cytokines are involved as mediator molecules in normal biologic processes, including growth and differentiation of hematopoietic, lymphoid, and mesenchymal cells. They also play an important role in orchestrating host defense mechanisms. Multiple cytokines function as a network in a synergistic and self-regulated manner.

TABLE 12-2.   EXAMPLES OF ORGAN-SPECIFIC AND SYSTEMIC AUTOIMMUNE DISEASES WITH KNOWN AUTOANTIGEN TARGETS

Disease	Organ	Examples of Known Autoantigens	Mechanism of Damage	Prevalence (%)
Organ-specific autoimmune diseases				
Thyroiditis (autoimmune)	Thyroid	Thyroglobulin and thyroid peroxidase	T cells/antibody	1.0–2.0
Pernicious anemia	Stomach	Hydrogen/potassium, intrinsic factor	T cells/antibody	1–2% in > 6-yr-old
Celiac disease	Small bowel	Transglutaminase	T cells/antibody	0.2–1.1
Graves' disease	Thyroid	Thyroid-stimulating hormone receptor	Antibody	0.2–1.1
Vitiligo	Melanocytes	Tyrosinase, tyrosinase-related protein-2	T cells/antibody	0.4
Type 1 diabetes	Pancreas β cells	Insulin, glutamic acid decarboxylase	Antibody	0.2–0.4
Multiple sclerosis	Brain/spinal cord	Myelin basic protein, proteolipid protein	T cells	0.01–0.15
Pemphigus	Skin	Desmogleins (e.g., desmoglein 1)	T cells	< 0.01–> 3.0
Hepatitis (autoimmune)	Liver	Hepatocyte antigens (cytochrome P450)	T cells/antibody	< 0.01
Myasthenia gravis	Muscle	Acetylcholine receptor	Antibody	< 0.01
Primary biliary cirrhosis	Liver bile ducts	2-Oxoacid dehydroxegenase complexes	T cells/antibody	< 0.01
Systemic autoimmune diseases				
Rheumatoid arthritis	Joints, lungs, heart, others	IgG, filaggrin, fibrin, others	T cells in joints?/antibody	0.8
Systemic lupus erythematosus	Skin, joints, kidney, brain, lungs, heart, others	Nuclear antigens (DNA, histones, ribo-nucleoproteins, others)	Antibody	0.1
Polymyositis/dermatomyositis	Skeletal muscles, lungs, heart, joints, others	Muscle antigens, aminoacyl-tRNA synthetases, other nuclear antigens	T cells/antibody	< 0.01

37. **Describe the role of cytokines in the pathogenesis of autoimmune disease.**
    Several control mechanisms are in place to protect against pathogenic cytokine effects. Among them are transient duration of expression of the cytokines and their receptors and the production of cytokine antagonists and inhibitors. Breakdown of the these mechanisms leads to unregulated action or inappropriate production of certain cytokines, resulting in pathophysiologic consequences (Table 12-3). Cytokines have the ability to translate diverse etiologic factors into pathogenic forces and to maintain the chronic phase of inflammation and tissue destruction. IL-1 and TNF have received the most attention as cytokines that can lead to tissue degradation. Both these cytokines induce the expression of a series of proteases and may inhibit the formation of extracellular matrix or stimulate excessive matrix accumulation.

TABLE 12-3. DEFECTS IN CYTOKINE PRODUCTION OR SIGNALING THAT CAN LEAD TO AUTOIMMUNITY

Cytokine or Protein	Defect	Result
Tumor necrosis factor α	Overexpression	Inflammatory bowel disease, arthritis, vasculitis
Tumor necrosis factor α	Underexpression	Systemic lupus erythematosus
Interleukin-1-receptor antagonist	Underexpression	Arthritis
Interleukin-2	Overexpression	Inflammatory bowel disease
Interleukin-7	Overexpression	Inflammatory bowel disease
Interleukin-10	Overexpression	Inflammatory bowel disease
Interleukin-2 receptor	Overexpression	Inflammatory bowel disease
Interleukin-10 receptor	Overexpression	Inflammatory bowel disease
Interleukin-3	Overexpression	Demyelinating syndrome
Interferon-γ	Overexpression in skin	Systemic lupus erythematosus
Transforming growth factor β	Underexpression	Systemic wasting syndrome and inflammatory bowel disease
Transforming growth factor β receptor in T cells	Underexpression	Systemic lupus erythematosus

38. **Give an overview of the factors contributing to autoimmune disease.**
    The triggers for autoimmune diseases are diverse and include immunologic, genetic, viral, drug-induced, and hormonal factors, acting singly or in combination. Because so many different factors contribute to specific autoimmune diseases, a universal panacea for pathologic autoimmunity is unlikely to be described. These factors are best subdivided into two categories, the genetic and environmental.

39. **How important are genetic factors in autoimmune disease?**
    Genetic factors exert the most significant influence on an individual's predisposition to autoimmune disease. This statement is supported by the significantly increased prevalence of autoimmune diseases among relatives of patients with autoimmune diseases as opposed to estimates from the general population. The greater disease concordance among monozygotic twins compared with dizygotic twins also suggests a strong influence of genetic factors on disease susceptibility.

40. **Give examples of important MHC gene products involved in antigen presentation.**
The most important MHC gene products involved in antigen presentation are the class I molecules (HLA-A, HLA-B, and HLA-C) and the class II molecules (HLA-DR, HLA-DQ, and HLA-DP). These surface markers are highly polymorphic with more than 275 allelic variants now sequenced to the DNA level. Class I and II molecules consist of a light chain and a heavy chain that combine to form a peptide-binding site; the bound peptide is then presented to T-cell receptors. Differences in amino acid sequence in the HLA molecule can result in variation in the shape of the binding site. This variation can lead to differences in binding affinity. Thus, genetic variation in HLA molecular structure generates profound effects on antigen presentation. These factors probably account for some association between HLA phenotype and certain autoimmune diseases.

41. **What other genetic factors may be involved in vulnerability to autoimmune disease?**
Defects in the structure and expression of cytokines and their receptors, polymorphisms in transporter genes, and interference with apoptosis genes and their polypeptide products also contribute to increased vulnerability to autoimmune disease.

42. **Discuss the importance of infection as an environmental factor involved in the development autoimmune disease.**
Among the major environmental risk factors, infection seems to be the most important. It can initiate an autoimmune disease by disrupting peripheral tolerance in ways that include exposure of self to the immune system through breakdown of vascular or cellular barriers; the occurrence of cell death by necrosis rather than apoptosis; "bystander" activation of macrophages and T lymphocytes, which can then provide costimulatory signals; and superantigen effects of bacterial products. Infection seems to trigger autoimmunity in people with a genetic predisposition.

43. **What is molecular mimicry?**
Molecular mimicry, whereby an antigen of a microorganism or a constituent of food that sufficiently resembles a self-molecule can induce a cross-reactive autoimmune response, has been thought of an alternative process. Despite some experimental evidence, this hypothesis has not been documented as leading to autoimmune disease in humans.

44. **Discuss other environmental factors in the development of autoimmune disease.**
Other environmental initiators of autoimmunity can act like infections (1) by causing tissue damage, such as sunlight in lupus erythematosus, or (2) by altering a host molecule sufficiently for it to become immunogenic, as in chemical or drug-induced autoimmune syndromes. Procainamide induces antinuclear antibodies and may sometimes also cause systemic lupus-like syndrome. Again, a permissive genetic background is also necessary in such circumstances.

45. **Explain the role of the internal environment in the development of autoimmune disease.**
Autoimmunity may arise entirely from within. An intracellular self-molecule may become in some way aberrantly expressed at the cell surface. Paraneoplastic autoimmune associations and hormonal disturbances are common examples.

46. **What are paraneoplastic autoimmune associations?**
The internal environment accounts for paraneoplastic autoimmune associations of cancers of the ovary, lung, and breast, in which an antigen associated with the tumor provokes autoimmune responses that damages structures such as cerebellar, motor, or sensory neurons; nerve terminals, as in the Lambert-Eaton myasthenic syndrome; or retinal cells. These syndromes reflect a misguided immune defense against the cancer since they usually precede overt expression of the cancer and even limit dissemination.

47. **How can hormones affect autoimmunity?**
Hormones have been implicated in the female predisposition to autoimmunity. Estrogen exacerbates systemic lupus erythematosus in murine models by altering B cell repertoire in the absence of inflammation. Autoimmune thyroid disease and type 1 diabetes sometimes erupt in the postpartum period. Effects of psychological stress that may act via neuroendocrine pathways are not well defined.

48. **Describe the mechanisms of immunologic tissue injury in different autoimmune diseases.**
Immune responses cause disease when they are directed against self-antigens. The various mechanisms by which tissue damage occurs include deposition of antibodies in tissue, T lymphocyte–mediated delayed-type hypersensitivity reactions, and direct killing of target cells by T lymphocytes.

49. **How are autoimmune diseases mediated by antibody production?**
   1. By production of antibodies directed against antigens in particular cells or tissues
   2. By deposition of antigen-antibody (immune) complexes in circulation in the vessel walls
      Davidson A, Diamond B: Autoimmune diseases. N Engl J Med 345:340–350, 2000.

50. **Which diseases result from targeting of cellular or extracellular antigens by antibodies?**
Diseases resulting from targeting of certain cellular or extracellular antigens by antibodies are usually limited to specific organs. Generally these antibodies are autoantibodies, but in some cases they may be directed against foreign antigens that may cross-react with some component of self tissue. Examples of such diseases include autoimmune hemolytic anemia, thrombocytopenic purpura, Graves' disease, myasthenia gravis, acute rheumatic fever, Goodpasture's syndrome, and pernicious anemia.

KEY POINTS: AUTOIMMUNE DISEASE

1. T cells are responsible for cell-mediated immunity.

2. Induction of peripheral B-cell tolerance is essential in maintaining immune surveillance against foreign antigens but not against self-antigens.

3. Central T-cell tolerance is the result of deletion of self-reactive T cells in the thymus.

4. Autoimmune diseases affect approximately 3–5% of the population.

5. Direct killing by cytotoxic T cells occurs primarily in cells infected by virus. Examples include hepatitis B– and coxsackie B–induced myocarditis.

51. **List the three mechanisms by which antibodies can cause disease.**
   - Opsonization and phagocytosis
   - Complement and Fc-receptor interaction
   - Initiation of abnormal physiologic responses

52. **Explain opsonization and phagocytosis.**
Antibodies can activate the complement system and thus opsonize the target cells, resulting in their phagocytosis. Autoimmune hemolytic anemia and thrombocytopenic purpura are two examples of diseases caused by this mechanism.

53. **Explain complement and Fc-receptor interaction.**

Antibodies can recruit the neutrophils and macrophages into the target tissues by binding with either the antibodies or attached complement proteins by Fc or complement receptors. This interaction results in release of byproducts that are chemotactic for leukocytes and also cause tissue damage and disease.

54. **How can antibodies cause abnormal physiologic responses?**

Antibodies may compete with physiologic proteins to bind with cellular receptors, thus interfering with the normal functioning of these receptors. Thus disease may result without actual tissue damage. Graves' disease and myasthenia gravis occur by this mechanism.

55. **How does deposition of antigen-antibody complexes in the circulation of vessel walls cause autoimmune disease?**

Immune complexes consist of an antigen, which may be self or foreign, linked to the antibody. These complexes are produced in the course of the normal immune process. They result in disease only when there is a problem with their clearance or when they are produced in excessive amounts. Clinical manifestations of the diseases caused by immune complexes depend on the site of their deposition in the target tissue and not on the source of the antigen. Therefore, these conditions tend to be systemic without any specific preference for any organ or tissue.

Davidson A, Diamond B: Autoimmune diseases. N Engl J Med 345:340–350, 2000.

56. **What are the most common sites of immune complex deposition?**

The most common sites of immune complex deposits are the capillaries in the renal glomeruli and the synovium. Such deposits may trigger a local inflammatory response, causing cell adhesion and increased vascular permeability. The pathogenesis of some diseases (e.g., systemic lupus erythematosus, polyarteritis nodosa, post-streptococcal glomerulonephritis) involve the deposition of immune complexes in blood vessel walls.

57. **Which diseases are triggered by T lymphocytes?**

Tissue injury due to T-cell activation usually involves a delayed-type hypersensitivity reaction or direct killing of target cells.

58. **Which cells are involved in delayed-type hypersensitivity reaction?**

The cells involved in delayed-type hypersensitivity reaction are the macrophages. They release cytokines, hydrolytic enzymes, nitric oxide, and reactive oxygen intermediates such as superoxide anion radicals and hydrogen peroxide molecules. Under the influence of various cytokines and growth factors, chronic delayed-type hypersensitivity ultimately results in fibrosis. Clinically, delayed-type hypersensitivity reaction plays an important role in the pathogenesis of diseases such as insulin-dependent diabetes mellitus, multiple sclerosis, and rheumatoid arthritis.

59. **How does direct killing occur?**

Direct killing by cytolytic T lymphocytes is seen mostly in cases in which the cells are infected by a virus. Direct killing occurs even if the virus itself does not have any cytopathic effect. Hepatitis B infection in humans results in liver inflammation as a result of such cytolytic T lymphocyte response. Another example in humans is myocarditis associated with coxsackie B virus.

60. **List the common organ-specific autoimmune diseases.**

1. Diseases resulting from immune response to a specific antigen in an organ:
   - Hashimoto's thyroiditis
   - Autoimmune anemias

- Goodpasture's syndrome
- Type 1 (insulin-dependent) diabetes mellitus
2. Diseases resulting from autoantibodies acting as antagonists or agonists of hormone receptors
   - Graves' disease
   - Myasthenia gravis

61. Discuss the salient features of Hashimoto's thyroiditis.

Hashimoto's thyroiditis is more common in middle-aged women and is characterized by production of antibodies and T lymphocytes reactive against thyroid antigens. Patients mount a delayed-type hypersensitivity reaction in the thyroid. The antibodies are produced mainly against thyroglobulin and thyroid peroxidase, which are involved in iodine uptake in the thyroid. The eventual results is hypothyroidism.

62. What causes autoimmune anemias?

Pernicious anemia results from production of autoantibodies against the intrinsic factor, which is a protein expressed in the intestinal epithelium that facilitates the absorption of vitamin B_{12}. This vitamin is essential for hematopoiesis. Other anemias result from antibody response against red blood cell antigens. These antigens induce activation of complement and eventually hemolysis. They may induce opsonization of red blood cells as well.

63. What is Goodpasture's syndrome?

Goodpasture's syndrome is caused by production of autoantibodies against basement membrane antigens of the kidney glomeruli and the alveoli of the lungs. The antibodies activate complement, causing tissue damage. The end results are a rapidly progressive glomerulonephritis in the kidney, intra-alveolar hemorrhage, and septal fibrosis in the lungs.

64. Explain the autoimmune mechanism of type 1 (insulin-dependent) diabetes mellitus.

The attack on insulin-producing beta cells in the pancreas is initiated by activated cytotoxic T lymphocytes (CTLs) that target specific islets for lysis. The CTL activity triggers the release of cytokines, which in turn stimulate the proliferation of activated macrophages and autoantibodies that are attracted to the site of inflammation. The autoantibodies, together with complement-mediated lysis as well as macrophage and CTL activity, are responsible for the overall destruction of pancreatic tissue and create the ensuing pathology. Type 1 diabetes may account for 5% to 10% of all diagnosed cases of diabetes.

65. Explain the basic autoimmune mechanism of Graves' disease.

Patients produce autoantibodies against the receptor for thyroid-stimulating hormone (TSH). This hormone, which is produced in the pituitary gland, induces the production of thyroid hormones. Binding of the autoantibodies to the receptor mimics the normal action of TSH, leading to an overproduction of thyroid hormones.

66. What causes myasthenia gravis? How common is the disease?

Myasthenia gravis is characterized by production of autoantibodies against acetylcholine receptors on the motor end-plates of muscles. The autoantibodies block the normal binding of acetylcholine to its receptor and induce complement-mediated degradation of the receptors. Myasthenia gravis occurs in about 5 people per 100,000 population.

67. Discuss the symptoms of myasthenia gravis.

Patients experience weakness that fluctuates with activity. It may be limited to the facial muscles, resulting in difficulty in chewing, swallowing, smiling, and talking. It especially affects the ocular muscles, causing ptosis. More severe cases may affect all of the skeletal or voluntary muscles, including those that control breathing, coughing, and arm and leg movements.

68. **List the common systemic autoimmune diseases.**
- Systemc lupus erythemtosus (SLE)
- Multiple sclerosis (MS)
- Rheumatoid arthritis
- Scleroderma

69. **Summarize the most important features of systemic lupus erythematosus.**
SLE typically appears in women aged 20–40 years. It is more common in African American and Hispanic women than in Caucasians. Patients have autoantibodies against several antigens, including DNA, histones, red blood cells, platelets, leukocytes, and clotting factors. Patients may develop glomerulonephritis, arthritis, and vasculitis.

70. **Describe the nature and cause of multiple sclerosis.**
MS most often is characterized by episodes of neurologic dysfunction followed by periods of stabilization or partial-to-complete remission of symptoms. A relapsing-remitting pattern is the most common manifestation. MS is caused by the production of autoreactive T cells that attack myelin of the central nervous system.

71. **Summarize the epidemiology of multiple sclerosis.**
In general, women are affected at almost twice the rate as men. Caucasians are more than twice as likely as others to develop the disease. MS is five times more prevalent in temperate climates, such as the northern United States, than in tropical regions. Children of patients with MS have a risk of developing the condition 10 times higher than the general population.

72. **What causes rheumatoid arthritis?**
Most patients produce a group of autoantibodies called rheumatoid factors, which react against the Fc region of IgG. These IgM autoantibodies bind circulating IgG molecules. The complexes are then deposited in the joints, inducing a type III hypersensitivity reaction, which leads to chronic inflammation. The predominant symptom is chronic inflammation of joints.

73. **In what population is rheumatoid arthritis most common?**
Rheumatoid arthritis is most common in women 40–60 years old.

74. **Summarize the most important features of scleroderma.**
The most common symptom is tightening of the skin, usually in hands, feet, and face. Other features include interstitial lung disease and pulmonary hypertension. The cause is not known, but a recent study suggests that in some cases the immune reaction is against fetal cells still circulating in the mother.

75. **Give the two basic strategies for management of autoimmune diseases.**
Management of autoimmune diseases has been directed toward either (1) managing the consequences of the condition (e.g., insulin replacement in patients with diabetes mellitus, joint replacement in patients with rheumatoid arthritis) or (2) suppressing the aberrant immune response.

76. **What are the goals of suppressing the aberrant immune response?**
This strategy may focus on a nonspecific immunosuppression with the main goal of preserving organ function or target specific molecules involved in the pathogenesis to minimize the risks associated with a shotgun approach. There has been significant advancement in terms of identifying such appropriate targets in different autoimmune diseases.

77. **What major advances have been made in the treatment of rheumatoid arthritis?**
Management of rheumatoid arthritis has undergone a major change since the benefits of instituting early treatment were recognized. Methotrexate remains the first-line immunosuppressive

agent; however, introduction of newer therapies targeting specific cytokines such as TNF-α and their receptors (e.g., interleukin 1 receptors) has greatly improved the outcome of treatment. Long-term safety of these agents, particularly with respect to infections, cancer, and other autoimmune diseases, remains to be ascertained.

78. **Summarize the approach to treatment of systemic lupus erythematosus.**
Because SLE is a highly heterogeneous disease, its management has depended on the clinical manifestations. Patients with mostly cutaneous involvement respond well to antimalarial agents such as hydroxychloroquine and chloroquine. At the other end of the spectrum, in patients with major organ involvement (e.g., brain, kidneys, lungs), immunosuppression with high doses of corticosteroids and other drugs such as cyclohosphamide, azathioprin, and mycophenolate mofetil is often necessary. Intravenous infusions of IgG have also been found to be useful in some cases resistant to conventional therapy. Therapy targeting cytokines and their receptors is still in its evolutionary phase; several clinical trials are under way.

79. **What advancements have been made in the treatment of multiple sclerosis?**
The availability of interferon β-1a and glatiramer acetate (copolymer I) has greatly improved the outcome of disease in a majority of patients. Some studies indicate that early use of interferon β-1a may be effective in delaying the onset of obvious clinical symptoms of MS. Glatiramer acetate, which is a nonspecific inhibitor or T lymphocytes in vitro, may also act by redirecting the type 1 response to a type 2 T cell response. Before the advent of these agents, symptomatic relief, with corticosteroids for acute exacerbations, was the mainstay of treatment.

80. **How is type 1 diabetes treated?**
Treatment options for type 1 diabetes have been limited to prevention of complications resulting from hyperglycemia. Therefore, most efforts have focused on patient education and maintaining uniform insulin level with the use of pumps and other devices. Studies looking into preventing or delaying the onset of type 1 diabetes using subcutaneous or oral insulin have not been successful.

WEBSITES

1. American Academy of Allergy, Asthma and Immunology: www.aaaai.org

2. National Library of Medicine: www.nlm.nih.gov

BIBLIOGRAPHY

1. Abbas A, Litchman AH (eds): Cellular and Molecular Immunology, 5th ed. Philadelphia, W.B. Saunders, 2003.
2. Davidson A, Diamond B: Autoimmune diseases. N Engl J Med 345:340–350, 2000.
3. Dighiero G, Rose NR: Critical self-epitopes are key to the understanding of self-tolerance and autoimmunity. Immunol Today 20: 423–428, 1999.
4. Germain RN: Autoimmune diseases. Nat Rev Immunol 2:309, 2002.
5. Hayakawa K, et al: Self-tolerance and autoimmunity. Science 285:113, 2000.
6. Kee BL, Murre C: Autoimmunity. Curr Opin Immunol 13:180, 2001.
7. Liu, Y-J, Banchereau J: Immunologist 4:55, 2000.
8. Mackay IR: Tolerance and autoimmunity. BMJ 321:93–96, 2000.
9. Marrack P, Kappler J, KotzinBL: Autoimmune disease: Why and where it occurs. Nature Med 7:899–905, 2001.

CHAPTER 13

FOOD ALLERGY AND INTOLERANCE

Suzanne S. Teuber, M.D.

1. **What is a food allergy?**
   An adverse reaction to food mediated by the immune system. It may be an IgE-mediated response (e.g., peanut-induced anaphylaxis) or non-IgE, cell-mediated disorders (e.g., celiac disease).

2. **What are the different types of food allergy syndromes?**
   See Table 13-1.

TABLE 13-1.   TYPES OF FOOD ALLERGY SYNDROMES

IgE-mediated
   Anaphylaxis (systemic reaction), mild to severe
   Food-dependent, exercise-induced anaphylaxis
   Food-pollen syndrome
   Food-induced asthma
   Contact urticaria

Mixed IgE-/non-IgE-mediated
   Atopic dermatitis

Non-IgE-mediated
   Allergic eosinophilic esophagitis/gastroenteritis
   Protein-induced enteropathy
   Celiac disease
   Protein-induced enterocolitis
   Protein-induced proctocolitis
   Dermatitis herpetiformis
   Heiner's syndrome
   Allergic contact dermatitis

---

3. **What are the causes of other adverse reactions to foods?**
   Some reactions can be due to toxic effects of microorganisms contaminating food or toxic plant or fungal components. Reactions due to pharmacologically active compounds, metabolic disorders, psychological factors, or unknown mechanisms are commonly called *food intolerance* reactions (Table 13-2).

4. **How common is food allergy versus food intolerance?**
   - 5–8% of children have a food allergy; about 2.5% of infants develop cow's milk allergy.
   - ~2% of adults have a food allergy confirmed by oral challenges. Many more exhibit a mild food allergy, termed oral allergy syndrome or pollen-food syndrome, that usually consists of

TABLE 13-2. FOOD INTOLERANCE REACTIONS

Toxic
Bacterial enterotoxins
Fungal toxins
Solanine
Ciguatera poisoning
Saxitoxin
Scombroid fish poisoning

Metabolic disorder/enzyme deficiency
Lactase deficiency
Phenylketonuria
Pancreatic insufficiency

Pharmacologic sensitivity
Caffeine
Histamine
Other vasoactive amines
Capsaicin
Alcohol
Methylxanthines

Psychological
Anorexia nervosa
Bulimia
Idiosyncratic food aversion

mild itching in the mouth with a food in the context of cross-reactive pollen allergens, but this condition is underreported. Studies suggest that 25–50% of adults with pollen allergy experience mild allergy to cross-reactive fruits or vegetables.

- About 1% of households in one United States telephone survey reported a peanut or tree nut allergy. A recent United Kingdom survey suggested a prevalence of 1.5% for peanut allergy.
- 25% of households report alteration of diet due to an unconfirmed "food allergy" or intolerance.
- Lactase deficiency is estimated to affect 25% of the United States population and up to 75% of the world's population.

Grundy J, Matthews S, Bateman B, et al: Rising prevalence of allergy to peanut in children: Data from two sequential cohorts. J Allergy Clin Immunol 110:784–789, 2002.

5. **How does IgE-mediated food allergy manifest clinically?**
A full spectrum of clinical signs and symptoms is possible (Table 13-3). Reactions often start immediately on contact with the food in the mouth or within the first 1–2 minutes in those with severe allergy. Reactions almost always begin within 30 minutes; less commonly the reaction may occur up to 2 hours later.

6. **What are the main foods involved in IgE-mediated allergies in children and adults in the United States?**
In **children,** studies using double-blind, placebo-controlled food challenges have shown that cow's milk, soy, egg, wheat, peanut, tree nuts, and fish are the most common food allergen

TABLE 13-3.	CLINICAL MANIFESTATIONS OF IGE-MEDIATED FOOD ALLERGY	
System	Possible Symptoms	Possible Signs
Skin	Itching, generalized	Flushing
	Itching of palms/soles	Urticaria
Ocular	Itching	Conjunctival injection
	Tearing	Periorbital swelling
	Swelling	
Upper respiratory	Itching of nose, palate, throat	Rhinorrhea
		Nasal obstruction
	Sensation of swelling	Stridor
	Difficulty speaking	
Lower respiratory	Shortness of breath	Wheezing
	Wheezing	Obstruction by spirometry
Gastrointestinal	Nausea	Vomiting
	Abdominal cramps	Hyperperistalsis
	Diarrhea	Diarrhea
Genital tract	Vaginal itching	
	Scrotal itching	
	Uterine cramping	
Cardiovascular	Light-headedness	Hypotension
	Difficulty walking	Arrhythmia
	Fainting	Tachycardia
Psychiatric	Fear	
	Sense of doom	

sources. In **adults,** peanuts, tree nuts, crustaceans, and fish are the most common food allergen sources.

7. **What factors may influence the prevalence of a particular food allergy?**
The prevalence of a particular food allergy depends on cultural and geographic considerations. For example, in Japan, buckwheat and rice allergy are important among children. In Scandinavian countries, fish allergy is more prevalent. In Israel, sesame allergy is the most common food associated with anaphylaxis in children. In Spain, fruit allergy, particularly peach, may be the most common food allergy.

8. **Are the main allergens in foods fats, carbohydrates, or proteins?**
Proteins. Many are glycoproteins, usually heat-stable.

9. **Give specific examples of protein food allergies.**
   - The main allergen in shrimp is a muscle protein called tropomyosin.
   - The main allergen in cow's milk is beta-lactoglobulin.
   - The main allergens in fish are proteins called parvalbumins, which control the calcium flux and are found only in fish and amphibians.
   - Both egg white and egg yolk contain allergens, although egg white appears to be more allergenic.

- The main allergens in peanuts, soy, and tree nuts are seed storage proteins called albumins, vicilins, and legumins.

10. **Do children outgrow IgE-mediated food allergies?**
New data suggest that about 10% of children with peanut allergy become tolerant by age 5–6 years; however, if they are not tolerant by then, the allergy appears to be persistent through adulthood. Approximately 85% of children allergic to milk, soy, and egg tolerate the implicated food by age 3–5 years. If the reaction was anaphylactic and the level of IgE antibody is high, the development of tolerance is less likely. (Most reactions to cow's milk are non-IgE-mediated GI reactions.) In general, if a child has a low level of IgE to a food, there is a greater chance of developing tolerance when rechallenged later compared with children with high IgE levels. Incremental food challenges are quite useful and allow liberalization of the diet after 1–3 years of avoidance. A child may still have a positive skin test or in vitro specific IgE assay and yet tolerate the food.

11. **Are food allergies acquired as an adolescent or adult outgrown?**
Food allergies that are acquired as a teen or as an adult do not seem to resolve.

12. **What is the most life-threatening kind of food allergy syndrome?**
IgE-mediated systemic reactions. A systemic reaction means that an allergic reaction develops distal to the immediate site of contact with the food. Someone who gets some itching in the mouth and throat when eating cantaloupe is said to have the oral allergy syndrome, which is believed to be a local reaction to the food. Someone who breaks out in generalized hives is having a systemic reaction. When a systemic reaction is severe, the term *anaphylaxis* is commonly used, but it is also correct to use the term when speaking about any systemic reaction. Modifiers of mild, moderate, or severe are often used in front of "systemic reaction" or "anaphylaxis." There are no widely accepted definitions of different grades of anaphylaxis, although a grading system has recently been proposed.
Ring J, Behrendt H: Anaphylaxis and anaphylactoid reactions: Classification and pathophysiology. Clin Rev Allergy Immunol 17:387–399, 1999.
Sampson HA: Anaphylaxis and emergency treatment. Pediatrics 11:1601–1608, 2003.

13. **What is the immediate cause of death from food allergy?**
Severe bronchospasm is frequently reported in the few available case series examining food allergy mortality. Symptoms can start out mild (hives) and then progress. Severe symptoms can persist for many hours before death. However, any of the following manifestations can result in death within minutes:
- Laryngoedema
- Oral angioedema blocking the airway
- Bronchospasm
- Hypotension/cardiovascular collapse

14. **What are the risk factors for death from anaphylaxis to foods?**
- Failure to administer epinephrine early in the reaction. Many patients do not have self-injectable epinephrine because of failure of physicians to prescribe epinephrine or their own failure to carry it with them or keep the prescription up to date. In addition, many states do not allow all levels of emergency medical technicians to administer epinephrine in the field.
- Underlying asthma
- Peanut, tree nut, or seafood allergy
- Adolescent or young adult (may be related to denial of symptom severity)
- History of previous severe reactions
- Failure to activate the emergency medical system after recognizing a reaction due to denial of its potential severity

- Failure to recognize biphasic anaphylaxis, which occurs when a systemic reaction initially seems to respond completely to therapy, only to recur within an hour or two.
- Patient taking beta blockers and perhaps ACE inhibitors may have more severe anaphylaxis.

15. **How many people die annually in the United States from food-induced anaphylaxis?**

    About 150 people are believed to die each year in the U.S. due to fatal food allergic reactions.

16. **Should I prescribe omalizumab to patients with a history of anaphylaxis to food?**

    No. Studies are currently under way to evaluate omalizumab, a monoclonal anti-IgE antibody, in the prevention of food-induced anaphylaxis. Only one study using anti-IgE therapy in peanut allergy has been published. This study used TNX-901, an antibody that is no longer in clinical development. In the published study, not all patients on active therapy achieved protection, but the majority in the high-dose arm were able to tolerate significantly more peanut protein (the mean threshold dose went from about half a peanut equivalent to almost nine peanuts).

    Leung DY, Sampson HA, Yunginger JW, et al: Effect of anti-IgE therapy in patients with peanut allergy. N Engl J Med 348:986–993, 2003.

17. **How is food allergy diagnosed?**

    A combination of history, physical examination, laboratory evaluation, skin prick testing, elimination diets, sometimes endoscopy and/oral food challenges (Fig. 13-1). The history, which is most important, should focus on the age of onset, symptoms, time between ingestion and reaction, reproducibility (do the reactions occur every time the food is eaten?), presence of atopic dermatitis, asthma, allergic rhinitis, or other atopy. The history should also focus on conditions that may be in the differential diagnosis of food allergy or intolerance, such as gastrointestinal conditions (hiatal hernia, pyloric stenosis, gallstones). Subsequent evaluation is driven by the suspected pathophysiology of the reported adverse reaction.

18. **What role do skin tests have in the evaluation of food allergy?**

    If an IgE-mediated disorder is likely, skin testing can be very useful.

    - A negative prick skin test with a high-quality extract has a high negative predictive value (95%) and suggests that the patient does not have an IgE-mediated food allergy to that allergen.
    - A positive skin test predicts a clinical reaction to a food only about 40% of the time. *Thus, the presence of IgE against a food does not equate with clinical food allergy.* Emerging data suggest that the size of a positive skin prick test may raise the positive predictive value of the test; i.e., a very large positive skin test (e.g., > 8mm) in suspected peanut or tree nut allergy is 95% predictive when supported by history.
    - There is a rare risk of systemic reaction to prick skin testing, especially in patients with a history of anaphylaxis to a food.
    - Intradermal skin testing should never be performed with foods because the false positive rate is even higher and there is a higher risk of systemic reactions in sensitive individuals (deaths have been reported).

    Clark AT, Ewan PW: Interpretation of tests for nut allergy in one thousand patients in relation to allergy or tolerance. Clin Exp Allergy 33:1041–1045, 2003.

    Sporik R, Hill DJ, Hosking CS. Specificity of allergen skin testing in children. Clin Exp Allergy 30:1540–1546, 2000.

19. **What role do in vitro specific IgE assays have in the diagnosis or management of food allergy?**

    Specific IgE assays (i.e., Pharmacia CAP-System FEIA) can be useful both in the diagnosis of food allergy and in predicting which pediatric patients may become tolerant of a food when followed over time. Only the Pharmacia CAP-System FEIA assay has been evaluated in this way.

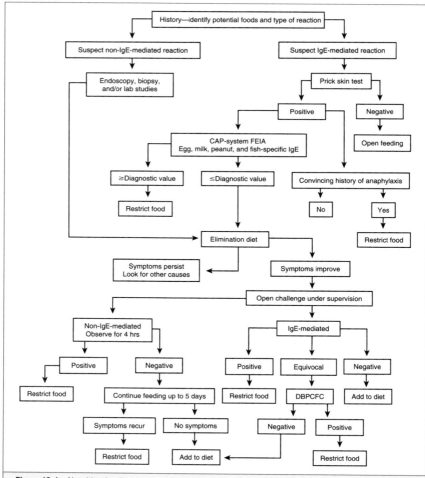

Figure 13-1. Algorithm for diagnosis of food allergy or intolerance. DBPCFC: double-blind, placebo-controlled food challenge. CAP: Pharmacia CAP-System FEIA. (From Sampson HA: Diagnosing food allergies in children. In Lichtenstein LM, Busse WW, Geha RS: Current Therapy in Allergy, Immunology, and Rheumatology, 6th ed. St. Louis, Mosby, 2004, p 149, Fig. 13-1.)

- The level of IgE cannot be used to predict severity of a reaction.
- There are more false negatives with in vitro assays than with skin prick tests. In a recent study of patients with a clear nut allergic history, 22% had a negative CAP, while 40% had misleading false-positive CAPs to nuts they were known to tolerate.
- CAP values over 15.0 kU/L may be highly predictive (> 95%) of food allergy when supported by the history for cow's milk, peanut, and tree nuts; over 20 kU/L for fish; and over 7.0 kU/L to egg for children over age 2, and > 2.0 kU/L for children under age 2.

- When re-evaluating a child with a previous history of cow's milk, egg or peanut allergy, if there has been no intervening clinical allergic reaction and CAP values at reassessment are < 0.5 kU/L for egg, < 7.0 kU/L for cow's milk, and < 5.0 kU/L for peanut, it is worthwhile to perform an incremental oral challenge with the food in question since it may now be tolerated.

  Clark AT, Ewan PW: Interpretation of tests for nut allergy in one thousand patients in relation to allergy or tolerance. Clin Exp Allergy 33:1041–1045, 2003.

  Sampson HA: The evaluation and management of food allergy in atopic dermatitis. Clin Dermatol 21:193–192, 2003.

21. How is an elimination diet performed?

Usually an elimination diet involves elimination of only one or two foods that are suspected by history and laboratory evaluation. However, in certain cases, severe food restriction and substitution with an elemental diet for 2–6 weeks may be indicated to see whether a chronic condition improves. For instance, a patient with severe atopic dermatitis or a patient with allergic eosinophilic gastroenteritis who may have a food allergy component may benefit from such a severe restriction. If improvement occurs, blinded food challenges can be performed to see which foods may be implicated. In gastrointestinal disorders, such as celiac disease, endoscopy and biopsies are coordinated with the elimination diet.

Sampson HA: Food allergy. Part 2: Diagnosis and management. J Allergy Clin Immunol 103:981–989, 1999.

22. What are oral food challenges?

Oral food challenges are performed with incremental doses of the food, starting with an amount half of that reported to be the minimum to provoke symptoms in published studies (e.g., milligram amounts in egg, peanut, tree nut, sesame, or seafood allergy and cow's milk as low as 0.1 mL). If 10 gm of dried food or around 60 gm of a wet food are ingested without reaction, it is highly unlikely that the patient is sensitive to the food.

- As noted above, if the skin test or in vitro CAP IgE level exceeds certain levels, oral challenges are unnecessary to confirm allergy.
- When diagnosis is uncertain, oral challenges are considered the gold standard in food allergy diagnosis because the history can be falsely positive in 60% of cases and the false-positive rate for skin tests or in vitro tests is about 50% (with the exception that history + high values are highly predictive of allergy).
- Challenges are very useful to follow children over time to see if they have become tolerant of a food. For example, a child about to start kindergarten who has a CAP value to peanut of 3.2 kU/L and has not had any accidental exposures to peanut in 3.5 years may now tolerate peanut.
- Challenges for IgE-mediated reactions should be performed only in a clinic or hospital setting with appropriate resuscitative equipment and trained personnel.

  Bock SA, Sampson HA, Atkins FM, et al: Double-blind placebo-controlled food challenge as an office procedure: A manual. J Allergy Clin Immunol 82:986, 1988.

23. What types of oral challenges are done?

- Open challenge: no blinding. Used in infants or children or after a negative double- or single-blind challenge in an adult.
- Single blind: the food is hidden in another food that the patient tolerates or in opaque capsules. The physician is aware of whether it is a placebo or actual food challenge.
- Double blind: a third party randomizes the placebo and actual food challenges.

24. When is a food patch test performed?

A food patch test can be performed when non-IgE-mediated food allergy contributing to atopic dermatitis or allergic eosinophilic esophagitis or gastroenteritis is suspected. Finn chambers are used to apply food extracts to the patient's back and the sites are read at 48 and 72 hours, as done in work-ups for allergic contact dermatitis caused by chemicals. More trials are needed, and the use of such testing with foods is not standardized but may be helpful.

Sampson HA: The evaluation and management of food allergy in atopic dermatitis. Clin Dermatol 21:193–192, 2003.

Spergel JM, Beausoleil JL. Mascarenhas M, Liacouras CA: The use of skin prick tests and patch tests to identify causative foods in eosinophilic esophagitis. J Allergy Clin Immunol 109:363–368, 2002.

25. **What is food-dependent, exercise-induced anaphylaxis?**
This systemic, IgE-mediated reaction occurs only when two criteria have been met: (1) ingestion of the implicated food and (2) vigorous exercise within several hours of eating the food. When the food is eaten without exercise or the patient exercises vigorously without previously eating the food, no clinical reaction occurs. The unique juxtaposition of eating the allergenic food with the physiologic and metabolic changes incurred by exercise results in mast cell activation. This condition has been studied in a double-blind fashion using treadmill tests. Increasingly, cases are being reported in which the exercise is mild to moderate, such as housework or a brisk walk.
- The disorder usually has an onset in young adulthood in atopic individuals.
- The foods implicated have included wheat, celery, fruit, peanut, fish and crustaceans. Wheat is the most common allergen implicated, however.

26. **Define oral allergy syndrome, also known as pollen/food syndrome.**
Itching, irritation, and mild swelling or urticaria in and/or around the mouth as part of an immediate reaction to a fresh fruit or vegetable is called oral allergy syndrome. The preferred term now is pollen/food syndrome because the symptoms are suspected to be due to cross-reactive allergens present in both a sensitizing pollen and the food. Up to 25–50% of pollen-allergic patients may manifest this syndrome to some degree.

27. **How is pollen/food syndrome diagnosed?**
In vitro specific IgE assays and skin prick tests with commercial fruit or vegetable extracts can return negative due to the labile nature of the heat-sensitive allergens. If the fresh fruit or vegetable is macerated and pricked with the skin prick test needle and then used to prick the patient's skin, an immediate wheal and flare reaction can often be demonstrated. This technique is called a "prick plus prick" skin test.

28. **How is pollen/food syndrome treated?**
Pollen/food syndrome is not usually life-threatening and usually does not require the prescription of self-injectable epinephrine. However, some cases progress to extensive oral, upper airway, or lower airway involvement. There is also concern that some cases of systemic food allergy (e.g., to tree nuts) may start with mild oral symptoms and evolve over continued exposures, implying that the symptoms were actually a mild systemic reaction rather than due to pollen cross-reactivity.

Usually, the involved food is an allergen source only when fresh, not cooked, since the involved proteins are normally heat-labile. For example, someone may tolerate celery in soup, but not fresh celery. Cross-reactive homologous proteins between fruits or vegetables and commonly allergenic pollens have been demonstrated.

29. **Can allergen immunotherapy be used to treat the pollen/food allergy syndrome?**
There is a case report of abatement of oral allergy syndrome after a course of immunotherapy for coexistent pollen allergy.

30. **What are some of the reported pollen/food cross-reactivities?**
See Table 13-4.

TABLE 13-4.	POLLEN/FOOD SYNDROME RELATIONSHIPS
Pollen	**Food**
Ragweed	Melons
	Bananas
	Cucumber
Birch	Apples
	Stone fruits (apricot, cherry, plum)
	Hazelnuts
	Carrot
Mugwort	Celery
	Carrot
	Some spices
Grass	Potato
	Tomato
	Peach

31. **Should someone with peanut allergy avoid all legumes?**
No. It is unusual, even in the setting of severe anaphylactic sensitivity, to be allergic to other legumes (Table 13-5). Rarely, in about 5% of cases, a patient may react clinically (often much less severely) to one or two other specific legumes. However, it is extremely common to show positive skin tests or in vitro specific IgE tests to other legumes, even though these foods are tolerated clinically.

TABLE 13-5.	CROSS-REACTIVITY RELATIONSHIPS IN IgE-MEDIATED FOOD ALLERGY
Food	**Cross-Reactivities**
Peanut	Very rarely soy, pea, or other bean
Cow's milk	Goat's milk, mare's milk, sheep's milk
Chicken egg	Other bird eggs
	Rarely chicken meat
Shrimp	Other crustaceans (lobster, crab, crayfish)
	Rarely molluscs (scallops, clam, oysters)
Fish	Other species, can be variable
Tree nuts	Other tree nuts, quite variable

32. **Can a child with egg allergy get the measles-mumps-rubella (MMR) vaccine?**
Yes. Most lots of MMR have no detectable egg protein. Even with detectable egg protein, children have tolerated the MMR vaccine in a 2-shot regimen: one-tenth of the dose is given, followed by the rest of the dose if there is no reaction in 30 minutes. With this protocol, there have been no significant systemic reactions to the vaccine.

33. **Can an adult with egg allergy get the flu vaccine?**
In most adults who report that they have egg allergy, no IgE against egg is discernible on tests. Egg allergy is usually outgrown in childhood, or patients may be describing an idiosyncratic intolerance reaction (e.g., bloating with eating a lot of egg). Generally, a careful history reveals that the patient ingests egg routinely in small amounts in baked goods. Such patients can be assured that the vaccine will be tolerated.

34. **Discuss food-induced asthma.**
Most reactions to foods that include bronchospasm as a symptom include other symptoms as well (e.g., lip swelling, oral itching, rhinorrhea, periorbital edema). However, in a small subset of patients with moderate-to-severe asthma, food allergy may contribute to the disease. This subset is to be distinguished from patients with systemic food allergy, who may have an asthmatic response on inhaling food particles (see question 36).

35. **How common is food-induced asthma?**
Among asthmatics in general, surveys have found that 20–60% of patients believed that certain foods were a trigger. Double-blind food challenges in one study, however, showed positive results (drop in FEV_1) in only about 2.5% of those who believed they had food-induced asthma in a population that included both adults and children. On the other hand, the prevalence of positive food challenges increased to 6–8% in unselected pediatric asthmatics.
Although the prevalence of food-induced asthma is lower than perceived by patients, if a food allergy is diagnosed, the possibility for clinical improvement after eliminating exposure to the specific food in a patient with chronic asthma is real.

36. **Can a person have an allergic reaction by just being near the food?**
Yes. Fatal cases of anaphylaxis have been described in which shrimp or crab was boiled and the airborne proteins (which have been documented and quantitated in cooking steam) elicited severe anaphylactic reactions. Such reactions are possible with any food that is cooked or handled in a way that produces respirable particles containing allergenic proteins.

37. **Is it true that people have had allergic reactions to peanuts on airplanes?**
Yes. People have had reactions to apparently airborne peanut dust on commercial airliners. The Food Allergy Network sponsored a survey that reported data about 31 people who had reported in-flight reactions to peanuts. Fourteen of these reactions were provoked by inhalation. Two subjects were given epinephrine during the flight. Peanut allergens have been detected in airplane air filters.

38. **Is there such a thing as a fatal kiss?**
You have to decide that one. It has not happened yet to our knowledge as a result of food allergy. However, it has been reported that patients with severe sensitivity to tree nuts, peanuts, or seafood may be so sensitive that residual protein in the mouth of someone who recently (within several hours) ate the food can transmit enough protein to cause an allergic reaction (usually mild, but a few cases have been severe).

39. **Summarize the clinical characteristics of allergic eosinophilic esophagitis or gastroenteritis.**
Clinical characteristics include abdominal pain, nausea, vomiting, failure to thrive, diarrhea, sometimes iron-deficiency anemia, heme-positive stools, and peripheral eosinphilia. Onset of symptoms may occur from infancy to young adulthood. Up to 50% of pediatric cases are related to food allergy and may show IgE to common foods like cow's milk or egg. These cases tend to resolve over 2–3 years. Only a fraction of adult cases respond to an elimination diet and are therefore food-related.

40. **What endoscopic findings are associated with allergic eosinophilic esophagitis or gastroenteritis?**
    Antral gastritis with eosinophilic inflammation is most common, along with small bowel involvement. Some patients have prominent esophagitis or colitis.

41. **Describe the diagnosis and treatment of allergic eosinophilic esophagitis or gastroenteritis.**
    Assay for IgE to foods by skin prick testing or the food patch test can be used to detect cell-mediated reactions to foods. Try eliminating all test-positive foods from the diet. Patients may need to use a trial period of an elemental formula diet. If symptoms are responsive, eliminate the offending foods permanently. Otherwise, corticosteroids may be needed. Patients have no apparent increase in long-term risk of malignancy.
    Spergel JM, Beausoleil JL, Mascarenhas M, Liacouras CA: The use of skin prick tests and patch tests to identify causative foods in eosinophilic esophagitis. J Allergy Clin Immunol 109:363–368, 2002.

42. **What are the clinical characteristics of food protein–induced enterocolitis?**
    Food protein-induced enterocolitis appears in infants from 1 day to 9 months after birth. It is not seen in breast-fed infants. Signs and symptoms include bloody diarrhea, emesis, failure to thrive, dehydration, fecal polymorphonuclear neutrophils (PMNs), leukocytosis, and ill appearance (infant may appear septic). The condition is outgrown.

43. **Summarize the endoscopic findings in infants with food protein–induced enterocolitis.**
    Endoscopic findings include diffuse colitis, crypt abscesses, chronic inflammation (sometimes with erosive gastritis), esophagitis, prominent eosinophilia, and mild-to-moderate villous atrophy.

44. **How is food protein–induced enterocolitis diagnosed?**
    Symptoms improve rapidly within a few days of restriction of the offending protein: usually cow's milk or soy, sometimes solid baby foods. Diagnosis can be confirmed by hospitalization for a protein challenge at least 2 weeks after the infant is stable on a hydrolyzed formula. The infant is fed 0.6 gm/kg body weight. Symptoms develop in less than 12 hours: leukocytosis, heme-positive and PMN-positive diarrhea, emesis (in some cases), and shock (rare).

45. **Summarize the treatment for food protein–induced enterocolitis.**
    Avoidance of the offending protein until about 18 months of age.

46. **Describe the clinical characteristics of food protein–induced proctocolitis.**
    Onset of symptoms occurs within 4 days to 4 months after birth. Breast-fed infants may also be affected. Signs and symptoms include a well-appearing infant with blood streaked or bloody stools, fecal PMNs, and (in some cases) peripheral eosinophilia. The condition is outgrown.

47. **What is the major endoscopic finding in food protein-induced proctocolitis?**
    Eosinophilic rectal inflammation, sometimes with colitis.

48. **How is food protein–induced proctocolitis treated?**
    Symptoms clear within several days of dietary manipulation. In breast-fed infants, maternal avoidance of cow's milk is indicated first, followed by avoidance of egg and soy. In formula-fed infants, a switch to a highly hydrolyzed hypoallergenic formula is indicated. Infants tolerate the offending protein by 9–12 months of age. No known long-term sequelae have been noted.

49. **What are the clinical characteristics of food protein-induced transient enteropathy?**
Food protein-induced transient enteropathy (excluding gluten enteropathy) appears from 2 to 18 months after birth. Offending proteins include cow's milk, soy, egg (rare), chicken, and fish. Signs and symptoms include anorexia, emesis, diarrhea, and the chronic sequelae of malabsorption. The condition is outgrown.

50. **What is the major endoscopic finding of food protein-induced transient enteropathy?**
Flattening of the small intestinal villi.

51. **Summarize the treatment of food protein-induced transient enteropathy.**
Avoidance of the offending protein, usually by switching formulas to a highly hydrolyzed hypoallergenic formula. Infants usually outgrow this disorder by 9–12 months of age. If the onset was later, the reintroduction of the protein should be later. No long-term sequelae have been reported.

52. **What is gluten enteropathy or celiac disease?**
It is an allergy to gluten, which is a collection of poorly water-soluble seed storage proteins present in the closely related cereals wheat, barley, and rye. Oats may be tolerated, according to recent data. Rice and corn are also tolerated.

53. **Describe the clinical characteristics of gluten enteropathy or celiac disease.**
Onset of symptoms may occur at any time from 6 months of age to adulthood. The condition is permanent; it is not outgrown. Classic signs and symptoms include malabsorption syndrome, iron deficiency anemia, folate deficiency, steatorrhea, diarrhea, metabolic bone disease, weight loss, and growth delay. Associated diseases include dermatitis herpetiformis, abdominal lymphoma, type 1 diabetes, IgA deficiency, recurrent apthous ulcers, hyposplenism, hypo- and hyperthyroidism, myasthenia, sarcoidosis, and cerebellar atrophy (rare).

54. **Discuss the endoscopic findings of gluten enteropathy.**
Endoscopic findings include small bowel villus flattening, crypt hyperplasia, intense lymphocytic infiltrates in the lamina propria, and many surface intraepithelial lymphocytes.

55. **How is gluten enteropathy diagnosed?**
In screening, a peroral capsule biopsy of the jejunum can be performed. To confirm the diagnosis, the biopsy results should improve on a gluten-free diet. In some cases, a repeat biopsy is necessary after a 3- to 6-month gluten challenge (daily gluten ingestion). Early diagnosis may be based on symptoms such as anemia, diarrhea, or weight loss or may be made during evaluation for an associated disease (in which case celiac disease may be diagnosed in absence of gastrointestinal symptoms). IgA antigliadin antibodies, IgA anti-endomysium antibodies, and anti-tissue transglutaminase antibodies are supportive of the diagnosis.

56. **What is the only treatment for gluten enteropathy?**
Strict dietary avoidance of gluten.

57. **Define dermatitis herpetiformis.**
Dermatitis herpetiformis is an intensely pruritic, bullous skin disease with small blisters in groups, usually on elbows, shoulders, knees, or buttocks. It is highly associated with gluten enteropathy.

58. **How is dermatitis herpetiformis diagnosed?**
Biopsy shows IgA and C3 deposited in a granular fashion in the tips of the dermal papillae. Almost all patients have an abnormal small bowel biopsy, although they are often asymptomatic.

59. **Summarize the treatment for dermatitis herpetiformis.**
Gluten avoidance normalizes the small bowel biopsy and often slowly improves the skin lesions (the process may take a year). Dapsone is often effective.

60. **Define Heiner's syndrome.**
Heiner's syndrome, also called Wilson-Heiner-Lahey syndrom, consists of the constellation of cow's milk protein–induced occult rectal blood loss, anemia, and hypoproteinemia with pulmonary infiltrates in infants or toddlers transitioned to cow's milk. The syndrome has been reported only in association with cow's milk, not with cow's milk formulas. Biopsy of the lung shows IgG, IgA, and C3 deposition with iron-laden macrophages. Pulmonary symptoms and signs may recur during childhood with subsequent cow's milk exposure.

61. **Discuss the relationship between food allergy and atopic dermatitis.**
In approximately 33% of children with chronic moderate-to-severe atopic dermatitis, food allergy is confirmed by double-blind, placebo-controlled food challenges. When the implicated foods are eliminated from the diet, the skin disease usually improves. The food allergy is usually *not* apparent to the child or the family until the disease has been brought under control by aggressive local therapy and double-blind, placebo-controlled food challenges are performed. A positive challenge often presents as a morbilliform rash in the areas usually affected by atopic dermatitis rather than an urticarial response, along with nausea or abdominal pain in about half and respiratory tract symptoms in slightly less than half of patients.

62. **Which foods are usually involved?**
Egg, cow's milk, peanut, soy, and wheat account for approximately 80% of positive double-blind challenges in published series. Children are usually sensitive to only one or up to three foods as confirmed by challenge, even though with skin tests or RAST many foods may test positive.

63. **Link sex with food allergy in four moves or less (akin to the Kevin Bacon game).**
Sex → condoms → latex allergy → cross-reactive foods.

64. **Why are some foods cross-reactive with natural rubber latex?**
Natural rubber latex is made from the sap of the *Hevea brasiliensis* tree, which by volume is composed of up to 30% cis-1,4-polyisoprene. The cis-1,4-polyisoprene is the naturally occurring plant hydrocarbon that is vulcanized into natural rubber. The hydrocarbon exists in the sap as part of liquid rubber particles, surrounded by lipids, phospholipids, and proteins. The associated proteins are not excluded from the rubber-making process and can be present in significant quantities in natural rubber end products, such as examination gloves. Patients with "latex allergy" are allergic to these *plant* proteins. It is not unexpected that some of these would cross-react with plant proteins from other sources.

65. **Which foods are most commonly reported to be cross-reactive with natural rubber latex?**
About 20% of patients with clinically evident latex allergy also have a fruit allergy:
- Most common: banana, avocado, kiwi, and chestnut.
- Also reported: potato, tomato, apple, apricot, celery, cherry, fig, melon, papaya, peach, and nectarine.

66. **Why are food allergens hard to avoid?**
In the United States, labeling laws for processed or prepackaged foods are strict. All food ingredients must be declared. However, some of the lesser food ingredients are allowed to be listed ambiguously, such as "hydrolyzed vegetable protein," "natural flavoring," or "spices." Highly food-allergic patients may know to be wary of processed and packaged foods with ambiguous ingredients, but even if the label is clear, the food may still harbor a hidden allergen (Table 13-6).

TABLE 13-6. REACTIONS TO HIDDEN ALLERGENS

Source of Allergen	Reason for No Declaration on Label
Trace ingredient	Not required by law to explicitly state source: spice, natural flavoring, other
Ingredient	Recent recipe change, labels not properly changed
Ingredient	Error in labels: same labels used for two or more processing plants even though recipes differ at the different sites
Contaminant	Contaminated at wholesale (e.g., tree nuts mixed)
Contaminant	Rehashing or reworking (e.g., a small amount of batter left over from a similar product is mixed with a large amount of fresh batter)
Contaminant	Traces of food allergen left on shared equipment contaminate the first products of the next batch (e.g., ice cream with peanuts contaminating a plain ice cream)
Source of Allergen	**Reason Consumer Missed the Allergen**
Ingredient	Listed on label, but not expected by patient (e.g., milk in canned tuna)
Ingredient	Listed on label, but an unfamiliar term was used (e.g., vitellin, ovomucoid, or livetin for egg)

All bets are off with restaurant foods! Fatal anaphylaxis to peanuts has occurred in an unsuspecting patron eating chili in a fast-food restaurant (it was the "secret ingredient") and in a college student eating eggrolls in which the ends were glued down with peanut butter. Contamination of utensils, cookware, or grills (shrimp/fish) can occur. Additionally, some restaurants may use gourmet, expellar-pressed peanut or tree nut oils in salad dressings that contain relevant allergens. Highly processed peanut oil has been shown to be tolerated in peanut-allergic individuals.

67. **Summarize the treatments for food allergy.**
    - Avoidance is currently the only definite approach to both IgE-mediated and non-IgE-mediated food allergy disorders.
    - Pollen immunotherapy or vaccination has been reported to cure a case of oral allergy syndrome.
    - Oral cromolyn sodium has not been effective as a prophylactic medication.
    - Infusion with monoclonal antihuman IgE may prove useful for patients with life-threatening food allergy who are at high risk for accidental ingestion (e.g., peanut allergy), but studies with the commercially available product, omalizumab, have not yet been performed (see question 16).

68. **What treatments may become available in the future?**
    Future peptide therapy with T-cell epitopes of food allergens or modified food allergens without the IgE-binding epitopes is possible, along with therapy with recombinant proteins that contain point mutations in the IgE-binding sites, rendering the protein unable to bind IgE. Such studies are under way in animal models.

69. **What should you do for a patient who comes to your office with a history of life-threatening IgE-mediated food allergy?**
    - Prescribe epinephrine for self-injection—enough for 2 injections, if needed.
    - Prescribe or instruct the patient to buy antihistamine in a liquid, chewable tablet, or rapidly dissolving tablet to be carried as an adjunctive treatment to epinephrine. Liquid is best, but some patients find it hard to carry.
    - Advise the patient to call 911 at the start of a reaction. No one should wait to see if it is "a bad one." The patient should carry a cell phone, if possible.
    - The patient needs to have an emergency plan at all times. Family members and friends need to be familiar with using epinephrine and how to call for help. If the patient is a child, the school needs to be involved. The Food Allergy Network has invaluable printed and audiovisual resources that can help with ensuring the safety of a child at school.
    - Advise the patient to obtain a MedicAlert bracelet or tag.
    - Give the patient information about how to read food labels, including alternative names for the food (e.g., casein, whey, and whey hydrolysate are all cow's milk), risk of ambiguous labels ("natural flavoring"), and risks of cross-contamination in processed foods and restaurants.
    - Link the patient with good resources:
      1. Food Allergy Network, 10400 Eaton Place, Suite 107, Fairfax, VA 22030-2208. Toll-free phone:1-800-822-2762 (www.foodallergy.org).
      2. American Academy of Allergy, Asthma and Immunology, 611 East Wells St., Milwaukee, WI 53202. Toll-free phone: 1-800-822-2762 (www.aaaai.org).
      3. American Dietetic Association, 216 West Jackson Blvd., Chicago, IL 60606-6995. Phone: 312-899-0040 (www.eatright.org)

70. **What can you do for patients who report subjective symptoms such as "brain fog" or joint pains after ingestion of a specific food?**
    Do not dismiss the symptoms. If you do not listen to patients' concerns, they may spend hundreds or thousands of dollars on unproven methods (see question 71). Double-blind, placebo-controlled food challenges with at least 2 placebos and 2 actual foods administered in the primary care physician's office are easy, without risk, reimbursable, and helpful to the patient. Such challenges are *highly* likely to prove that there is no relationship between the food and the symptoms. Use either capsules with the dried food inside or food hidden in a vehicle of mashed potatoes, applesauce, or a smoothie. Make sure to include the amount of the food that the patient believes has caused reproducible reactions and make sure that you and your staff cannot taste any difference between the hidden food challenge and the placebo challenge. The patient should ingest the challenges in the office and then go home and keep a diary of symptoms. A challenge is positive only if both placebos are negative and both hidden target food challenges are positive for the subjective symptoms.

71. **Why are unproven methods often used or sought for food allergy diagnosis and treatment?**
    Unproven methods to diagnose "food allergy" are sometimes applied by alternative medicine practitioners to people with chronic illnesses or conditions for which the etiology is unknown or for which medical management has been unsatisfactory. In addition, some people believe that certain subjective symptoms, such as fatigue, are related to certain foods or unknown foods and thus seek this type of evaluation or treatment.
    Teuber SS, Porch-Curren C: Unproved diagnostic and therapeutic approaches to food allergy and intolerance. Curr Opin Allergy Clin Immunol 3:217–221, 2003.

72. **List examples of unproven methods.**
    - Provocation-neutralization
    - Four-day rotation diet or rotary diversified diet
    - Applied kinesiology testing or muscle-response testing

KEY POINTS: IGE-MEDIATED FOOD ALLERGY

1. The presence of IgE to a food does *not* equate to clinical reactivity to a food.

2. Patients who have had only mild systemic allergic reactions to foods may develop life-threatening anaphylaxis the next time they accidentally ingest the food and should thus be referred to an allergist to design an anaphylaxis action plan.

3. Risk factors for death from food-induced anaphylaxis include delayed or no use of self-injectable epinephrine, history of asthma, and allergy to peanut, tree nut, or seafoods.

4. About 10% or more of children with peanut allergy may become tolerant by school age; thus it is worthwhile to reevaluate such children.

5. Avoidance is currently the only available treatment.

6. Food-dependent, exercise-induced anaphylaxis may be overlooked in the differential diagnosis of anaphylaxis because the amount of exercise required can be minimal.

- Electrodermal testing
- Food immune complex assay testing
- IgG RAST or food-specific IgG assays
- In vitro cell assays

72. **Explain provocation-neutralization.**
This method is used by some physicians to "diagnose" and then "treat" non-IgE-mediated "food allergy." It has been shown in two double-blind trials to be ineffective for diagnosis. Food extracts of various dilutions are either injected intradermally or given under the tongue, and subjective symptoms over the next 10–20 minutes are recorded. If a symptom occurs (e.g., sleepiness), a different dilution of the food extract is given (either higher or lower) until the symptom is gone. The dose of food extract that correlates with resolution of the symptom is called the neutralizing dose. Patients are then instructed to take the neutralizing dose sublingually or by injection prophylactically before exposure, after exposure for "treatment," or on a regular basis.

73. **What is the 4-day rotation diet or rotary diversified diet?**
This diet has been promoted in the belief that foods are better tolerated if food groups are rotated completely so that foods from one group are eaten only every 4–5 days. For example, milk may be consumed every 4 days. No clinical trials substantiate this difficult-to-follow diet. Such a diet has been promoted by some health care practicioners to be used for subjective reactions (fatigue, weakness, arthralgias) purportedly due to foods.

74. **How is applied kinesiology testing or the muscle-response test supposed to work?**
Muscle strength in one arm is measured while vials containing the various food are held in the patient's opposite hand. A drop in strength indicates "allergy" to the food. A blinded study has shown that results are nonreproducible.

75. **Explain the so-called rationale behind electrodermal testing.**
Skin conductance is measured by placing one electrode in the patient's hand and another to various acupuncture points in the legs. A glass vial containing an allergen (food or environmental) is placed on an aluminum plate in the circuit. If "allergy" is present, a drop in electrical conductance is measured. This method has been disproved in controlled studies.

76. **What is food immune complex assay testing?**

Normal people have been shown to have circulating immune complexes to commonly ingested foods, and even breast milk can contain immune complexes with food. The intestinal mucosa is not impermeable, and small quantities of food proteins circulate in the blood, which may become part of an immune complex that leads to elimination of the foreign protein. It has not yet been shown that any clinical diseases result from this process; such assays should be considered experimental only.

77. **Explain IgG RAST or food-specific IgG assays.**

It is normal to produce some IgG and especially IgA to the foods that we commonly eat. When subclasses of IgG were described, there was great interest in IgG4 as a marker for food allergy, but it has now been shown that normal people produce IgG4 to foods without clinical symptoms. Extremely high levels of IgG to food proteins, which can be visualized by the naked eye in a precipitin assay, are possibly involved in the pathogenesis of food-induced pulmonary hemosiderosis, as seen with cow's milk ingestion and in case reports with egg and pork. However, there is no proof of IgG antibody involvement in other types of adverse reactions to foods.

78. **What are in vitro cell assays?**

Currently advertised assays use a cell sorter to assess leukocyte or platelet cell volume after a blood sample has been applied to curvettes containing freeze-dried food extracts. The use of such assays is not supported by the available literature.

79. **Can food allergies be prevented?**

It is not clear whether food allergies in high risk-families (i.e, atopy in both parents or history of severe atopic dermatitis or food allergy in a sibling) can be prevented, but studies suggest that by following certain dietary exclusions, the onset of disorders may be delayed and the severity may be decreased.

80. **Give examples of possible prevention strategies.**

- Consider maternal avoidance of peanut, tree nuts, shrimp, and fish in the last trimester of pregnancy as investigational only. Consider maternal avoidance of cow's milk, peanut, tree nuts, shrimp, and fish during breast feeding another investigational measure.
- Strongly encourage breast-feeding for at least one year.
- If supplemented, or when weaning, use extensively or partially hydrolyzed hypoallergenic formulas. There is not enough evidence to support the recommendation for extensive hydrolysates over partial hydrolysates.
- Delay solids until 6 months.
- Delay cow's milk and egg until over 12 months.
- Delay peanut, tree nuts, crustaceans, and fish until over age 3 years or perhaps longer.

Osborn D, Sinn J: Formulas containing hydrolysed protein for prevention of allergy and food intolerance in infants. Cochrane Database Syst Rev 4:CD003664, 2003.

81. **Which food additives have been reported to cause adverse reactions?**

Food additives were targeted in the 1970s and 1980s as common precipitants of urticaria and asthma in adults and children and of hyperactivity in children (Table 13-7). With the exception of sodium metabisulfite as a precipitant of asthma and/or anaphylaxis, well-designed trials have recently exonerated many of the additives in common use, such as monosodium glutamate and aspartame.

Geha RS, Beiser A, Ren C, et al: Review of alleged reaction to monosodium glutamate and outcome of a multicenter double-blind placebo-controlled study. J Nutr 130:1058S–1062S, 2000.

Stevenson DD: Monosodium glutamate and asthma. J Nutr 130:1067S–1073S, 2000.

TABLE 13-7.	ROLE OF FOOD ADDITIVES IN ALLERGIC REACTIONS		
Additive	Role	Purported Reactions	Supported by Adequate Clinical Trials?
Sulfites	Preservative Antibrowning	Asthma, anaphylaxis	Yes
MSG	Flavor enhancer	Chinese restaurant syndrome	Not supported (rare mild symptoms to *high* doses given without food; no symptoms when given with food)
		Asthma	Not supported
		Urticaria	Not supported
Aspartame	Sweetener	Urticaria	Not supported
Tartrazine	Food dye	Urticaria	A few rare cases supported
		Asthma	Not supported
		Hyperactivity in children	Rare, only 2–3% of suspected cases (only two trials)
Other food dyes		Urticaria	Only a few cases reported
		Hyperactivity in children	Not well studied
BHA/BHT	Preservative	Urticaria	Only a few cases reported
Parabens	Preservative	Urticaria	Only a few cases reported
Benzoates	Preservative	Urticaria	Only a few cases reported

WEBSITES

1. Food Allergy Network: www.foodallergy.org

2. American Academy of Allergy, Asthma and Immunology: www.aaaai.org

3. American Dietetic Association: www.eatright.org

BIBLIOGRAPHY

1. Bock SA, Sampson HA, Atkins FM, et al: Double-blind placebo-controlled food challenge as an office procedure: A manual. J Allergy Clin Immunol 82:986, 1988.

2. Clark AT, Ewan PW: Interpretation of tests for nut allergy in one thousand patients in relation to allergy or tolerance. Clin Exp Allergy 33:1041–1045, 2003.

3. Geha RS, Beiser A, Ren C, et al: Review of alleged reaction to monosodium glutamate and outcome of a multi-center double-blind placebo-controlled study. J Nutr 130:1058S–1062S, 2000.

4. Grundy J, Matthews S, Bateman B, et al: Rising prevalence of allergy to peanut in children: Data from two sequential cohorts. J Allergy Clin Immunol 110:784–789, 2002.

5. Leung DY, Sampson HA, Yunginger JW, et al: Effect of anti-IgE therapy in patients with peanut allergy. N Engl J Med 348:986–993, 2003.

6. Metcalfe DD, Sampson HA, Simon RA (eds): Food Allergy: Adverse Reactions to Foods and Food Additives, 2nd ed. Blackwell Science, Cambridge, 1997.

7. Morisset M, Moneret-Vautrin DA, Kanny G, et al: Thresholds of clinical reactivity to milk, egg, peanut and sesame in immunoglobuline E-dependent allergies: Evaluation by double-blind or single-blind placebo-controlled oral challenges. Clin Exp Allergy 33:1046–1051, 2003.

8. Osborn D, Sinn J: Formulas containing hydrolysed protein for prevention of allergy and food intolerance in infants. Cochrane Database Syst Rev 4:CD003664, 2003.

9. Ring J, Behrendt H: Anaphylaxis and anaphylactoid reactions: Classification and pathophysiology. Clin Rev Allergy Immunol 17:387–399, 1999.

10. Sampson HA: Anaphylaxis and emergency treatment. Pediatrics 11:1601–1608, 2003.

11. Sampson HA: Food allergy. Part 1: Immunopathogenesis and clinical disorders. J Allergy Clin Immunol 103:717–728, 1999.

12. Sampson HA: Food allergy. Part 2: Diagnosis and management. J Allergy Clin Immunol 103:981–989, 1999.

13. Sampson HA: The evaluation and management of food allergy in atopic dermatitis. Clin Dermatol 21:193–192, 2003.

14. Sicherer SH: Food allergy. Lancet 360:701–710, 2002.

15. Spergel JM, Beausoleil JL, Mascarenhas M, Liacouras CA: The use of skin prick tests and patch tests to identify causative foods in eosinophilic esophagitis. J Allergy Clin Immunol 109:363–368, 2002.

16. Sporik R, Hill DJ, Hosking CS. Specificity of allergen skin testing in children. Clin Exp Allergy 30:1540–1546, 2000.

17. Stevenson DD: Monosodium glutamate and asthma. J Nutr 130:1067S–1073S, 2000.

18. Teuber SS, Porch-Curren C: Unproved diagnostic and therapeutic approaches to food allergy and intolerance. Curr Opin Allergy Clin Immunol 3:217–221, 2003.

19. Zeiger RS: Current issues with influenza vaccination in egg allergy. J Allergy Clin Immunol 110:834–840, 2002.

CHAPTER 14

INSECT ALLERGY

Rahmat Afrasiabi, M.D.

1. **What is the overall prevalence of sting reactions in adults and children?**
   3.3% of adults and 0.4% to 0.8% of children develop systemic reaction following stings.

2. **Of people who develop systemic reaction following insect stings, what percentage have skin or radioallergosorbent test (RAST) evidence of sensitization?**
   26% of people who have been stung by Hymenoptera have RAST or skin test evidence of sensitization. Venom sensitization is rather common following a sting, occurring in 30–40% of those who had recently been stung. However, this figure may change, depending on the time interval between sting and testing. Persons stung more than 3 years before testing have a 15–20% rate of positive skin or RAST tests, suggesting that sensitization is often transient.
      Golden DBK, Hamilton R, Lictenstein LM: Insect sting allergy with negative venom skin test responses. J Allergy Clin Immunol 107:897–901, 2001.

3. **Describe the natural history of a positive skin test or RAST in asymptomatic adults with a history of bee sting and no systemic reaction.**
   - The prevalence of positive skin test, RAST test, or both in adults with no history of systemic reaction to stings ranges from 15% to 25%.
   - The mean conversion rate to a negative skin test after 4 years is 45%
   - 33% become skin test-negative after 2.5 years
   - 80% become negative after 6–8 years.
   - Venom specific IgE remains positive in 30–40% after 2.5 to 6.8 years, even when skin tests become negative.
   Reisman RE: Studies of the natural history of insect sting allergy. Allergy Proc 10:97–101, 1989.

4. **Outline the relevant taxonomy of Hymenoptera.**
   Hymenoptera is the order, which contains four families: Vespidae (yellow jacket, hornets, paper wasps), Apidae (bees), Halictidae (sweet bees), and Formicidae (ants).

5. **List the major features of vespid venoms.**
   - Vespid venoms are immunologically similar.
   - Dol a 5 is the most potent allergen.
   - Their phospholipases do not cross-react with honeybee venom. Phospholipases are the dominant allergens in wasps, whereas hyaluronidases are related to allergens in bee venom.

6. **What should you know about asymptomatic adult sensitization to Hymenoptera venom?**
   It is common but transient and disappears at the rate of 12% per year.

7. **What is the risk of a systemic reaction on a subsequent sting of a Hymenoptera in asymptomatic, sensitized adults with positive skin test?**
   17%. The risk may be higher than 17% if a positive skin test persists for years.

8. **Is the frequency of sting reactions different in atopic versus nonatopic people?**
The frequency of sting reactions does not differ among atopic, nonatopic, or unselected populations; however, the frequency of venom sensitivity on skin testing is greater in people who have skin test sensitivity to inhalant allergens.

9. **Summarize the factors that affect the frequency and risk of insect sting allergy.**
   - Risk of exposure is clearly the most important factor. For this reason children and adults who work or play outdoors and beekeepers and their families are at higher risk of insect sting allergy.
   - Agricultural and fruit-belt regions of the country have larger populations of honeybees, whereas Polistes wasp sensitivity is more frequent in the central Gulf Coast regions such as Texas and Louisiana.
   - Multiple stings increase the risk of allergy, as do repeated stings in close proximity only weeks apart.

   Golden DBK: Epidemiology of allergy to insect venoms and stings. Allergy Proc 10:103–107, 1989.

10. **Is the pattern of venom skin test and RAST results different?**
The RAST is negative in approximately 20% of skin test–positive people. However, approximately 10% of RAST-positive people have negative skin tests.

11. **How many people die from insect sting allergy each year in the United States?**
An estimated 40–50 people die each year from insect sting allergy. However, this figure may not reflect the real number of deaths because in many unrecognized and unsuspected cases the cause of death may be attributed to myocardial infarctions or cerebrovascular accidents.

12. **What is the fate of people with a history of insect sting allergy on subsequent stings?**
Their fate is somewhat unpredictable and varies considerably. Only 30–60% of sting-allergic patients have systemic reactions when deliberately challenged, even though the nonreactors may react to subsequent stings.
The frequency of recurrent systemic sting reactions in children is considerably lower. Children whose prior systemic reaction is only cutaneous have only a 10% incidence of a subsequent systemic reaction, and the incidence of more severe reaction with respiratory or circulatory symptoms is 0.4%.

13. **Summarize the natural history of a large local reaction.**
The recurrence rate appears to be high. A history of a large local reaction does not predict progression to systemic reaction. The eventual risk of anaphylaxis in such people ranges from 5% to 10%. The factors favoring systemic reaction include multiple stings and repeat stings within a few weeks.

14. **What is the true incidence of immediate hypersensitivity to *Triatoma*?**
The true incidence of immediate allergic reaction to *Triatoma* is unknown; however, a questionnaire survey by the California State Health Department found a 5% incidence of allergic reactions to *Triatoma* in Mariposa County.

15. **What are the common names for *Triatoma*?**
Kissing bug and cone-nosed bug.

16. **What are the most commonly encountered species of *Triatoma* in the United States?**
There are 10 *Triatoma* species in the United States. However, only six species are likely to be encountered in the continental United States:
   - *T. lecticularius*
   - *T. gerstaeckeri*

- *T. protracta*
- *T. sanguisuga*
- *T. rubida*
- *T. recurva*

17. **What is the primary host of *T. protracta*?**
The wood rat (genus *Neotoma*).

18. **List the features of *T. protracta* that have clinical and practical significance.**
- *T. protracta* lives in the nest of its primary host, the wood rat.
- Each summer the adult bugs discur. It is during this time that bites are common.
- *T. protracta* generally flies when the air temperature is above 20°C (65°F) and usually does not fly more than 1 mile. The flights are primarily nocturnal.
- The insects are attracted by light to houses.
- Most bites occur when the host is asleep.
- In a nonallergic person, the bite is painless.
- The sensitive person usually wakes up with symptoms of impending anaphylaxis.

19. **What is the source of *Triatoma* antigens?**
Salivary gland secretions.

20. **Where in the United States are fire ants ubiquitous?**
In the Southeastern United States and along the Gulf Coast.

21. **What is the major characteristic feature of a fire ant sting?**
Sterile pustule.

22. **Describe mosquitoes and allergic reactions to their bites.**
There are 13 genera and 150 species of mosquitoes (Culicidae) found in the United States and Canada. Most reports describe local reactions. In few published case reports, extensive local skin reactions, fever, and delayed systemic symptoms were described. Two of the three patients studied had positive skin test and elevated IgE to whole body extract. Using immunoblotting techniques, genus-specific and species-specific IgE antibodies to *Aedes* and *Culex* mosquitoes have been shown in the sera of mosquito-sensitive persons.

23. **Describe common systemic symptoms following Hymenoptera stings.**
Systemic reactions, which occur up to 4 hours after the sting, are defined as immediate reactions. Symptoms are generalized and manifest at sites remote from the sting. They may include generalized pruritus, urticaria, and laryngeal edema with feeling of tightness in the throat or closing feeling of throat and upper respiratory airway, bronchospasm with wheezing, and shortness of breath. Other symptoms include abdominal cramping, nausea and/or vomiting, and vascular collapse.

24. **Which of the Hymenoptera species leaves its stinger at the site of the sting?**
Honeybee. However, in 4–8% of cases, vespid stingers and venom sacs also evulse.

25. **Describe the clinical presentations of delayed reactions after Hymenoptera stings.**
- Usually occur more than 4 hours following sting
- Progressive swelling and erythema at the sting site
- Serum sickness-like reactions
- Guillain-Barré syndrome
- Glomerulonephritis
- Influenza-like symptoms, including fever, myalgia, and shaking chills, 8–24 hours after a honeybee sting

KEY POINTS: INSECT ALLERGY

1. Patients must carry their Epi-Pen kits at all times.

2. Patients should be provided with avoidance strategies not only for stinging insects, but also for kissing bugs.

3. There are three types of local reactions to fire ants: wheal and flare reactions, sterile pustules, and large local reactions.

4. Honey bees classically leave their stinger at the site of the sting, but occasionally vespid stingers and venom sacs also evulse.

26. **Describe the biochemical nature of allergens in honeybee, vespids, and fire ants.**
    Venom allergens are all proteins, and most of them are enzymes. The most important allergens of honeybee are:
    - APIM I, which is phospholipase A2
    - APIM II, which is hyaluronidase
    - APIM III, which is melittin
    - APIM IV, which is acid phophatase

27. **Describe the biochemical nature and allergens of vespids.**
    - DOLM I, which is phospholipase A
    - DOLM II, which is hyaluronidase
    - DOLM III, which is acid phosphatase
    - DOLM IV, which is the common name of antigen 5

28. **List the antigens of the fire ant.**
    SOLI I, SOLI II, and SOLI III; the SOLI II antigen is phospholipase.

29. **What tests are available to evaluate patients with a clinical history of systemic reaction to Hymenoptera?**
    Both skin and RAST tests are available for diagnosis. The lyophilized preparations of honeybee, wasps, yellow jacket, yellow hornet, and white-faced hornet are commercially available. Bumblebee venom has extensive cross-reactivity with honeybee venom. The person with a history of systemic allergic reaction to bumblebee can be identified by honeybee skin test. The scratch test using venom concentration of 1 μg/mL is used for screening. If the initial scratch tests are negative with venom concentrations ranging from 1 ng/mL to 1 μg/mL, intradermal skin tests are performed. The skin test should also include a positive control (using histamine) and a negative control (using diluent).

30. **Describe the sensitivity, specificity, and clinical application of skin and RAST tests.**
    The skin test is more rapidly available and more sensitive than the RAST. The RAST test is negative in approximately 20% of skin test–positive patients. However, in 10% of subjects the RAST test may be positive with a negative skin test. The recommendation is to do both tests in patients with a strong history of systemic reaction and a negative skin test. Between 8% and 25% of people with sting sensitivity have negative skin test at venom concentrations below 14 gm/ml.

31. **How early can you proceed with these tests following a systemic reaction? Is there a waiting period after an anaphylactic reaction?**
Skin and RAST tests may be done at 2 weeks or later following anaphylaxis. Because of the consumption of specific IgE during anaphylaxis episodes, these tests are unreliable immediately after an episode of anaphylaxis. If the tests are negative at 2 weeks after an episode of anaphylaxis, they may be repeated four weeks later.

32. **Describe the geographic distribution of imported fire ants.**
There are two major imported fire ants; the black fire ant (*Solenopsis richteri*), which is a native of Argentina and Uruguay, and the red fire ant (*Solenopsis invecta*), originally a native of Argentina, Paraguay, and Brazil. Historically they appear to have entered the United States through Mobile, Alabama. Fire ants are common in the southern United States. Recent reports show that their habitat is expanding westward. They have been recently spotted in Arizona, California, and New Mexico.

Kemp SF, Deshazo RD, Moffitt JE, et al: Expanding habitat of imported fire ant (*Solenopsis invicta*): A public health concern. J Allergy Clin Immunol 105:683–691, 2000.

33. **List the three types of local reactions to fire ant stings.**
1. Wheal-and-flare reactions
2. Sterile pustule
3. Large local reaction

34. **How are fire ant stings treated?**
The pustules occur within 24 hours after the sting and are pathognomonic for fire ant sting. No known treatment can effectively prevent the pustules or accelerate their resolution.

35. **Summarize the symptoms of systemic reactions to fire ant stings.**
Symptoms range from generalized urticaria, angioedema, pruritus, and erythema to life-threatening reactions of bronchospasm, laryngeal edema, or hypotension. Toxic reactions including seizures, mononeuritis, serum sickness, nephrotic syndrome, and worsening of preexisting cardiopulmonary conditions have been reported.

36. **How common are episodes of anaphylaxis after fire ant stings?**
The exact incidence of anaphylaxis to fire ants is not known. Surveys have reported that from 0.6% to 16% of people who are stung have anaphylactic reactions. The anaphylaxis may occur hours after the sting. To date, more than 80 fatal cases of anaphylaxis have been attributed to fire ants.

37. **Who is at risk for systemic reactions to fire ant stings?**
Systemic reactions usually occur in people who have been sensitized through prior stings; however, some people without a prior history of fire ant stings develop anaphylaxis after their first exposure. It appears that such people have been sensitized by prior exposure to *Vespula* (yellow jacket) venom. Both clinical and laboratory evidence support cross-reactivity between *Vespula* and *Solenopsis* venom.

Kemp SF, Deshazo RD, Moffitt JE, et al: Expanding habitat of imported fire ant (*Solenopsis invicta*): A public health concern. J Allergy Clin Immunol 105:683–691, 2000.

38. **Describe the composition of fire ant venom.**
95% of fire ant venom is composed of water-insoluble alkaloids that have cytotoxic, hemolytic, antibacterial, and insecticidal properties and are primarily 2.6 di-substituted piperindines. These alkaloids are the cause of sterile pustules but do not induce IgE responses. The water-soluble proteins of *Solenopsis invecta* venom contain four major allergic proteins, SOLI I–IV. SOLI-I has phospholipase A and B and some immunologic cross-reactivity activity with vespid venoms.

Two-thirds of the venom proteins are comprised of SOLI-II, which does not have any immunologic cross-reactivity with other hymenoptera venoms. SOLIli-III is a member of antigen 5 families of venom proteins without consistent cross-reactivity with vespid antigen-5.

39. **How is reaction to fire ant venom confirmed?**
The commercially available venoms of imported fire ants, unlike Hymenoptera, contain significant and stable amounts of venom allergens. Skin test, enzyme-linked immunosorbent assay (ELISA), and RAST can be used to confirm a history of systemic reaction to imported fire ant. Several studies found the venom RAST test to be superior to whole-body RAST. The venom ELISA has similar sensitivity.

40. **Discuss the role of immunotherapy in prevention of reactions to fire ant stings.**
Immunotherapy with whole body extract of imported fire ant has been done in the past 30 years by injecting a dilution of whole body venom on a weekly basis, with a gradual increase in dose until reaching a maintenance dose of 0.5 mL of 1:10 dilution of the 1:10 weight/volume stock whole-body venom. Maintenance doses are usually given every 4–6 weeks.

41. **Describe protective strategies for people with a history of sting sensitivity to Hymenoptera.**
    - Avoid wearing bright and light-colored clothes that attract bees.
    - Avoid wearing scents and perfumes. ·
    - Wear gloves and long pants while working in their gardens.
    - Avoid drinking out of uncovered, opened soda cans left outside.
    - Wear shoes, long pants, or slacks when walking in grass fields.
    - Use insecticides especially designed to kill Hymenoptera.

42. **What advice do you give to patients with a history of anaphylaxis to _Triatoma_ to minimize exposure to kissing bugs?**
See Table 14-1.

43. **What methods can be used to control imported fire ants?**
    - Basic methods are broadcast applications, individual mound treatments, or both.
    - Chemical barriers and spot treatments may be helpful.
    - Broadcast applications using a bait containing a slow-acting toxicant (hydramethylnon) should be dissolved in an attractant food source such as soybean oil. Corn grits that have absorbed the toxicant-containing oil are an easily broadcast carrier.
    - Because the toxicant is a slow-acting chemical, it allows enough time for the worker ants to feed the queen and other ants before the worker ants die.
    - This method leads to the eventual demise of the colony because the queen either dies or no longer produces eggs.

44. **List the three most important steps in the treatment of anaphylaxis following an insect sting.**
    1. Epinephrine
    2. Epinephrine
    3. Epinephrine

45. **How much epinephrine should be used in adults and children?**
    - 0.3 mL of 1:1000 for adults
    - 0.3 of 1:2000 for children weighing less than 30 kg

46. **What epinephrine-containing kits are available to treat anaphylaxis?**
    1. Ana-kit contains a syringe preloaded with two 0.5-mL doses of 1:1000 epinephrine, along with chewable antihistamine tablets, tourniquet, and alcohol swab. One of the problems is

TABLE 14-1. STRATEGIES TO MINIMIZE EXPOSURE TO KISSING BUGS

1. Trap wood rats in the immediate vicinity (100 yards) in rural settings and certainly in a dwelling if a wood rat nest is found.
2. Check attic, basements, and crawl spaces for wood rat nests.
3. If a nest is found, trap the rat, destroy the nest, and treat area with malathion 2% emulsifiable concentrate.
4. Block wood rat access to structures with one-fourth-inch hardware cloth; check periodically.
5. Weather-strip all doors and windows that are open.
6. Be sure that pet doors close with no openings greater than one-sixteenth of an inch.
7. Do not bring outdoor furniture into the house; you may bring *Triatoma* with it.
8. Use gravity flap covers on the outside of exhaust ports for fans and air conditioners.
9. Keep outdoor lighting to a minimum.
10. Curtains should be drawn in lighted rooms at night.
11. Do not use ultraviolet insect traps.
12. Inspect dark, quiet area (along baseboard, behind curtains, in furniture, in closets) weekly during *Triatoma* season (mid-spring to mid-fall).
13. Scrutinize sleeping area. Bedding should be inspected each evening before retiring. A bed net (available from outdoor/sporting goods stores) is the best exclusionary device while sleeping and should be tucked in at all times.
14. Except in known cases of infestation, insecticides are of little value. Safe levels of residual insecticides do not immediately prevent *Triatoma* from gaining access and biting.
15. Do not attempt to destroy the entire local wood rat population; this approach is ineffective. Consider seasonal (spring and fall) dusting of local wood rats with carbaryl 2% dust to control insects.

that patients frequently take the tablets first and wait until the symptoms worsen before taking the epinephrine.

2. EpiPen and EpiPen Jr, Epi-EZ-Pen and Epi-EZ-Pen Jr, which contain 0.3 mL of 1:1000 and 1:2000 epinephrine and 0.3 mL of 1:1000 and 1:2000 epinephrine, respectively. These devices are easier to use and practical. However, only single dosing is available.
3. Other available kits include min-I-Jet, Anahelp, and Fastjekt.

47. How do you instruct the patient to use the EpiPen and Epi-EZ-Pen?
All patients should be instructed how to use the EpiPen and the Epi-EZ-Pen, which includes a practice pen. The patient should be instructed not to mistake and use the practice pen for treatment of anaphylaxis. The pharmacist should also further train patients. Fatalities have been reported as a result of patients not knowing how to use the EpiPen. Patients should be advised to carry an epinephrine kit with them all the time. The kits should be stored at room temperature and protected from exposure to sunlight.

48. Describe step-by-step management of anaphylaxis after insect sting.
Table 14-2 outlines the six steps in management of anaphylaxis due to insect sting. In addition, all patients should be given written instruction on insect avoidance, prescription for epinephrine

with several refills and instructions on how to use it as well as a referral to the pharmacist to provide training. Referral to an allergist for follow-up evaluation should be arranged.

49. **Is immunotherapy indicated for children with a history of urticaria as the only manifestation of systemic reaction to hymenoptera stings?**

No. To answer this and similar questions, a natural history study was designed at Johns Hopkins University. Two hundred forty-two children ages 3–16 years, whose only reactions were mild generalized reactions (cutaneous angioedema and or urticaria), were randomly assigned to two groups. One group (68 children) received venom immunotherapy. The second group (174 children) received no treatment. Only 1 (1.2%) of 84 stings in the children receiving venom

---

TABLE 14-2.   SIX STEPS IN THE TREATMENT OF INSECT STING ANAPHYLAXIS

1. Aqueous epinephrine 1:1000 (1 mg/mL) should be administered intramuscularly in a dose of 0.01 mg/kg of body weight up to a maximum of 0.3 mL. If hypotension exists, lower the dose (1–5 4 µg/kg) using 1:10,000 (0.1 mg/mL) preparation, which can be given intravenously by infusion.

2. Parenteral H_1 antihistamine, usually diphenhydramine, is commonly administered. The use of antihistamines as the only treatment of urticaria and cutaneous angioedema, which appears to have become a common practice in many emergency departments, should be discouraged. Epinephrine should be used for these milder forms of anaphylaxis and is highly effective in reversing itching and urticaria.

3. The combination of H_1 and H_2 antihistamines may be more effective in the treatment and prevention of histamine-induced falls in diastolic blood pressure.

4. Glucocorticoids should be used systemically. Their use upregulates the beta receptors and also interferes with arachidonic acid metabolism, with a decrease in synthesis of leukotrienes and prostaglandins. Their use may also be effective in preventing late-phase reactions. Patients should be informed about the potential risks of parenteral use of steroids, including avascular necrosis of the head of femur, which may lead to hip replacement.

5. Intravenous glucagon at the dose of 504 µg/kg as an intravenous bolus should be administered for the treatment of anaphylaxis in the patients who are taking beta blockers, because they do not usually respond to routine doses of epinephrine. Persistent hypotension may respond to intravenous glucagons, which has the unique property of activating adenyl cyclase independently of beta receptors, leading to an increase in intracellular cyclic adenosine monophosphate (cAMP). However, because of its vasodilator property, it can sometimes lead to hypotension.

6. Patients whose only manifestations are urticaria and cutaneous angioedema may be discharged after clearance of these symptoms. They should be prescribed an epinephrine kit and instructed how to use it in case of recurrence of symptoms because of the biphasic nature of some of anaphylactic reactions. Patients who present with significant bronchospasm or hypotension or who live in areas far away from a medical care facility should be admitted to the hospital or kept for observation for 8–12 hours before discharge.

immunotherapy caused a mild systemic reaction. Eighteen (9.2%) of 196 stings in untreated children produced systemic reactions; none of these reactions were more severe than their original sting reactions. The study concluded that immunotherapy was of little medical benefit.

50. **Is there any indication for evaluation and immunotherapy for a large local reaction following Hymenoptera sting?**
    In most patients presenting with large local reactions as the only manifestation after a sting, venom-specific IgE antibodies are demonstrable. A very small group of these patients develop anaphylaxis after future stings; therefore, skin or RAST test and immunotherapy are not indicated.

51. **How effective is the immunotherapy for Hymenoptera?**
    - The rate of protection varies, depending on the maintenance dose and whether the immunotherapy is for vespids or honeybees.
    - At the usual maintenance dose of 100 μgm, 98% of the adults and children on vespid immunotherapy have clinical protection.
    - The clinical protection for honeybee is reported to be at 80%.
    - Clinical protection is reduced at lower maintenance doses. At a maintenance dose of 50 μgm, clinical protection for adults following sting challenge drops to 79%.

52. **When can immunotherapy for Hymenoptera safely be discontinued?**
    The decision to continue or discontinue immunotherapy should be individualized.
    - A repeat sting reaction is seen in 22% of patients who stop immunotherapy after 1–2 years.
    - The risk of an allergic reaction dropped from a 50–60% level to 2% in patients on maintenance therapy.
    - The risk of sting reaction remains less than 10% in the first few years after cessation of 5 or more years of venom immunotherapy.
    - The negative skin test and live sting challenges are not absolute predictors of no field-sting systemic reaction.
    - A new survey study indicates an ongoing 10% chance of reacting each time the patient is stung, with commutative risk after discontinuation of immunotherapy as high as 20% or more over 10–20 years.
    - The frequency of reaction in the first 5 years off venom therapy was reported as no different from the frequency in patients in their second 5 years off immunotherapy.
    - The mean 7-year cumulative risk of a systemic reaction to sting off venom immunotherapy in a survey of 113 patients was reported to be 14.2% and reached 16.2% at 10 years off of venom immunotherapy.
    Golden DBK, Kagey-Sobotka A, Lichtenstein LM: Survey of patients after discontinuing venom immunotherapy J Allergy Clin Immunol 105:385–390, 2000.

53. **How safe is the immunotherapy for Hymenoptera?**
    Systemic reactions do occur during venom immunotherapy. Up to 12% of people on venom immunotherapy have allergic reactions during the treatment, both during build-up and during maintenance. The systemic reactions are more common with honeybee and wasp immunotherapy.

54. **What safety precautions should be implemented during venom immunotherapy?**
    - Patients should be advised to stay in the office for 30 minutes following injection.
    - Patients should sit in the visible part of the office under supervision.
    - Patients should avoid using the bathroom after they receive their injections, because if they develop serious reaction and faint, they may not be accessible for treatment.
    - Patients should be advised to carry their epinephrine-kit when they come for immunotherapy.

55. **What are the indications for venom immunotherapy?**
Adults who have experienced a systemic reaction, including urticaria, cutaneous angioedema, respiratory symptoms, and cardiovascular collapse with positive skin or RAST test.
Children with respiratory symptoms and cardiovascular collapse.

56. **Should the decision to administer venom immunotherapy be individualized?**
Yes. The decision should take into account many factors, including medical, financial, and logistic considerations.

57. **Is immunotherapy available for *Triatoma*?**
Successful immunotherapy for *T. protracta*–induced anaphylaxis has been reported for 5 patients who were treated with 1000 units of maintenance dosage developed by Saxon and colleagues at UCLA. The 5 patients showed excellent protection at 28 to 33 weeks of therapy during bite challenges. All patients had a local reaction similar to positive skin test reaction during bite challenges. Skin test reactivity was not lost while the patient showed excellent protection without systemic reaction after bite challenges.

The standardized antigen was developed by RAST-inhibition assay, which was defined as the amount of antigen that inhibited 50% of the maximum binding of 10 μL of the reference serum and equal to 0.4 units. The antigens were extracted from salivary gland of *Triatoma* colonies.

Rohr AS, Marshall NA, Saxon A: Successful immunotherapy for *Triatoma protracta*-induced anaphylaxis. J Allergy Immunol 73:369–375, 1984.

WEBSITE ⊕

Asthma and Allergy Foundation of America: www.aafa.org

BIBLIOGRAPHY

1. Adkinson NF Jr, Yunginger JW, Busse WW, et al (eds): Middleton's Allergy: Principles and Practice, 6th ed. St. Louis, Mosby, 2003.

2. American Academy of Allergy, Asthma and Immunology: Allergy and Immunology Medical Knowledge Self-assessment Program, 3rd ed. American Academy of Allergy, Asthma and immunology, American College of Physicians, 2003.

3. Golden DBK: Epidemiology of allergy to insect venoms and stings. Allergy Proc 10:103–107, 1989.

4. Golden DBK, Kagey-Sobotka A, Lichtenstein LM: Survey of patients after discontinuing venom immunotherapy. J Allergy Clin Immunol 105:385–390, 2000.

5. Golden DBK, Hamilton R, Lictenstein LM: Insect sting allergy with negative venom skin test responses. J Allergy Clin Immunol 107:897–901, 2001.

6. Kemp SF, Deshazo RD, Moffitt JE, et al: Expanding habitat of imported fire ant *(Solenopsis invicta)*: A public health concern. J Allergy Clin Immunol 105:683–691, 2000.

7. Reisman RE: Studies of the natural history of insect sting allergy. Allergy Proc 10:97–101, 1989.

8. Rohr AS, Marshall NA, Saxon A: Successful immunotherapy for *Triatoma protracta*-induced anaphylaxis. J Allergy Immunol 73:369–375, 1984.

CHAPTER 15

DRUG HYPERSENSITIVITY AND ALLERGY

Bruce T. Ryhal, M.D.

1. **Distinguish between drug hypersensitivity and adverse drug reaction.**
   Drug hypersensitivity usually refers to an immune-mediated drug hypersensitivity reaction (IDHR). The IDHRs constitute a subset of the broad category of adverse drug reactions (ADRs). Most ADRs are not hypersensitivity responses; instead, they represent a side effect, an overdose, a drug-drug interaction, or other effect related to the dose or pharmacology of the medication. IDHRs differ from drug intolerance or idiosyncratic reactions, which are mediated by nonimmune processes of physiology or metabolism. Defining a drug reaction as a possible hypersensitivity response guides plans for further diagnosis and treatment of an affected patient.

2. **What important clinical characteristics help to define an IDHR?**
   - The symptoms and signs should correspond to possible mechanisms of immune damage.
   - The reaction generally should not occur early on first exposure to a medication, because specific immunologic memory for a drug usually does not exist before the drug's first administration.
   - The reaction should manifest again on re-exposure to the drug, and the response triggered after the second exposure should typically be more rapid in onset.
   - The involved drug should have a chemical structure capable of eliciting an immune response.
   - Because immunity is variably specific, the reaction should not be a universal, dose-dependent pharmacologic effect of the drug.

      Adkinson NF, Essayan E, Gruchalla R et al: Task Force Report: Future research needs for the prevention and management of immune-mediated drug hypersensitivity reactions. J Allergy Clin Immunol 109:S461–S478, 2003.

      Bernstein IL, Gruchalla RS, Lee RE et al (eds): Disease management of drug hypersensitivity: A practice parameter. Ann Allergy Asthma Immunol 83:665–700, 1999.

3. **Is there a distinction between drug allergy and drug hypersensitivity?**
   Drug allergy has such a variety of meanings, depending on the context, that some authors have suggested abandoning medical use of the term. In allergy and immunology specialty textbooks, allergy usually means IgE-mediated, or immediate-type, hypersensitivity. In many general medical texts and journals, *drug allergy* may be used interchangeably with *drug hypersensitivity*. In institutional medical charts, *drug allergy* is commonly used to mean almost any ADR. In lay usage, the word "allergy" can denote many types of real or suspected untoward reaction. The more precise specialty definitions apply in this chapter (Fig. 15-1). These distinctions are not merely academic but can have consequences for clinical evaluation and management.

4. **How does an anaphylactoid reaction differ from anaphylactic reactions?**
   Anaphylactic reactions involve specific IgE-mediated mast cell and/or basophil degranulation with mediator release. Clinical findings include urticaria, angioedema, bronchospasm, and hypotension. **Anaphylactoid reactions** may clinically simulate anaphylaxis and involve mast cells, but they do not involve specific IgE and therefore are not true drug allergic reactions. Anaphylactoid events may occur after first exposure to a drug.

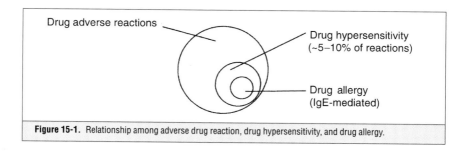

Figure 15-1. Relationship among adverse drug reaction, drug hypersensitivity, and drug allergy.

5. **What is the difference between desensitization and a graded challenge?**
In order to be desensitized, a patient must show evidence, usually by a positive skin test, of prior sensitization. **Desensitization,** therefore, applies most accurately to the reduction of IgE-mediated hypersensitivity. **Graded challenge** is the term used to describe the practice of administering incremental doses of a drug to a patient with some other suspected type of adverse drug reaction. Increasingly, however, desensitization is used to denote a form of graded challenge (as in aspirin desensitization) involving physiologic processes that may not include IgE.

6. **What mechanisms of immune damage have been associated with drug hypersensitivity?**
The Gell and Coombs classification of human hypersensitivity provides models for understanding immunologic drug reactions. **Type I** reaction is IgE-mediated and constitutes an immediate hypersensitivity response. **Type II** hypersensitivity involves antibody-mediated cytotoxicity. Immune complex reactions are termed **type III.** Cell-mediated immunity causes **type IV** hypersensitivity. For the majority of suspected IDHRs, the exact mechanism of involvement of the immune system is not fully known, and some drug reactions may involve multiple pathways.

7. **Describe the pathogenesis of type I hypersensitivity reactions.**
Type I hypersensitivity reactions are true drug allergies. They are elicited by the binding of some form of the drug to specific IgE attached to Fcε receptors on mast cells. Degranulation and activation of the mast cell occur with release of histamine and other preformed and newly synthesized mediators of inflammation. Clinical findings include urticaria, angioedema, bronchospasm, and anaphylaxis.

8. **Describe the proposed mechanism for type I reactions.**
The proposed mechanism involves a multiple-step process. The first step is a period of exposure to the drug in a manner likely to favor a Th2 response and IgE production. During this period the drug enters into an appropriate antigen-presenting cell (APC) for processing. High-molecular-weight protein drugs may be directly processed, whereas low-molecular-weight drugs usually require haptenization to proteins and peptides to be recognized as antigenic (or allergenic). In the APC endosome compartment, drug-peptide fragments are bound to newly synthesized major histocompatibilty complex (MHC) class II molecules and transported to the cell surface. The MHC-antigen complexes at the cell surface are presented with costimulatory molecules on the APC to CD4+ T cells, which produce cytokines, such as interleukin (IL)-4, that stimulate IgE production by B cells.

9. **Give examples of agents that may cause type I reactions.**
Beta-lactams such as penicillin that can bind to human proteins and create allergenic haptens are the most common cause of type I drug hypersensitivity. Other drugs that may produce this type of reaction include proteins, generally of large molecular weight, such as:
- Antithymocyte globulin
- Chymopapain

- Heterologous antiserum
- Insulin
- Protamine
- Recombinant granulocyte-macrophage colony-stimulating factors (GM-CSF)
- Streptokinase
- Tetanus toxoid

10. **Describe the mechanism of a type II hypersensitivity reaction.**
    Toxicity due to type II hypersensitivity is caused by antibodies directed against antigens on or
    near the cell surface. Specific antibodies are necessary to initiate this form of cytotoxic reaction,
    but in contrast to type I reactions, the antibodies are typically of the IgG or IgM class.

11. **Give examples of type II reactions.**
    A major example of type II reaction is Coombs'-positive hemolytic anemia, in which penicillin
    exposure results in the production of antibodies directed against penicillin-coated erythrocytes,
    causing lysis of the cells. Other examples are:
    - Granulocytopenia due to phenothiazines and sulfonamides
    - Immune-induced thrombocytopenia due to sulfonamides, quinidine or heparin
    - Methacillin-induced interstitial nephritis
    - Methyldopa-induced immunohemolytic anemia

12. **What determines the clinical manifestations of type II reactions?**
    The clinical manifestations of type II reactions depend largely on which target cell is involved.

13. **Describe the clinical and pathologic features of a type III hypersensitivity
    reaction.**
    Type III hypersensitivity involves damage resulting from immune complex deposition in tissue
    and blood vessels. Antibodies are usually of the IgG or IgM class and arise with ongoing
    exposure to the drug. Antigen-antibody complexes are created which may activate
    complement.

14. **Give examples of a type III reaction.**
    Medications such as heterologous antiserum and other proteins with a long half-life in the body
    may elicit a type III reaction. The clinical manifestations typically resemble serum sickness (skin
    rash, fever, lymphadenopathy, and arthralgia) and occur between 1 and 3 weeks after drug
    administration. Penicillin and cefaclor have been associated with a serum sickness-like illness,
    although the mechanism of this syndrome appears to be more complex and, in the case of cefa-
    clor, seems not to involve significant antigen-antibody reactions.

15. **Describe the proposed pathogenesis of a type IV hypersensitivity reaction.**
    In type IV hypersensitivity, or delayed hypersensitivity, cell-mediated cytotoxicity is responsible for
    the various clinical symptoms. Both CD4+ and CD8+ T cells mediate type IV responses. The pro-
    posed mechanism involves binding of drug haptens to intracellular or extracellular proteins for
    presentation by MHC molecules to drug-specific T cells. Subsequent cytokine release by T cells,
    together with the production of other mediators of cytotoxicity, creates the inflammatory response
    that is seen in conditions such as delayed-type hypersensitivity skin disease. Subtypes of the
    delayed hypersensitivity response may account for a variety of IDHRs, including maculopapular
    erythematous (morbilliform) eruptions, pustular exanthems, and some bullous reactions.

16. **Give examples of a type IV reaction.**
    Examples of delayed hypersensitivity include contact dermatitis induced by:
    - Ethylenediamine
    - Neomycin

- Topical anesthestics
- Topical antihistamines
- Topical corticosteroids

Pichler WJ: Delayed drug hypersensitivity reactions. Ann Intern Med 139:683–693, 2003.

17. **What mechanisms of drug hypersensitivity may exist outside the Gell and Coombs' classification?**

Multiple mechanisms have been proposed to explain the many drug reactions that have suspected immunologic characteristics but do not fit into any of the type I through type IV classifications.

The innate immune system, which has lesser specificity, may augment some drug reactions and may not need prior exposure to the drug or its metabolites to be activated. The innate system has pattern recognition receptors that protect the body against a broad range of foreign substances with certain characteristic structures. Innate immunity activated by a concomitant infectious process, such as a viral illness, has been proposed to modulate the immunologic response to drugs.

Syndromes that mimic systemic autoimmunity, such the procainamide-induced lupus-like syndrome, represent another pathway of damage. An autoimmune form of hepatitis is associated with anti-cytochrome P450 autoantibodies induced by drugs such as halothane.

Some nonpeptide drugs, such as penicillin and sulfamethoxazole, can be presented to T cells through association with MHC independently of covalent processing, but the precise clinical significance of this finding is still under investigation.

18. **Describe the most important methods for arriving at a clinical diagnosis of a suspected hypersensitivity drug reaction.**

The medical history and physical exam are the most important tools for arriving at a diagnosis of IDHR. Confusion often results when multiple drugs have been administered and a reaction has occurred. A complete list of all medications taken by patient and the time and dates of administration must be recorded. Information should be collected about the patient's prior reactions and any previous exposure to the suspected medications. Knowledge of the pharmacology and side effects of the drugs as well as the general risk of hypersensitivity for each drug taken is important. The patient's individual risk for drug hypersensitivity should be assessed. Alternative causes, such as infection, should be excluded. The physical exam can help define the type of reaction, which then can be correlated with the time course of administration of the various drugs to suggest a plausible cause and mechanism. Limited diagnostic testing is available for most drug reactions.

19. **Who is at risk for drug hypersensitivity?**

Several categories of patients may be at greater risk for drug hypersensitivity. The elderly are more susceptible to adverse drug reactions in general, and females are more likely to acquire autoimmune problems than males. Patients who have had previous immune reactions to one or more drugs may be at greater risk, especially if they have reacted to a chemically similar medication. Higher-risk patients may show genetic variation in drug metabolic enzymes. Patients with concomitant viral infections are more likely to develop hypersensitivity. A common example is the morbilliform rash often seen in patients with mononucleosis who are given amoxicillin. Patients with AIDS also have more drug-induced morbilliform cutaneous reactions, typically occurring 1 to 2 weeks into treatment with the drug and especially with sulfonamides. Atopy by itself does not appear to be a risk factor for sensitization to nonprotein drugs.

Strom BL, Schinnar R, Apter AJ: Absence of cross-reactivity between sulfonamide antibiotics and sulfonamide nonantibiotics. N Engl J Med 349:1628–1635, 2003.

20. **How does method of delivery affect the risk for hypersensitivity reactions?**

Topical administration is the most likely to result in sensitization; oral ingestion is the least likely to cause an immune reaction; and parenteral delivery is intermediate in risk of sensitization.

21. **Name the dematologic syndromes that can result from drug hypersensitivity.**
     Drug reactions are most commonly heralded by skin changes, partly because they are the most
     noticeable and partly because the skin is an active metabolic and immunologic organ. Clinical
     syndromes include:
     - Cutaneous vasculitis
     - Eczema
     - Erythema multiforme, Stevens-Johnson syndrome, toxic epidermal necrolysis
     - Erythema nodosum
     - Erythroderma (exfoliative dermatitis)
     - Fixed drug eruptions
     - Lichenoid eruptions
     - Morbilliform rashes
     - Photoallergic reactions
     - Urticaria/angioedema

     Beltrani VS: Cutaneous manifestations of adverse drug reactions. Immunol Allergy Clin North
     America 18:867–895, 1998.

22. **What are the causes and characteristics of drug-induced urticaria?**
     Drug-induced urticaria is due to release of mast cell mediators and occurs most often because
     of a type I hypersensitivity reaction, although type III and pseudoallergic reactions may also
     result in this syndrome. Lesions are typically erythematous wheals that are pruritic and blanch
     on pressure. The lesions are evanescent and usually vanish and/or relocate within 24 hours.
     Angioedema, or soft tissue swelling, may occur with an urticarial reaction and, when present, is
     often most visible on the face and perioral region. Severe, systemic mast cell mediator release
     results in anaphylaxis; thus, urticarial reactions are of significant concern.

23. **Give examples of drugs that may induce urticaria.**
     Examples of medications likely to induce urticaria include many of the drugs that cause type I
     hypersensitivity. Aspirin and related drugs can cause an urticarial rash, presumably through
     leukotriene mechanisms not involving specific immunity.

24. **Describe the clinical features of drug-induced morbilliform reactions.**
     Drug-induced morbilliform reactions are among the most common of all drug reactions. The
     morbilliform rashes typically begin on the trunk as small maculopapular, blanching areas of
     erythema and may spread to involve the limbs. The palms and soles are often spared. Pruritus
     is variable. The lesions can become confluent. The rash usually develops within 1–3 weeks of
     initiating a drug, and medications that have been used for a long time (months or years) in the
     patient are rarely suspect.

25. **How are morbilliform reactions treated?**
     Some of these reactions may resolve despite continued use of the drug, but this course of action
     is not riskless, because some more-serious reactions may have a morbilliform initial appear-
     ance. Most cases resolve with symptomatic treatment and discontinuation of the drug.

26. **How are erythema multiforme, Stevens-Johnson syndrome, and toxic
     epidermal necrolysis (TEN) related to drug hypersensitivity?**
     These three diseases share certain clinical and pathologic features. Ten to 20% of cases of
     erythema multiforme are attributed to drug reactions. Erythema multiforme may begin early
     after drug administration and manifests as erythematous target lesions with central bullae. The
     individual lesions are nonblanching, have varying shapes, and persist in a specific location for
     1 week or more instead of relocating, like urticarial lesions, within 24 hours. Erythema multiforme
     major involves multiple mucosal surfaces in addition to the skin and presents with more
     systemic symptoms.

Patients with **Stevens-Johnson syndrome** have purpuric macules and blisters with prominent trunk and face involvement.

TEN presents with fever, diffuse erythema, and edema evolving into widespread bullae formation with skin detachment. It is thought that drugs cause most cases of TEN. A proposed immune mechanism accounting for TEN is keratinocyte apoptosis mediated by Fas (CD95) and Fas ligand (FasL).

Roujeau JC, Stern RC: Severe adverse cutaneous reactions to drugs. N Engl J Med 331: 1272–1285, 1994.

27. **Which medications may be associated with these three reactions?**
    - Allopurinol
    - Anticonvulsants
    - Barbiturates
    - Nonsteroidal anti-inflammatory drugs (NSAIDs)
    - Penicillins
    - Sulfonamides

28. **How does drug-induced erythroderma differ from TEN?**
    Drug-induced erythroderma may be confused with TEN but is usually a less severe disease. Diffuse erythema with scaling and exfoliation occurs in the erythroderma syndrome, although full-thickness epidermal detachment is not found. Many drugs, including vancomycin, sulfonamides, and penicillins, may cause exfoliative dermatitis. Erythroderma has been referred to as red-man syndrome, although the term "red man" is also used to describe the immediate and transient histamine flush caused in some patients by vancomycin infusion. In contrast to TEN, erythroderma may respond to corticosteroid treatment.

29. **What are fixed drug eruptions?**
    Fixed drug eruptions are typically well-circumscribed, erythematous papules and plaques that recur at the same site each time a drug is administered. The lesions are commonly found around the oral, anal, and genital areas and often occur less than 8 hours after re-administration of a drug. They may be pruritic or cause a burning dysesthesia. The characteristic recurrence at a specific site suggests immunologic memory, perhaps related to skin T cells.

30. **Which drugs that may cause fixed eruptions?**
    - Acetaminophen
    - Barbiturates
    - NSAIDs
    - Oral contraceptives
    - Phenolphthalein
    - Sulfonamides

KEY POINTS: DRUG HYPERSENSITIVITY/ALLERGY

1. A drug reaction exhibiting memory, specificity, and a plausible mechanism of immune damage is suggestive of an immune-mediated drug hypersensitivity reaction (IDHR).

2. A thorough drug history is the most important step in determining the cause of a suspected drug hypersensitivity/allergy reaction.

3. Very limited testing is available for most suspected drug hypersensitivity reactions.

4. Treatment of an IDHR nearly always involves stopping the suspected drug.

31. **Describe the characteristics of drug allergy–associated eczema.**
   The clinical syndrome of drug-induced eczema occurs most commonly with topical administration of a drug, although systemic administration may cause some cases. Eczema consists of disrupted skin with varying degrees of erythema, vesiculation, scaling, and thickening.

32. **How may drugs cause eczema?**
   Many drugs may cause contact dermatitis with eczema after topical administration, presumably through type IV hypersensitivity mechanisms. Medications that may cause eczema through systemic administration include penicillin, bleomycin, and gold.

33. **Are lichenoid eruptions associated with drug hypersenstitivity?**
   Lichenoid drug eruptions are rashes that clinically resemble lichen planus. The drug-induced lesions are well-circumscribed, violaceous or red papules with occasional scaling. They may appear after several months of drug administration.

34. **Which drugs have been associated with lichenoid eruptions?**
   - Antimalarials
   - Beta blockers
   - Captopril
   - Dapsone
   - Furosemide
   - Gold
   - Methyldopa
   - Penicillamine
   - Sildenafil
   - Thiazides

35. **Is drug hypersensitivity involved in photoallergic responses?**
   Light-induced rashes may be of several types. Photoirritant or phototoxic dermatitis is nonimmune in etiology and usually occurs rapidly after administration of the drug followed by sun exposure. Examples of phototoxic drugs include tetracyclines, phenothiazines, and NSAIDS. A photoallergic response, which occurs after a period of sensitization, is often delayed in onset and resembles a contact dermatitis.

36. **Give examples of photoallergic reactions.**
   Examples include the pruritic, inflammatory skin reactions seen on light-exposed areas after administration of medications such as:
   - Fluoroquinolones
   - Griseofulvin
   - Phenothiazines
   - Sulfonamides
   - Thiazides

37. **What systemic syndromes are associated with drug hypersensitivity?**
   Anaphylaxis may be seen after drug exposure and is a systemic syndrome consisting of urticaria, bronchoconstriction, and hypotension. True anaphylaxis is due to a type I hypersensitivity reaction and usually occurs within minutes (rarely hours) of exposure to a drug.
       Drug-induced systemic lupus-like syndromes may occur after use of hydralazine or procainamide. Clinical symptoms resolve promptly when these medications are discontinued.
       Various forms of vasculitis can occur due to drug hypersensitivity and may be systemic or limited to the skin. Drug-induced urticarial vasculitis is similar to urticaria in appearance, but the skin lesions are more persistent. Drugs can also cause the syndrome of hypersensitivity vasculitis, which affects postcapillary venules and causes nonblanching, purpuric papules (palpable

purpura) that are most numerous on the lower extremities. Henoch-Schönlein purpura may also be triggered by medications.

38. **Which drugs may be associated with vasculitis?**
    - Amiodarone
    - Granulocyte colony-stimulating factor
    - Penicillins
    - Propylthiouracil
    - Sulfonamides
    - Thiazides

39. **Do drugs cause hypersensitivity reactions that predominantly affect a single organ system?**
    Single organ systems other than the skin may be the main focus of a drug hypersensitivity reaction. Selected examples are listed in Table 15-1.

TABLE 15-1. HYPERSENSITIVITY REACTIONS AFFECTING A SINGLE ORGAN SYSTEM		
Target Organ	**Clinical Findings**	**Drugs**
Lungs	Pneumonia with eosinophilia	Penicillin
		Nitrofurantoin
		NSAIDs
		Sulfonamides
	Alveolar or interstitial infiltrates	Methotrexate
		Melphalan
Kidney	Interstitial nephritis	Methacillin
		Sulfonamides
	Membranous glomerulonephritis	Allopurinol
		Gold
Liver	Hepatitis	Halothane
		Sulfonamides
	Hepatitis with cholestatic jaundice	Phenothiazines

40. **What types of diagnostic testing are available to evaluate drug reactions?**
    Only limited testing is available for most IDHRs. Some studies may be helpful to confirm a clinical diagnosis. Tests in common use include:
    - Drug challenge
    - Epicutaneous, intradermal, and patch skin testing
    - In vitro antibody testing with RAST and/or ELISA
    - Autoantibodies including Coombs' test and antiplatelet antibodies
    - Tests for immune complexes or complement activation including C3, C4, cryoglobulins, and C1q binding assays
    - Serum β-tryptase
    - Skin biopsy

41. **What tests have limited availability or are used only for research?**
    - Cytotoxic testing
    - In vitro lymphocyte transformation
    - Isolation of specific T-cell clones
    - Leukocyte histamine release assays

42. **Give an overview of testing for hypersensitivity reactions.**
    Testing can be used in some instances to confirm or to exclude a specific immune mechanism. Although testing can demonstrate lack of sensitization at a particular point in time, the risk of sensitization at a later date cannot entirely be excluded.

43. **Describe the uses and limitations of testing for type I hypersensitivity reactions.**
    A suspected type I clinical reaction with anaphylaxis can be confirmed by an elevated serum β-tryptase, although this test does not identify the causative agent. For a limited number of drugs, the risk of a type I reaction can be determined by epicutaneous and intradermal skin testing. Skin testing has clear predictive value for type I immune reactions due to penicillin, insulin, chymopapain, tetanus toxoid, protamine, and streptokinase. Although occasionally used to test other drugs such as cephalosporins, the negative predictive value for these substances is not accurately known. The negative predictive value is critical because it represents the likelihood that a negative test will correlate with safe administration of the drug. Skin testing is inaccurate for most drugs that are not high-molecular-weight protein drugs. In vivo metabolites and hapten-protein conjugates may cause an adverse reaction even though skin testing of the native drug does not. Skin testing may also give false positive results, because many drugs act as irritants, even at dilute concentrations. Radioallergosorbent (RAST) or enzyme-linked immunosorbent (ELISA) tests are also available to quantitatively assay IgE antibody to some drugs. These tests may be less sensitive than skin tests but can be used in patients who cannot stop antihistamines or who have dermographism.

44. **Describe the uses and limitations of testing for type II hypersensitivity reactions.**
    Type II hypersensitivity reactions can be evaluated in the laboratory with tests for autoantibodies such as Coombs' and antiplatelet antibodies, although these tests will not confirm the involvement of a specific drug.

45. **What tests may be used for type III hypersensitivity reactions?**
    Type III reactions may show abnormalities on measurement of C3, C4, cryoglobulins, and C1q binding assays.

46. **What tests may be used for type IV hypersensitivity reactions.**
    Type IV hypersensitivity, when due to contact dermatitis, can be tested with specific patch testing. Lymphocyte proliferation testing and isolation of specific T-cell clones are research tools for evaluating type IV reactions.

47. **What investigative options may be used if specific testing for a drug is not available?**
    If specific testing is not available, the clinician can discontinue all or selected drugs and observe the results. Once the clinical symptoms have resolved, a graded drug challenge is an optional procedure.

48. **How is a drug challenge used to test and treat patients?**
    An incremental or graded drug challenge can help determine whether a patient will have an adverse reaction to a specific drug. A graded drug challenge is based on the assumption that

small doses of a medication are less likely to have major toxic effects than full doses. Incremental drug challenge is not true desensitization because no immune sensitization is demonstrated before the challenge. In fact, if sensitization is proven, such as with a positive skin test, a desensitization protocol should be used instead. Usually, desensitization protocols involve more drug dilutions and are more cautious than graded challenges. A graded challenge should not be attempted where the drug is suspected to have caused mucocutaneous bullous skin disease, TEN, or vasculitis, since these disorders are associated with considerable morbidity and mortality. Protocols for graded challenge are available for many drugs including sulfonamides, aspirin, NSAIDs, acyclovir, zidovudine, pentamidine, and penicillamine. Depending on the severity of the possible reaction, required monitoring for a challenge may vary from an ICU setting to a carefully observed office environment. The patient's historical reaction to the medication and the likelihood of known reactions to the drug can help estimate risk.

49. **What is the role of penicillin testing in the evaluation of a patient with a history of a penicillin reaction?**
Penicillin skin testing is the model for much of drug hypersensitivity testing. As with all immediate hypersensitivity skin testing, penicillin skin tests are predictive of IgE-mediated reactions only. Serum sickness-type reactions, hemolytic anemia, and nonurticarial rashes are not excluded by a negative test.

50. **How is penicillin testing performed?**
To achieve maximum predictive value, testing must be performed with both major and minor determinant materials. Major determinant mix is available commercially as PrePen, which is benzylpenicilloyl-polylysine, and will detect only about 80% of penicillin-sensitized patients. The remainder of sensitized patients will have significant IgE-mediated reactions only to minor determinant mix, which is not available commercially in the United States. Benzylpenicillin (penicillin G) is used as the sole minor determinant test in many centers. If minor determinant mix is synthesized and used according to published protocols, nearly 99% of skin test-negative patients can be administered penicillin safely. Active components of synthesized minor determinant mix include benzylpenicilloate and benzylpenilloate. For all testing reagents, a prick test is performed and followed by intradermal testing if the prick test is negative.

Macy E, Richter PK, Falkoff R, et al: Skin testing with penicilloate and penilloate prepared by an improved method: Amoxicillin oral challenge in patients with negative skin test response to penicillin reagents. J Allergy Clin Immunol 100:586–591, 1997.

Saxon A, Beall GN, Rohr AS, et al: Immediate hypersensitivity reactions to beta-lactam antibiotics. Annal Internal Med 107:204–215, 1987.

51. **How can testing evaluate possible hypersensitivity reactions to muscle relaxants, local anesthetics, and agents used in general anesthesia?**
Both hypersensitivity and pseudoallergic reactions can occur during local and general anesthesia. Often it is difficult to determine the cause since multiple drugs are administered during these procedures. Protocols are available for testing anesthetic agents and muscle relaxants (neuromuscular agents). The protocols for anesthetic agents represent a combination of skin testing and graded challenge, because specific IgE has not been demonstrated for most of these drugs. Although specific IgE has been found for some muscle relaxants, skin tests to these medications tend to have low predictive value. Good negative predictive values for skin testing of local anesthetics allow patients with negative results to receive these agents safely.

52. **What types of treatment are available for drug hypersensitivity?**
In nearly all cases, the suspected drug should be discontinued. Some rare cases that constitute only minor reactions, such as morbilliform rashes, can be treated through if no substitute medication is available. However, a morbilliform eruption may be the initial manifestation of potentially fatal reactions such as TEN. In general, treatment is directed at the presenting symptoms,

such as urticaria or anaphylaxis. Desensitization for some medications can allow continued use of the drug. TEN requires special attention, and most patients are managed the same as those with major burns. Systemic corticosteroids are harmful in advanced TEN. At least one uncontrolled report suggests that infusion of intravenous immune serum globulin (IVIG) may be effective for TEN.

Viard I, Wehrli P, Bullani R, et al: Inhibition of toxic epidermal necrolysis by blockade of CD95 with human intravenous immunoglobulin. Science 282:490–493, 1998.

53. **What types of drugs can be substituted for a medication that has caused a hypersensitivity reaction?**
The therapeutic indication for a drug often persists despite the need for withdrawal of the medication. Cross-reactivity between structurally similar drugs can be anticipated; therefore, structurally unrelated drugs are the preferred substitute. Oral forms of substitute drugs are usually safer and less likely to cause sensitization.

54. **Can other beta-lactams or cephalosporins be used in penicillin-allergic patients?**
Closely related beta-lactams, such as amoxicillin or ampicillin, should not be used in penicillin-allergic patients. Carbapenems (such as imipenim) are cross-reactive with penicillin. Monobactams (such as aztreonam) generally do not cross-react. Use of cephalosporins in penicillin skin test–positive patients poses an estimated 4% risk of reaction, and the safest course is to use a desensitization protocol if a cephalosporin is necessary for such patients. Skin testing for cephalosporins has unclear predictive value. Patients who give a vague history of a nonanaphylactic reaction to penicillin and have never been penicillin skin-tested probably have a less than 1% risk of reacting to a cephalosporin. First- and second-generation cephalosporins are more likely than third-generation drugs to cause allergic reactions in penicillin-sensitive individuals.

55. **When is drug desensitization appropriate?**
When substitution is impossible and the drug is necessary, drug-allergic patients may undergo a desensitization protocol.

56. **How is drug desensitization achieved?**
Extremely dilute solutions (such as a 10,000-fold dilution) of drug are administered initially, with a gradual increase in concentration and amount. A successful protocol results in antigen-specific mast cell desensitization, and full concentrations of the drug may then be given. Oral desensitization is the safest route. After desensitization, the drug must be continually administered until the required course is completed. Return of clinical sensitivity can occur on cessation of the drug. Penicillin desensitization has been the most successful. Protocols termed desensitization have been published for sulfonamides and aspirin, although these are more accurately called graded challenges.

Adkinson NF: Drug allergy. In Middleton E, Reed CE, Ellis EF, et al (eds): Allergy: Principles and Practice, 5th ed. St. Louis, Mosby, 1998, pp 1212–1224.

Patterson R, DeSwarte RD, Greenberger PA, et al: Drug Allergy and Protocols for Management of Drug Allergies, 2nd ed. Providence, Oceanside Publications, 1995.

57. **What is a pseudoallergic reaction?**
A pseudoallergic reaction has the clinical manifestations of an immediate hypersensitivity reaction but without involvement of IgE. Some medications, such as opiates, radiocontrast media (RCM), and vancomycin, can cause direct histamine release. Other drugs, such as the angiotensin-converting enzyme inhibitors, act through kinin mechanisms and may cause angioedema and cough. Other pathways that produce pseudoallergic responses include complement activation (protamine), leukotriene synthesis (aspirin and NSAIDs), and irritant bronchospasm (sulfites).

58. **Why is the anaphlylactoid reaction to RCM in high risk patients prevented by pretreatment rather than desensitization?**
Because radiocontrast materials can cause release of mast cell mediatiors without involvement of specific IgE, a densensitization protocol does not prevent RCM reactions and skin testing is not helpful. Patients who require RCM and who have had a previous reaction to RCM should receive pretreatment with corticosteroids and antihistamines to decrease the risk of an adverse reaction. Use of nonionic contrast materials can also decrease the likelihood of mast cell activation in individuals at risk.

59. **What are the clinical and biochemical characteristics of salicylate reactions?**
Salicylates cause pseudoallergic/anaphylactoid reactions in some people through inhibition of cyclooxygenase (COX) and through subsequent changes in prostaglandin and leukotriene production. Skin testing is not helpful in determining patients at risk since no specific IgE is involved. Weak inhibitors of COX, such as acetaminophen and salsalate, are better tolerated in aspirin-sensitive patients, although cross-sensitivity may occur, especially at high doses. The manufacturer's labeling on COX-2 inhibitors includes a warning for cross-sensitivity with aspirin. Preliminary studies indicate that the risk for cross-reactivity between aspirin and COX-2 inhibitors is much less than with older NSAIDs, and this finding would be predicted on theoretical grounds. A graded challenge, which is often called desensitization, can render aspirin-sensitive patients tolerant.

   Szczeklik A, Stevenson DD: Aspirin-induced asthma: Advances in pathogenesis, diagnosis and management. J Allergy Clin Immunol 111:913–921, 2003.

60. **What types of immune-mediated drug hypersensitivity reactions have been associated with bioengineered pharmaceuticals?**
Bioengineered drugs tend to be high-molecular-weight structures built on a protein scaffold and are expected to be highly immunogenic and sometimes allergenic. Choosing therapeutic synthetic molecules with a structure that is close to or identical with normal human proteins has reduced but not eliminated these risks. Recombinant proteins may act as antigens to stimulate an IDHR, or they may exert an adverse immunopharmacologic effect by interacting directly with the immune system in an exaggerated imitation of their normal function in the body. Table 15-2 summarizes ADRs to bioengineered drugs. In addition, nearly all recombinant protein drugs have been associated with a nonspecific or morbilliform rash in a subpopulation of patients.

61. **How is drug hypersensitivity related to drug metabolism?**
The risk of hypersensitivity may depend on alterations in an individual patient's drug metabolism. An example is anticonvulsant hypersensitivity syndrome, which is characterized by fever, maculopapular rash, and lymphadenopathy. Eosinophilia and diffuse inflammation of the liver and kidney also may be present. This syndrome may follow, within weeks to months, the administration of aromatic anticonvulsants such as phenytoin, carbamazepine, lamotrigine, and phenobarbital. Susceptibility to this type of hypersensitivity disorder may be due to the presence of a defined alteration in drug metabolism. Increased risk of immunologic damage has been proposed to increase with metabolic variation in the biotransformation of other drugs as well (Table 15-3).

   Gruchalla R: Drug metabolism, danger signals, and drug-induced hypersensitivity. J Allergy Clin Immunol 108:475–488, 2001.

   Montanaro A: Sulfonamide allergy. Immunol Allergy Clin North Am 18:843–850, 1998.

   Vittorio CC, Muglia JJ: Anticonvulsant hypersensitivity syndrome. Arch Intern Med 155:2285–2290, 1995.

62. **Discuss the link between drug toxicity and immunity.**
The link between toxicity and immunity may be the contribution of reactive metabolites of a drug to the formation of an immunogenic product. This product may trigger the specific immune

TABLE 15-2.   REACTIONS TO BIOENGINEERED DRUGS

Drug Category	Drug	Type of IDHR or Immunopharmacologic Adverse Effect
Immunostimulant biologic response modifiers	Interferon alfa-2b	Anti-drug antibodies
		Flu-like illness
		Neutropenia
	Interferon beta-1b	Anaphylactoid reaction
		Flu-like illness
		Neutropenia
		Urticaria
	Interferon gamma-1b	Antidrug antibodies
		Fever
	Interleukin-2	Bullous dermatitis
		Flu-like illness
Immunosuppressive biologic response modifiers	Alefacept	Anaphylaxis
		Lymphopenia
		Urticaria/angioedema
	Anakinra	Flu-like symptoms
		Neutropenia
	Etanercept	Antidrug antibodies
		Autoantibodies
		Urticaria
Other biologic response modifiers	Erythropoietin	Antierythropoietin antibodies with pure red cell aplasia
		Urticaria
	G-CSF	Leukocytoclastic vasculitis
	GM-CSF	IgE anti-drug antibodies
Monoclonal antibodies	Infliximab	Anaphylaxis
		Autoantibodies
		Infusion reaction
	Omalizumab	Anaphylaxis
	Trastuzumab	Anaphylaxis
		Infusion reaction
		Pulmonary infiltrates

G-CSF = granulocyte colony-stimulating factor, GM-CSF = granulocyte-macrophage colony-stimulating factor.

system ("drug-hapten model") or else activate the innate immune system ("danger model"), which could proceed to modulate a more complex adaptive immune response. Pharmacogenetic screening for metabolic variants with microarray technology may someday decrease the incidence of IDHRs.

TABLE 15-3.	DRUG HYPERSENSITIVITY RELATED TO DRUG METABOLISM		
Drug	Clinical Syndrome	Metabolic Alteration	Reactive Metabolite
Anticonvulsants	Anticonvulsant hypersensitivity syndrome	Hereditary deficiency of epoxide hydrolase	Arene oxides
Sulfamethoxazole	Skin rash	Slow *N*-acetylation or decreased glutathione	Sulfamethoxasole hydroxlyamine
Cefaclor	Serum sickness-like reaction	Hereditary variation in cefaclor metabolism	Cefaclor metabolites
Procainamide	Drug-induced lupus	Slow acetylators	Hydroxlamino-procainamide

63. **After receiving a medication, can a patient have a hypersensitivity reaction that is not due to the active drug or its metabolites?**
Excepients, preservatives, and contaminants can cause a hypersensitivity response. For example, pharmaceutical components such as gelatin, egg proteins, and benzylalkonium chloride have been associated with drug allergy.

64. **What is the responsibility of the health care professional to report drug hypersensitivity?**
As a category of adverse drug reaction, *serious* drug hypersensitivity reactions may be reported through MedWatch (1-800-FDA-1088), the FDA medical products reporting system. Except for adverse events associated with vaccines, reporting is voluntary at the federal level for health professionals. However, reports are encouraged since underreporting of reactions is a major concern. Some states and local agencies may have additional reporting requirements.

WEBSITES

1. American Academy of Allergy, Asthma and Immunology: www.aaaai.org

2. National Library of Medicine: www.nlm.nih.gov

BIBLIOGRAPHY

1. Adkinson NF: Drug allergy. In Middleton E, Reed CE, Ellis EF, et al (eds): Allergy: Principles and Practice, 5th ed. St. Louis, Mosby, 1998, pp 1212–1224.

2. Adkinson NF, Essayan E, Gruchalla R et al: Task Force Report: Future research needs for the prevention and management of immune-mediated drug hypersensitivity reactions. J Allergy Clin Immunol 109:S461–S478, 2003.

3. Beltrani VS: Cutaneous manifestations of adverse drug reactions. Immunol Allergy Clin North America 18: 867–895, 1998.

4. Bernstein IL, Gruchalla RS, Lee RE et al (eds): Disease management of drug hypersensitivity: A practice parameter. Ann Allergy Asthma Immunol 83:665–700, 1999.

5. Borish L, Tilles SA: Immune mechanisms of drug allergy. Immunol Allergy Clin North Am 18:717–729, 1998.

6. Dykewicz MS: Drug allergy. In Slavin RG, Reisman RE (eds): Expert Guide to Allergy and Immunology. Philadelphia, American College of Physicians, 1999, pp 127–160.

7. Gruchalla R: Drug metabolism, danger signals, and drug-induced hypersensitivity. J Allergy Clin Immunol 108:475–488, 2001.

8. Kalish RS, Askenase PW: Molecular mechanism of CD8+ cell-mediated delayed hypersensitivity: Implications for allergies, asthma and autoimmunity. J Allergy Clin Immunol 103:192–199, 1999.

9. Leyva L, Torres MJ, Posadas S, et al: Anticonvulsant-induced toxic epidermal necrolysis: Monitoring the immunologic response. J Allergy Clin Immunol 105:157–165, 2000.

10. Macy E, Richter PK, Falkoff R, et al: Skin testing with penicilloate and penilloate prepared by an improved method: Amoxicillin oral challenge in patients with negative skin test response to penicillin reagents. J Allergy Clin Immunol 100:586–591, 1997.

11. Montanaro A: Sulfonamide allergy. Immunol Allergy Clin North Am 18:843–850, 1998.

12. Patterson R, DeSwarte RD, Greenberger PA, et al: Drug Allergy and Protocols for Management of Drug Allergies, 2nd ed. Providence, Oceanside Publications, 1995.

13. Pichler WJ: Delayed drug hypersensitivity reactions. Ann Intern Med 139:683–693, 2003.

14. Roujeau JC, Stern RC: Severe adverse cutaneous reactions to drugs. N Engl J Med 331:1272–1285, 1994.

15. Strom BL, Schinnar R, Apter AJ: Absence of cross-reactivity between sulfonamide antibiotics and sulfonamide nonantibiotics. N Engl J Med 349:1628–1635, 2003.

16. Szczeklik A, Stevenson DD: Aspirin-induced asthma: Advances in pathogenesis, diagnosis and management. J Allergy Clin Immunol 111:913–921, 2003.

17. Viard I, Wehrli P, Bullani R, et al: Inhibition of toxic epidermal necrolysis by blockade of CD95 with human intra-venous immunoglobulin. Science 282:490–493, 1998.

18. Vittorio CC, Muglia JJ: Anticonvulsant hypersensitivity syndrome. Arch Intern Med 155:2285–2290, 1995.

HYPERSENSITIVITY PNEUMONITIS AND ALLERGIC BRONCHOPULMONARY ASPERGILLOSIS

Robert D. Watson, Ph.D., M.D.

CHAPTER 16

HYPERSENSITIVITY PNEUMONITIS

1. **By what other names is hypersensitivity pneumonitis (HP) known?**

   HP is also known as extrinsic allergic alveolitis. In addition, there are many types of HP, known by many different names, depending on the antigen or dust involved. The classic form is called farmer's lung.

2. **What are the causative agents of HP?**

   Fine biologic dusts or small chemicals, which can be inhaled into the smallest airways, initiate the immune response that is responsible for HP. These biologic, organic dusts contain materials that are antigenic, and the small chemicals may become haptens when combined with proteins (Table 16-1). Other sources of HP antigen include medicines (e.g., amiodarone, gold, procarbazine, minocycline, chlorambucil, sulfasalazine, beta-adrenergic blockers) and soybean hulls in veterinary feed.

   Patel AM, Ryu JH, Reed CE: Hypersensitivity pneumonitis: Current concepts and future questions. J Allergy Clin Immunol 108:661–670, 2001.

3. **Who gets HP?**

   HP usually develops after prolonged and/or intermittent exposure to antigens, at high or low levels, through numerous occupations or hobbies. Atopy is not a risk factor. Although uncommon, HP can occur in young children. The most common antigens are birds, but molds and methotrexate are also reported. Of interest, smokers are less susceptible to HP.

   Fan LL: Hypersensitivity pneumonitis in children. Curr Opin Pediatr 14:323–326, 2002.

4. **Is HP a new disease?**

   No. The first description of HP was in 1713 by Ramazzini, the father of occupational medicine. Farmer's lung was described in England in 1932.

5. **What is the prevalence of HP?**

   In the past, the prevalence of farmer's lung in an agricultural community ranged from 2.3% to 8.6%. Fortunately, the prevalence has been reduced with changes in farming methods. In people with high exposure to contaminated air conditioning systems, the prevalence is 15–60%; in pigeon breeders, it is 6–21%.

   Fink JN, Zacharisen MC: Hypersensitivity pneumonitis. In Middleton E, et al (eds): Allergy, Principles and Practice, 5th ed. New York, Mosby, 1998, pp 994–1004.

6. **How does HP present?**

   There are two main clinical presentations for HP: acute and chronic. A subacute description is sometimes used and can be helpful. The presentations and prognoses are quite different. This concept is key to understanding HP.

TABLE 16-1.   HYPERSENSITIVITY PNEUMONITIS ANTIGENS

Antigen	Disease	Source
Bacteria (including mainly thermophilic *Actinomycetes* and other aquatic bacterial species)	Farmer's lung	Moldy hay, grain, compost
	Bagassosis, composter's lung	Moldy sugar cane, moldy residential compost
	Ventilation pneumonitis	Humidifier/air conditioner
	Mushroom worker's lung	Mushroom compost
	Machine worker's lung	Metalworking fluid aerosols
	Humidifier lung	Cool mist humidifiers
	Detergent worker's lung	Detergent enzymes
Fungi (including *Aspergillus, Alternaria, Penicillium, Pullularia Trichosporon, Cryptostroma,* and *Rhodotorula* species)	Woodworker's lung	Moldy wood dust
	Suberosis	Moldy cork dust
	Cheese worker's lung	Cheese mold
	Sequoiosis	Moldy wood dust
	Summer-type HP	Japanese house dust
	Maple bark stripper's disease	Wet maple bark
	Malt worker's lung	Moldy barley dust
Animal proteins (including avian, bovine, porcine, rat, and mollusk shell proteins)	Bird breeder's disease	Pigeon, duck, turkey, parakeet
	Laboratory worker's lung	Rat urine
	Oyster shell lung	Shell dust
Insect proteins (including *Sitophilus granarius* and silkworm larvae)	Wheat weevil disease	Infested wheat flour
	Sericulturist's lung disease	Cocoon fluff
Amebae	Ventilation pneumonitis	Contaminated ventilation system
Chemicals (including toluene diisocyanate [TDI], diphenylmethane diisocyanate [MDI], phthalic anhydride, and trimetallic anhydride)	Paint refinisher's disease	Urethane, paint catalyst
	Bathtub refinisher's disease	Urethane, paint catalyst; resin, adhesive, foam
	Epoxy resin worker's lung	Epoxy resin
	Plastic worker's lung	Plastics industry

7. **Describe the acute presentation of HP.**
    The acute presentation is more dramatic, with fever up to 40°C, chills, fatigue, headache, and myalgia as well as respiratory signs and symptoms. Leukocytosis is common. Clinically,

patients appear to have acute pneumonia until it is recognized that the symptoms resolve within 24 hours of removal from the antigen exposure (usually in the workplace) and recur within 4–6 hours of re-exposure. Antigen levels are typically high.

8. **Describe the chronic presentation of HP.**
The chronic form is much more insidious and difficult to diagnose. Systemic symptoms include nonspecific malaise, anorexia, weight loss, fatigue, and weakness. Typically, the antigen exposure is prolonged and at a lower level, such as having a bird or two in the home. Patients are believed to have had subclinical disease for years before the damage becomes apparent. The chronic form can also be the culmination of repeated acute episodes.

9. **Are there only two presentations for HP?**
The **subacute** form is between the acute and chronic forms, with progressively worsening fatigue, dyspnea, and cough over a period of days to weeks. The systemic findings of the acute form are not always present.

10. **What questions should be asked about the patient's occupation, home, and hobbies if HP is considered?**
Temporal patterns such as:
- Improvement after vacations, possibly weekends away from home, work, or hobbies
- How long has the exposure taken place
- Worsening symptoms with reintroduction to a particular environment.
See also Table 16-2 for types of exposures.

TABLE 16–2. ENVIRONMENTAL EXPOSURES IN HYPERSENSITIVITY PNEUMONITIS
■ Pet and other animal exposures, particularly birds
■ Flood- or water-damaged environment
■ Presence of humidifiers, dehumidifiers, evaporative coolers, or vaporizers
■ Occupational or hobby exposure to organic dusts or chemicals
■ Use of feather or down clothing or bedding
■ Presence of visible mold in home or work environments
■ Methods in place to reduce exposures

11. **Discuss the main physical findings in patients with HP.**
Patients with **acute** HP appear ill. They have dry cough, dyspnea, and chest tightness. Bilateral crackles can be heard, suggesting a clinical diagnosis of acute pneumonia.

Patients with **chronic** HP present with progressive exertional dyspnea, but minimal physical findings are seen until they have late, severe disease. Late findings include cyanosis, dyspnea, and crackles.

12. **What are the main x-ray findings in HP?**
The chest x-ray may be normal or show nodular infiltrates in the acute form and diffuse fibrosis in the chronic form. During an acute attack, the chest x-ray may show soft, patchy densities in

both lung fields. These parenchymal densities often coalesce. Between episodes, the chest x-ray may be normal in acute HP.

13. **Summarize the role of CT scans in HP.**
In subacute and chronic HP, the CT scan is more useful than conventional chest x-rays. The CT scan also helps to distinguish chronic HP from idiopathic pulmonary fibrosis and sarcoidosis. In chronic HP, the CT scan findings include ground-glass opacities, centrilobular nodules, and a bronchocentric pattern of emphysema. In end-stage disease, the chest x-ray may show diffuse fibrosis, including parenchymal contracture or honeycombing.

14. **What spirometry findings are associated with HP?**
In acute HP the typical pulmonary function abnormality is decreased volume, or restriction. In some patients there is dual phase, with a drop in flow rates like an early asthmatic response, followed by a late response. Unlike the late asthmatic response, in the late HP response a decreased volume is found rather than decreased flow rate. In chronic HP, a mixed pattern can be found, with obstruction and/or restriction.

15. **How else can you distinguish HP from asthma?**
Arterial blood gasses can further differentiate asthma from HP, because carbon monoxide diffusing capacity (DLCO) is decreased in HP. Because both asthma and HP can express an early and a late response after exposure, performing spirometry before and after exposure may be of limited usefulness in distinguishing asthma from HP. Hypoxemia is worsened by exercise in HP. Hypoxemia and hypercapnia, even at rest, may be found in late disease.

16. **What are the main diseases to consider in the differential diagnosis of HP?**
The differential diagnosis also depends on the clinical presentation. Initially, the acute form with systemic symptoms presents like acute pneumonia. Later, when a temporal pattern is noticed, other illnesses such as building-related illness, organic dust toxic syndrome (ODTS), and occupational asthma need to be considered. These illnesses are much more common than HP. (ODTS illnesses are pulmonary disorders without fever or abnormal chest x-ray findings. They are caused by heavy exposures to organic dusts and toxins.)

17. **How does the differential diagnosis differ in the chronic form of HP?**
In chronic HP, other disorders with restrictive lung disease and fibrosis need to be considered, such as sarcoid disease, eosinophilic granuloma, and the idiopathic interstitial pneumonias.

18. **Explain the role of an industrial hygienist in HP.**
The role of the industrial hygienist is to analyze the suspected environment for the presence of HP antigens or other triggers and to recommend environmental changes or other avoidance measures that minimize production of or exposure to these antigens.

19. **Describe the pathophysiology of HP.**
HP includes a spectrum of lymphocytic and granulomatous interstitial and alveolar filling disorders. Inflammatory cells include mainly lymphocytes, macrophages, plasma cells, and some neutrophils. Macrophages with foamy cytoplasm, surrounded by mononuclear cells, may be specific for HP. Later, interstitial fibrosis with honeycombing, as in idiopathic pulmonary fibrosis, is found. Hilar adenopathy and systemic organ involvement are not part of HP.

20. **What immunologic parameters are involved in HP?**
Although both cell-mediated and humoral immunity are involved, the immunology is not understood. IgE is not thought to be important. IgG is probably involved in all patients, although some patients have specific elevations in IgA or IgM. We do not know whether complement has a significant role, although IgG, which is pivotal in HP, fixes complement. Complement levels do not

decrease in HP as in immune complex-mediated diseases, and immune complexes have not been found in bronchoalveolar lavage fluid (BAL). We also do not understand which regulatory or cell-mediated functions promote HP in the presence of specific antibody.

21. **Do macrophages play a role in HP?**
CD8+ cytotoxic T lymphocytes are elevated and probably have an important regulatory role involving alveolar macrophages. These macrophages appear to be directly involved in the pathogenesis of HP.

22. **Which is responsible for HP: the exposure or the patient?**
Both host and antigen factors appear to be necessary:
■ Many persons with exposure develop specific antibody, without any identifiable illness.
■ Antigen must be of a small enough size to penetrate the smallest airways, and must be present at higher levels intermittently or at lower levels chronically to cause disease.

23. **What tests should be considered for the evaluation of patients with HP?**
Pulmonary function testing, including spirometry, blood gasses, lung volumes, diffusion capacity, and possibly exercise challenge, should be done in patients suspected of having HP. Peripheral blood leukocytosis is common, usually without eosinophilia. The search for antigens is based on the exposure history. Depending on the environment, different antigens are suspected, and the search may involve an industrial hygienist. Several laboratories offer a "hypersensitivity panel" to screen for precipitins (usually IgG) directed against the most common HP antigens. The tests are done by Ouchterlony gel diffusion or enzyme-linked immunosorbent assay (ELISA).

24. **Are skin tests helpful in the evaluation of HP?**
Allergy skin tests are not helpful. Other skin tests have not been consistently useful and have no significant advantages over serologic methods for identification of antigen-specific IgG. These skin tests demonstrate an Arthus reaction, which detects antigen, IgG antibody, and complement complexes and occurs in 4–6 hours.

25. **Are invasive tests needed for the diagnosis of HP?**
Although other tests are usually adequate for a diagnosis, lung biopsy may be needed to diagnose the cause of pulmonary fibrosis. Needle biopsies are generally inadequate, since large biopsy samples are needed. Immunofluorescent studies may detect antigen, even in late-stage HP. Bronchoalveolar lavage (BAL) is not diagnostic because findings in symptomatic and nonsymptomatic patients overlap.

26. **Are the serologic tests diagnostic of HP?**
A positive IgG antibody is not diagnostic of HP, nor does a negative test exclude HP:
■ Inadequate testing materials can be responsible for a negative test.
■ A positive test confirms exposure to antigen, but not the presence of disease. Positive results are also found in 50% of exposed people without disease. A positive test is important to support the clinical suspicions, indicating sufficient exposure to generate an immune response.

27. **Discuss the major and minor diagnostic criteria for HP.**
Major criteria: symptoms compatible with HP, evidence of exposure to appropriate antigen, chest x-ray or high-resolution CT scan findings, lymphocytosis on BAL (if performed), HP histology (if biopsy done), and positive natural challenge by history.
Minor criteria: bibasilar rales, decreased diffusing capacity, and arterial hypoxemia.
Schuyler M, Cormier Y: The diagnosis of hypersensitivity pneumonitis. Chest 111:813–816, 1997.

28. **What test is pathognomonic for HP?**
Neither the hypersensitivity panel nor any other test is pathognomonic for HP.

29. **What is needed to make the diagnosis of HP?**
   A high index of suspicion! The diagnosis is confirmed by the elimination of symptoms and prevention of recurrences after complete removal from the suspected antigen. As such, identification of the causative antigen is a critical part of the diagnosis. Inhalation challenge and BAL are not usually required.
   Using the diagnostic criteria, the diagnosis may be confirmed with four of the major criteria and at least two of the minor criteria, and if other diseases with similar symptoms are ruled out.

30. **How is HP treated?**
   Avoidance of the identified antigen is an essential part of the treatment of HP. This strategy can involve the use of air filters, dust masks, removal of the antigen from the environment, or removal of the patient from the environment. Identification of the antigen may also help prevent the development of HP in coworkers.

KEY POINTS: HYPERSENSITIVITY PNEUMONITIS

1. A high index of suspicion and an early diagnosis allow a good prognosis and should prevent progression to end-stage disease.

2. The acute and chronic forms differ in presentations and prognoses.

3. A detailed exposure history to identify causative triggers is required.

4. Hypersensitivity serologies (specific IgG) are helpful but not diagnostic per se.

5. Systemic corticosteroids and avoidance of antigen are the main treatments.

31. **What medicines are used to treat HP?**
   Patients with acute HP usually respond dramatically to systemic corticosteroids, starting at prednisone doses of 60–80 mg/day. However, *corticosteroids must not be used as a substitute for avoidance measures because they do not prevent the progression of the disease to irreversible pulmonary fibrosis.* The dose and duration of treatment depend on the individual clinical and laboratory response. Typically, larger doses are continued for 2–3 weeks, then slowly tapered over a period of 4–6 months. Bronchodilators are generally not helpful but may be tried in the early part of an acute episode.

32. **How do patients with HP respond to treatment?**
   In early HP, patients with acute disease respond well to avoidance measures. However, once sensitized, small doses of antigen can trigger flares. Chronic HP may not respond to corticosteroids or even avoidance measures. Some patients require prolonged low-dose prednisone, but the response is variable. In some patients the disease can progress even after rigorous avoidance measures are instituted, and all patients should be monitored for several years. Desensitization is not indicated because the disease is not IgE-mediated.

33. **How is treatment of HP monitored?**
   Clinical and laboratory parameters are followed, including spirometric, radiologic, and blood gas studies. Serology is not useful for monitoring treatment because antibody levels persist for many years.

34. **If prednisone works, why not inhaled corticosteroids?**
Efficacy has not been shown with inhaled corticosteroids, but higher doses, as are possible with the newer products, have not yet been adequately studied.

35. **Discuss the prognosis of HP.**
With early diagnosis and institution of antigen avoidance measures, the prognosis is excellent. In such patients, removal of antigen usually reverses the damage. In chronic HP, the damage is irreversible and may progress even with antigen avoidance. Often patients with chronic HP do not respond well to corticosteroids.

36. **What are the predictors of a poor prognosis?**
A poor response after 6 months of prednisone suggests a poor prognosis, as does the presence of clubbing. Most deaths, although uncommon in HP, occur in the chronic presentation but can also occur in the acute presentation.

ALLERGIC BRONCHOPULMONARY ASPERGILLOSIS

37. **What clinical presentation suggests allergic bronchopulmonary aspergillosis (ABPA)?**
ABPA should be considered in patients with chronic, refractory asthma, particularly if they are steroid-dependent, and in patients with cystic fibrosis (CF).

38. **What are the causative agents of ABPA?**
Aspergillus is a common mold with over 150 species. *A. fumigatus* is the agent involved in over 80% of ABPA, although other species, such as *A. niger, A. flavus*, and *A. terreus* can also be involved. The spores are 2.0–3.5 microns in diameter, allowing deposition into the smaller airways. Healthy lungs, however, can clear these spores.

39. **Where do you find *Aspergillus* molds?**
Aspergillus molds are ubiquitous and, like other molds, are commonly found in moist environments of organic materials. They can be found in agricultural environments, such as hay, soil, and compost, and indoors in damp areas and bird excrement. *Aspergillus* is thermotolerant, growing at temperatures ranging from 15° to 53° C. The optimal temperature is 37°C.

40. **What other diseases are associated with *Aspergillus*?**
Aspergillus-allergic asthma, allergic *Aspergillus* sinusitis, chronic necrotizing pneumonia, hypersensitivity pneumonitis, invasive aspergillosis, and aspergilloma. The patient's genetics and immune responses determine whether these diseases occur upon exposure.

41. **What is the prevalence of ABPA?**
Up to 10% of patients with CF may have ABPA. In one study, 15% of children fulfilled the criteria for ABPA. Six percent of asthmatic patients with a positive *Aspergillus* skin test have ABPA. Occupation and geographical regions are important because of the distribution of the *Aspergillus* molds. Sometimes, in retrospect, the onset of ABPA in childhood is suspected.
  Chetty A, Menon RK, Malviya AN: Allergic bronchopulmonary aspergillosis. India J Pediatr 49:203–205, 1982.

42. **Is ABPA a new disease?**
No. Hinson first described it in 1932.
  Hinson KFW, Moon AJ, Plummer NS: Bronchopulmonary aspergillosis: A review and report of eight new cases. Thorax 7:317–333, 1952.

43. **List the stages of illness in ABPA.**
    - Acute
    - Remission
    - Exacerbation
    - Steroid-dependent
    - End-stage fibrosis

44. **Describe the characteristics of the acute stage.**
    Patients with acute disease have a typical clinical presentation of asthma with extremely elevated IgE levels, eosinophilia, pulmonary infiltrates, and *Aspergillus*-specific IgG and IgE. They respond to prednisone.

45. **Describe the remission stage.**
    The asthma is under control, and the chest x-ray is normal. IgE levels are still elevated but closer to normal. *Aspergillus*-specific IgG and IgE may be normal. Remission may last for many years.

46. **What is the exacerbation phase of ABPA?**
    The exacerbation phase is a repeat of the acute phase and is recognized when serum IgE increases, usually by more than double. Systemic symptoms such as dyspnea, fever, myalgia, and sputum production are not uncommon. This phase also responds to prednisone and is treated like the acute phase.

47. **At what phase is the diagnosis of ABPA usually made?**
    The steroid-dependent phase. The disease flares when tapering of the corticosteroid dose is attempted. IgE levels can be extremely high (over 30,000 ng/ml) and may remain above 5,000 ng/ml without disease activity, but they can also be normal. Chest x-ray findings usually show bronchiectasis, but not consistently. Earlier diagnosis requires a very high index of suspicion.

48. **Why is early diagnosis of ABPA important?**
    Early diagnosis is important before the development of irreversible late-stage disease, which is usually preventable with treatment.

49. **How does the end-stage fibrosis phase differ from the other stages?**
    End-stage patients have irreversible lung damage that may progress to respiratory failure. Serologic findings are variable. Spirometry shows irreversible obstruction and restriction. Patients present with shortness of breath, cyanosis, cor pulmonale, rales, and sometimes clubbing.

50. **What are the main physical findings in the earlier stages of ABPA?**
    In earlier stages, patients typically present with an asthma-like picture of wheeze, shortness of breath, chest tightness, and tenacious, often brown mucus plugs, which are sometimes blood-streaked. The asthma is not necessarily severe; however, patients do not respond to less aggressive asthma treatments and require systemic corticosteroids.

51. **What are the main x-ray findings in the earlier stages of ABPA?**
    In the earlier stages, intermittent pulmonary infiltrates are found on the chest x-ray. They can help differentiate between an asthma attack and a flare of ABPA. The chest x-ray can also show consolidation, which is much more remarkable than would be expected from the clinical presentation.

52. **What are the main x-ray findings in the later stages of ABPA?**
    In later stages, irreversible radiologic findings include central bronchiectasis and pulmonary fibrosis. Central bronchiectasis is suggestive of ABPA but may require a CT scan for detection.

CT scan has generally superceded bronchography, which was widely used in the past. Mucoid impaction is common.

53. **Describe the pathophysiology of ABPA.**
Much is not known about the pathophysiology. Clearly, however, ABPA is not an infection with *Aspergillus* per se; it results from immunologic responses to the mold that colonizes the airway. These responses include activation of CD4+ Th2 and CD3+ T lymphocytes and B lymphocytes.

54. **Does the elevated IgE cause ABPA?**
In ABPA, the *Aspergillus*-specific IgE and total IgE are much higher than in asthma. Specific IgE and IgG are elevated and presumed to be relevant. Of particular interest is why most atopic patients with *Aspergillus* exposure develop specific IgE but do not develop ABPA. A possible mechanism in the development of ABPA is a modification of the cellular immune response and/or immune regulators by *Aspergillus* toxins or binding proteins. A shift towards Th2 production may cause increased immunoglobulin production.

55. **What tests should be considered for the evaluation of suspected ABPA?**
If suspected clinically, the diagnosis is confirmed serologically and radiologically. Initial tests may include allergy skin testing for *Aspergillus*, total IgE, and a chest x-ray. If these tests support the diagnosis of ABPA, further tests, such as those listed in the diagnostic criteria, should be done. They include *Aspergillus*-specific IgG and IgE serologies, complete blood count with eosinophil count, and possibly sputum analysis with culture and staining.

KEY POINTS: ALLERGIC BRONCHOPULMONARY ASPERGILLOSIS

1. Consider the diagnosis in steroid-dependent asthma patients and particularly in patients with cystic fibrosis.

2. Expectoration of tenacious, thick, often brown mucous plugs, sometimes with streaks of blood, is not uncommon.

3. Initial testing could include skin testing for aspergillus, total IgE, and a chest x-ray, which often shows recurrent infiltrates.

4. Further testing to consider for the diagnosis of ABPA include aspergillus IgE and IgG serologies, complete blood count (markedly elevated eosinophil count), and possibly a chest CT scan.

5. Early aggressive use of systemic corticosteroids can usually prevent the progression to end-stage disease.

56. **Can *Aspergillus* be isolated from the sputum?**
Yes, although after corticosteroid treatment *Aspergillus* may not be found in up to 40% of patients. *Aspergillus* isolation from sputum is not diagnostic, although repeatedly positive cultures warrant further evaluation of ABPA.

57. **What is the differential diagnosis of ABPA?**
The main diagnosis to consider in a child with asthmatic symptoms and recurrent pneumonia is cystic fibrosis. Other diagnoses include parasitic infections such as visceral larval migrans, Churg-Strauss vasculitis, and eosinophilic pneumonia.

58. **What are the diagnostic criteria for ABPA?**
See Table 16-3.

TABLE 16-3.   AMERICAN DIAGNOSTIC CRITERIA FOR ABPA

1   Asthma
2. Immediate cutaneous reactivity to *A. fumigatus* (or mixed *Aspergillus* species)
3. Precipitating IgG antibodies to *A. fumigatus*
4. Elevated total IgE (> 1000 ng/mL)
5. Elevated IgE antibodies to *A. fumigatus*. The level should be double that found in patients with *Aspergillus*-related atopic disease, such as allergic rhinitis or asthma.
6. Central bronchiectasis
7. Infiltrates on chest x-ray, but they may be absent between flares of ABPA.
8. Eosinophilia coincident with chest x-ray infiltrates, but this finding may not be present while on corticosteroids.

---

59. **How is the diagnosis of ABPA established?**
There is no worldwide consensus on the diagnosis of ABPA. It has been suggested that the first five criteria in Table 16-3, plus one other, are necessary to confirm the diagnosis.

60. **What are the criteria for the diagnosis of ABPA in patients with CF?**
Proposed criteria for the diagnosis of ABPA in CF include:
- Clinical deterioration
- *Aspergillus* IgE, either by skin test or serological test
- Elevated serum IgE (>1000 ng/ml)
- *Aspergillus* IgG
- Change in chest x-ray
There is also a suggestion to check the total IgE annually. If it is elevated (> 500 ng/mL), check for *Aspergillus*-specific IgE, by skin test or serological test.

61. **Describe the treatment of ABPA.**
The mainstay of ABPA treatment remains oral corticosteroids. A usual treatment regimen is prednisone, 0.5 mg/kg/day for 1–3 weeks, then changed to alternate day doses for 2–3 months. After the serum IgE has diminished by two-thirds, the prednisone is tapered and possibly discontinued.

62. **How is treatment of ABPA monitored?**
Total serum IgE is measured frequently, often monthly initially, and less often as the disease stabilizes. Monitoring is useful to aid in both tapering the prednisone dose and identifying ABPA flares. Serial spirometry and chest x-rays are also useful.

63. **How do you distinguish between an asthma attack and a flare of ABPA?**
With difficulty, particularly in cystic fibrosis. An asthma attack associated with a marked increase in IgE (at least double) and pulmonary infiltrates on chest x-ray suggests an ABPA flare. Patients with these findings need more aggressive treatment with systemic corticosteroids.

64. **If ABPA is a fungal related disease, shouldn't antifungal treatment help?**
Leon and Craig reviewed the medical literature related to the use of antifungals in the treatment of ABPA. A small controlled study by Stevens showed a significant clinical improvement with

itraconazole. Wark et al. showed an anti-inflammatory effect of itraconazole in a controlled study of stable ABPA. Thus, it is not clear whether the benefit is from an antifungal effect. Antifungals may be a reasonable adjunctive treatment, particularly in patients requiring high-dose steroids.

Leon EE, Craig TJ: Antifungals in the treatment of allergic bronchopulmonary aspergillosis. Ann Allergy Asthma Immunol 82:511–516, 1999.

Stevens DA: A randomized trial of itraconazole in allergic bronchopulmonary aspergillosis. N Engl J Med 342:756–762, 2000.

Wark PAB, Hensley MJ, Saltos N, et al: Anti-inflammatory effect of itraconazole in stable allergic bronchopulmonary aspergillosis: A randomized controlled trial. J Allergy Clin Immunol 111:952–957, 2003.

65. **How important is fungal avoidance?**
Of interest, although attempts to eliminate *Aspergillus* have not proved helpful, natural or experimental challenges are known to induce severe immediate and delayed responses. Exposure to high levels of *Aspergillus* should be avoided, although complete avoidance is practically impossible. This strategy may also prevent disease in family members.

66. **What about other treatments of ABPA?**
Oral corticosteroids are still the recommended treatment. Inhaled corticosteroids have not been shown to consistently prevent ABPA recurrences, although the newer, high-dose inhaled corticosteroids need further investigation. Inhaled corticosteroids are used for treatment of the asthma associated with ABPA. Avoidance of asthma triggers, whether mold or otherwise, is important for asthma control. *Aspergillus* immunotherapy is not recommended.

67. **What is the prognosis of ABPA?**
With the exception of end-stage ABPA, the prognosis is favorable if the disease is treated and monitored aggressively. Progression of the disease can usually be prevented with the early use of systemic corticosteroids, although the disease can flare, even after years of remission.

WEBSITE

American Lung Association: www.lungusa.org

BIBLIOGRAPHY

1. American Thoracic Society/ European Respiratory Society international multidisciplinary classification of the idiopathic interstitial pneumonias: Am J Respir Crit Care Med 165:277–304, 2002.

2. Chetty A, Menon RK, Malviya AN: Allergic bronchopulmonary aspergillosis. India J Pediatr 49:203–205, 1982.

3. Cockrill BA, Hales CA: Allergic bronchopulmonary aspergillosis. Annu Rev Med 50:303–316, 1999.

4. Daroowalla F and Raghu G: Hypersensitivity pneumonitis. Compr Ther 23:244–248, 1997.

5. Fan LL: Hypersensitivity pneumonitis in children. Curr Opin Pediatr 14:323–326, 2002.

6. Fink JN, Zacharisen MC: Hypersensitivity pneumonitis. In Middleton E, et al (eds): Allergy, Principles and Practice, 5th ed. New York, Mosby, 1998, pp 994–1004.

7. Greenberger PA: Allergic bronchopulmonary aspergillosis. J Allergy Clin Immunol 110(5):658–692, 2002.

8. Greenberger PA: Allergic bronchopulmonary aspergillosis, allergic fungal sinusitis, and hypersensitivity pneumonitis. Clin Allergy Immunol 16:449–467, 2002.

9. Hinson KFW, Moon AJ, Plummer NS: Bronchopulmonary aspergillosis: A review and report of eight new cases. Thorax 7:317–333, 1952.

10. Knutsen AP, Mueller KR, Hutcheson PS, Slavin RG: Serum anti-*Aspergillus fumigatus* antibodies by immunoblot and ELISA in cystic fibrosis with allergic bronchopulmonary aspergillosis. J Allergy Clin Immunol 93:926–931, 1994.

11. Krasnick J, Meuwissen HJ, Nakao MA, et al: Hypersensitivity pneumonitis: problems in diagnosis. J Allergy Clin Immunol 97:1027–1030, 1996.

12. Leon EE, Craig TJ: Antifungals in the treatment of allergic bronchopulmonary aspergillosis. Ann Allergy Asthma Immunol 82:511–516, 1999.

13. Patel AM, Ryu JH, Reed CE: Hypersensitivity pneumonitis: Current concepts and future questions. J Allergy Clin Immunol 108:661–670, 2001.

14. Patterson R, Roberts M: Classification and staging of allergic bronchopulmonary aspergillosis. In Patterson R, Greenberger P, Roberts M (eds): Allergic Bronchopulmonary Aspergillosis, Providence RI, Oceanside Publications, 1995.

15. Sansores R, Salas J, Chapela R, et al: Clubbing in hypersensitivity pneumonitis, its prevalence and possible prognostic role. Arch Intern Med 150:1849–1851, 1990.

16. Schuyler M, Cormier Y: The diagnosis of hypersensitivity pneumonitis. Chest 111:813–816, 1997.

17. Seltzer JM: Building-related illness. J Allergy Clin Immunol 94:351–362, 1994.

18. Stevens DA: A randomized trial of itraconazole in allergic bronchopulmonary aspergillosis. N Engl J Med 342:756–762, 2000.

19. Viswanath PK, Banerjee B, Greenberger PA, Fink JN: Allergic bronchopulmonary aspergillosis: challenges in diagnosis. Medscape Respiratory Care 3(6), 1999.

20. Wark PAB, Hensley MJ, Saltos N, et al: Anti-inflammatory effect of itraconazole in stable allergic bronchopulmonary aspergillosis: A randomized controlled trial. J Allergy Clin Immunol 111:952–957, 2003.

21. Yoshizawa Y, Miyake S, Sumi Y, et al: A follow-up study of pulmonary function tests, bronchoalveolar lavage cells, and humoral and cellular immunity in bird fancier's lung. J Allergy Clin Immunol 96:122–129, 1995.

22. Zacharisen MC: Hypersensitivity pneumonitis: knowing what to look for. J Resp Dis 20:523–533, 1999.

CHAPTER 17

PRIMARY IMMUNODEFICIENCY

Pearl A. Barzaga, M.D.

1. **What are the differences between primary and secondary immunodeficiency diseases?**
   Congenital or primary immunodeficiencies are disorders in which the genetic defect is *intrinsic* to the cells and tissues of the immune system. In contrast, secondary immunodeficiencies are disorders of the immune system in which the defect is secondary to an *extrinsic* cause.
   Examples of secondary immunodeficiency diseases are malnutrition, malignancy, chemotherapy, corticosteroids, splenectomy, nephrotic syndrome, liver cirrhosis, and viral infection such as measles or HIV.

2. **Name the four major components of the immune system.**
   1. Humoral (B-cell lymphocyte) or antibody-mediated immunity
   2. Cellular (T-cell lymphocyte) immunity or cell-mediated immunity
   3. Phagocyte system
   4. Complement system

3. **What is the most common immunodeficiency among the four major components of the immune system?**
   Fifty to 65% of primary immunodeficiency disorders are attributed to a **humoral** or **B-cell defect,** and 5–10% of immunodeficiencies are T-cell disorders. A combined immunodeficiency involving both B-cell and T-cell dysfunction accounts for 20–25% of immunodeficiency disorders. The less common phagocytic disorders and complement disorders account for 10–15% and less than 2% of immunodeficiency diseases, respectively.

4. **Describe the common clinical presentations of primary immunodeficiency diseases.**
   1. There is increased susceptibility to infections, opportunistic pathogens, or organisms with low virulence. The infections may be recurrent, unusually severe, or complicated and may persist despite appropriate treatment.
   2. Autoimmune, inflammatory, hematologic, or malignant disorders such as systemic lupus erythematosus, inflammatory bowel disease, dermatitis, idiopathic thromobcytopenic purpura, autoimmune hemolytic anemia, and lymphoma are commonly associated.
   3. Failure to thrive, chronic diarrhea, and malabsorption.
   4. Severe reaction or infection with live vaccinations (e.g., vaccine-acquired poliomyelitis, bacille Calmette-Guérin infection).
   5. Family history of immunodeficiency or early death in childhood.
   6. Anatomic or physiologic features suggestive of a syndrome complex.
      Ballow M: Primary immunodeficiency disorders: Antibody deficiency. J Allergy Clin Immunol 109:581–591, 2002.
      Bonilla FA, Geha RS: Primary immunodeficiency diseases. J Allergy Clin Immunol 111:S571–S581, 2003.

5. **Name the most common organisms seen in patients with T-cell defects.**
   See Table 17-1.

TABLE 17-1. COMMON ORGANISMS ASSOCIATED WITH DIFFERENT DEFENSE SYSTEM IMMUNODEFICIENCIES

	Antibody Deficiency	Cellular Deficiency	Phagocyte Defect	Complement Deficiency
Clinical scenario	Recurrent sinopulmonary infection Sepsis Aseptic meningitis Chronic diarrhea Autoimmune disease Increased malignancy	Disseminated, opportunistic, and viral infections Dermatitis Thrush Chronic diarrhea Failure to thrive Increased malignancy	Lymphadenitis Cellulitis Gingivitis Liver and lung abscess Osteomyelitis	Encapsulated organism sepsis, meningitis, autoimmune disease
Bacteria	*S. pneumoniae* *S. aureus* *H. influenzae* *P. aeruginosa* *N. meningitides* *M. hominis* *U. urealyticum* *Salmonella*	Pyogenic bacteria *Salmonella typhi* *Campylobacter*	*S. aureus* *P. aeruginosa* *S. typhi* *S. marcescens* *Klebsiella* *B. cepacia* Enteric bacteria	Pyogenic bacteria *N. meningitidis* especially
Virus	Enteroviruses Poliovirus Echo virus Coxsackie Adenovirus	EBV, CMV, HSV, RSV Adenovirus Measles Vaccinia Molluscum contagiosum	None	None

Fungi	None	*C. albicans* *P. carinii* *A. fumigatus* *H. capsulatum* *C. immitis*	*C. albicans* *P. carinii* *A. fumigatus*	None
Mycobacteria	None	Nontuberculous BCG	Nontuberculous BCG	None
Protozoa	*G. lamblia*	*Cryptosporidia*		None

EBV = Epstein-Barr virus, CMV = cytomegalovirus, HSV = herpes simplex virus, RSV = respiratory syncytial virus, BCG = bacille Calmette-Guerin.

6. **Name the most common organisms seen in patients with B-cell or antibody defects.**
   See Table 17-1

7. **Which lymphocyte type predominates in the peripheral blood?**
   Fifty to 70% of the peripheral blood lymphocytes are T-cell lymphocytes, and 5–15% are B-cell lymphocytes.
   Buckley RH: Primary immunodeficincy diseases due to defects in lymphocytes. N Engl J Med 343:1313–1324, 2000.

8. **List the screening tests used to evaluate a patient suspected of immunodeficiencies.**
   See Table 17-2

9. **What advance tests can be ordered for further evaluation of immunodeficiency?**
   See Table 17-2

10. **Describe the clinical features of severe combined immunodeficiency (SCID).**
    SCID is a rare and fatal disease with severe deficiencies of both T- and B-cell function. Common features include:
    1. Early presentation during first few months of life
    2. Chronic diarrhea
    3. Failure to thrive
    4. Erythoderma or skin rash
    5. Absent tonsils, lymph nodes, and small thymus
    6. Viral and opportunistic infections *(Pneumocystis carinii, Candida albicans)*
    7. Bacterial infections (sepsis, pneumonia, otitis media)
    8. Overwhelming infection with live vaccinations
    9. Graft-versus-host disease (GVHD) from maternal lymphocytes or nonirradiated blood products

11. **Describe the laboratory features of severe combined immunodeficiency (SCID).**
    Lymphopenia within hours of birth is an **absolute indication for evaluation of SCID** because it is a pediatric emergency. Early diagnosis of SCID is crucial for survival. Laboratory features include:
    1. **Lymphopenia** (absolute lymphocyte count [ALC] < 2000/mm^3 as a newborn)
    2. Reduced circulating CD3+ T cells on flow cytometry
    3. Absent-to-low proliferative mitogen response
    4. Absent-to-low serum immunoglobulin and antibody response

12. **Name the most common genetic defect in SCID.**
    The most common form of SCID is X-linked **common gamma (γ) chain deficiency** of the inter-leukin (IL)-2 receptor that is mapped to the Xq13 locus and accounts for 44% of SCID cases. The γ chain is a common subunit shared by the IL-2 receptor and several other cytokine receptors (IL-4, IL-7, IL-9, IL-15, and IL-21).

13. **What is the treatment of choice for SCID?**
    Bone marrow transplant is the preferred treatment for SCID. There is a greater than 95% survival rate if patients with SCID are transplanted with HLA-identical or haploidentical bone-marrow donors within the first 3.5 months of life. Without treatment, SCID is otherwise fatal by the first year of life secondary to infections.

TABLE 17–2.   INITIAL SCREENING, SECONDARY AND TERTIARY LABORATORY TESTING FOR IMMUNE FUNCTION EVALUATION

	Screening	Secondary Testing	Tertiary Testing
Antibody	Quantitative immunoglobulins:	Immunoglobulin subclass[‡]	Molecular studies for genetic defects
	IgG, IgM, IgA, IgE	B-lymphocyte enumeration: CD19, CD20	Bacteriophage ΦX174 neoantigen
		Specific antibody response*	
		Isohemagglutinin IgM to ABO antigens	
		In vitro mitogen proliferation[§]	
Cellular	CBC (absolute lymphocyte count)	T-lymphocyte enumeration: CD2, CD3,	Molecular studies for genetic defect (CD154, γc)
	PA/lateral chest x-ray for thymic	CD4, CD8, CD16, CD56	ADA, PNP enzyme
	shadow	In vitro mitogen proliferation[§]	FISH 22q11
	HIV serology	MHC I, II enumeration	Cytokine production
	Delayed-type hypersensitivity test[∞]		NK cell cytotoxity (K562)
			Tetramer studies
Phagocyte	CBC (Neutrophil count)	CD18, CD15s (LAD)	Mutation analysis (gp91)
	Nitroblue tetrazolium dye test	Bone marrow aspirate	STAT 1 or 4 phosphorylation (IFNγ-IK12)
		Neutrophil granule morphologic evaluation	Phagocytosis
		Dihydrorhodamine assay	Intracellular/bactericidal killing assay
			Chemotaxis

(continued)

TABLE 17–2. INITIAL SCREENING, SECONDARY AND TERTIARY LABORATORY TESTING FOR IMMUNE FUNCTION EVALUATION *(continued)*

	Screening	Secondary Testing	Tertiary Testing
Complement	Total hemolytic complement (CH50)	Complement components quantitative and functional analysis	
		AH 50**	
Other	Sweat chloride	Nasal mucosal biopsy	
	α_1-Antitrypsin	Imaging for transesophageal fistula	

± Interpret with caution since clinical significance unclear.
* Pre- and post-antibody titers to tetanus toxoid, diphtheria toxoid, pneumovax, HIB, menomune vaccination may be used.
§ B-cell response: LPS (lipopolysaccharide) *E. coli;* PWM (pokeweed mitogen) T-cell response: PHA (phytohemagglutinin), ConA (concanavalin-A).
∞ Delayed type hypersensitivity skin test using *Candida,* tetanus, diphtheria, mumps, histoplasma, trichophyton, tuberculin PPD.
** If factor D or properdin deficiency suspected.

14. **Name the second most common molecular defect in SCID.**
    Autosomal recessive SCID caused by **adenosine deaminase (ADA) deficiency** accounts for
    16% of cases and is the second most common molecular defect. ADA is involved in purine
    metabolism, and the lack of ADA results in accumulation of toxic metabolites.

KEY POINTS: COMMON FEATURES IN SEVERE COMBINED IMMUNODEFICIENCY

1. Severe lymphopenia

2. Early presentation during first few months of life

3. Absent tonsils and lymphoid tissue

4. Bacterial, viral, and opportunistic infections

5. T-cell and B-cell immunodeficiency

---

15. **Describe the unique features of ADA-deficient SCID compared with other SCID defects.**
    Patients with ADA-deficient SCID are profoundly lymphopenic with an ALC < 500/mm^3. They
    have chondro-osseous dysplasia of the costochondral junction and apophysis of the iliac bone.
    The vertebral bodies reveal a "rachitic rosary" ribcage, abnormal bony pelvis, and "bone-in-bone"
    appearance on radiographs. Weekly enzyme replacement therapy with polyethylene glycol-ADA
    can be given, but provides less immunocompetence compared to bone marrow transplantation.

16. **What are the clinical manifestations of purine nucleoside phosphorylase (PNP) deficiency?**
    This autosomal recessive disorder encoded on chromosome 14q13 is another enzyme
    deficiency related to the purine salvage pathway. Lymphopenia is severe (ALC < 500 mm^3), but
    unlike patients with ADA deficiency, patients with PNP deficiency have a low but present
    T-cell function and normal numbers of B cells and natural killer (NK) cells. There are no associ-
    ated skeletal abnormalities. PNP-deficient patients are not only susceptible to infection but also
    have a high incidence of lymphoreticular malignancies and autoimmune disease. Neurologic
    complications range from ataxia to spastic diplegia and mental retardation. There are no associ-
    ated skeletal abnormalities. Prognosis is poor.

17. **Describe the genetic causes of SCID and other combined cellular immunodeficiencies including their lymphocyte phenotypes.**
    The common γ chain defect of the IL-2 receptor is an X-linked SCID disorder. A defect in JAK3, a
    signaling molecule associated with the common γ chain receptor, has an identical phenotype but
    is autosomal recessive. Other cytokine defects include the IL-7α receptor that is important for
    T-cell signaling or IL-2α receptor (CD25). A defect in receptor gene recombination includes a
    mutation in RAG1, RAG2, or the DNA repair enzyme, artemis. Abnormal nucleotide salvage path-
    ways are due to ADA or PNP deficiency. T-cell receptor (TCR) signaling defects include ZAP-70,
    CD45, p56^{lck}, CD3δ, or CD3ε mutations. A mutation in TAP1, TAP2, or the multi-subunit com-
    plex responsible for MHC-II promotion results in the lack of MHC-I or MHC-II expression. (See
    Table 17-3.)
    Ming JE, Stiehm ER, Graham JM: Genetic syndromes associated with immunodeficiency.
    Immunol Allergy Clin North Am 22, 2002.

18. **Summarize the genetic defects in severe combined and cellular immunodeficiencies.**
    See Table 17-3.

TABLE 17–3.	SUMMARY OF THE GENETIC DEFECTS AND PHENOTYPES OF SEVERE COMBINED AND CELLULAR IMMUNODEFICIENCIES		
Genetic Defect	**Inheritance**	**Chromosome**	**Flow Cytometry**
Cytokine defects			
γc	X	Xq13	T-B+NK-
JAK3	AR	19p13	T-B+NK-
IL-2α Receptor	AR	11p13	T↓B+NK+
IL-7α Receptor	AR	5p13	T-B+NK+
B-cell receptor/T-cell receptor rearrangement			
RAG 1 or 2	AR	11p13	T-B-NK+
Artemis	AR	10p13	T-B-NK+
Purine nucleotide metabolism			
ADA	AR	20q13-ter	T-B-NK-
PNP	AR	14q13.1	T↓B+NK+
TCR signaling			
ZAP-70	AR	2q12	CD8-B+NK+
CD3δ	AR	11q23	CD3↓B+NK+
CD3ε	AR	11q23	CD3↓B+NK+
p56lck	AR		T+B+NK+
CD45	AR		T-B +NK↓or T+B+NK+
MHC-I defect			
TAP 1 or TAP 2	AR	6q21.3	CD8-B+NK+
MHC-II defect			
CIITA	AR	16p13	CD4-B+NK+
RFXANK	AR		
RFX5	AR	1q21	
RFXAP	AR	13q	
Other			
Reticular dysgenesis	AR		T-B-NK-myeloid

19. **Name the disorder of a newborn with a congenital heart defect, hypocalcemia, and absent thymus.**
    DiGeorge syndrome is associated with dysmorphogenesis of the third and fourth brachial pouches. The defects are associated with neonatal tetany and complications related to congenital heart defects during the first 24 hours of life. The degree of T-cell deficiency is variable and depends on the amount of thymic hypoplasia involved. Opportunistic infections are seen in patients with severe T-cell defects, but patients with partial DiGeorge syndrome rarely have

immunologic sequelae. Immunoglobulin levels are normal or elevated and are secondarily affected with poor antibody function or low serum IgA. Facial dysmorphism is also common.

20. **How is DiGeorge syndrome diagnosed?**
DiGeorge syndrome is a T-cell deficiency due to a **chromosome 22q11 deletion** that can be detected by **fluorescent in situ hybridization (FISH).** The defect may be due to monosomy, autosomal dominant, or sporadic transmission. Variations of the "22q11 deletion syndrome" in addition to DiGeorge syndrome include velocardiofacial syndrome, Spritzen syndrome, CATCH 22 syndrome (**c**ardiac defects, **a**bnormal facies, **t**hymic hypoplasia, **c**left palate, and **h**ypocalcemia), and CHARGE anomaly (**c**oloboma, **h**eart disease, **a**tresia choanae, **r**etarded growth and development, **g**enital hypoplasia, and **e**ar anomalies or deafness). Studies suggest that the defect may be due to a mutation in the TBX-1 transcription factor gene (*T-box*).

KEY POINTS: COMMON FEATURES OF DIGEORGE SYNDROME

1. T-cell immunodeficiency with variable B-cell deficiency

2. Absent or hypoplastic thymus

3. Hypoparathyroidism

4. Congenital heart malformation (tetralogy of Fallot, interrupted aortic arch type B, truncus arteriosus, right-sided heart anomalies)

5. Facial dysmorphisms (hypertelorism, low-set ears, micrognathia, short upper lip philtrum, anti-mongoloid eye slant)

21. **What is Omenn's syndrome?**
Omenn's syndrome is a **partial defect in the *RAG1* or *RAG2*** gene that results in:
- Generalized erythroderma or desquamation
- Diarrhea
- Hepatosplenomegaly
- Generalized lymphadenopathy
- Hypereosinophilia
- Markedly elevated serum IgE
- Overwhelming infections

22. **Name the triad in Wiskott-Aldrich syndrome (WAS).**
Eczema, thrombocytopenia with small platelets, and **recurrent sinopulmonary infections** due to immunodeficiency are known as the WAS triad. However, the triad occurs in only one-third of cases. Twenty percent of patients have only thrombocytopenia at birth. Moderate-to-severe eczema appears by 1 year of age. Infections are due to encapsulated bacteria such as *Streptococcus pneumoniae* and *Haemophilus influenzae*, but opportunistic infections with *Pneumocystis carinii* and viruses also occur. Bleeding, infection, malignancy, and vasculitis are the major causes of death before teenage years.

23. **What is the defect in WAS?**
WAS is a combined T-cell and B-cell disorder encoded on Xp11 as an X-linked recessive trait. The **WAS protein** is crucial for cytoskeletal regulation and actin polymerization of hematopoietic

cells and lymphocytes. Patients without the WAS protein have loss of T-cell surface microvilli, decreased platelet size, and defective T-cell function. Carriers of the WAS mutation can be detected by non-random X-chromosome inactivation. Prenatal diagnosis of WAS may be obtained by chorionic villous sampling or amniocentesis.

24. **Summarize the treatment for WAS.**
Bone marrow transplant before the age of 5 years from HLA-identical siblings or from matched unrelated donors is the preferred treatment. Intravenous immunoglobulin (IVIG), antibiotics, and splenectomy may also be indicated.

25. **A child who is wheelchair-bound by age 12 may have what immunodeficient disease?**
Ataxia-telangiectasia, an autosomal recessive disorder associated with (1) oculocutaneous telangiectasia, (2) progressive cerebellar ataxia, and (3) recurrent sinopulmonary infections. The ataxia appears when the child starts to walk and progresses to wheel-chair confinement by age 10–12 years. Dysphagia and other neurologic symptoms are common features. There is a 15% incidence of lymphoreticular tumors. An **elevated alpha-fetoprotein level** is seen in 95% of patients. No effective treatment is currently available for ataxia-telangiectasia, and most patients die from infection, malignancy, or progressive neurologic sequelae.

26. **Describe the immunodeficiency seen in ataxia-telangiectasia.**
Cell-mediated immunity is impaired but not absent (as seen in patients with SCID). Opportunistic infections are not observed. Further evaluation demonstrates a T-cell lymphopenia with a selective decrease in CD4+ subsets, poor mitogen response, and cutaneous anergy. Dysgammaglobulinemia is characterized by a low IgA in 50–80% of the patients with normal IgG but depressed IgG2 levels. IgM levels are normal, although in monomeric form, and IgE levels are also low.

27. **What is the underlying defect in ataxia-telangiectasia?**
The ***ATM*** **(ataxia-telangiectasia mutated)** gene on chromosome 11q22-23 is a protein kinase responsible for apoptosis, cell cycle homeostasis, and **DNA repair**. A defect in the ATM gene results in a failure to halt the cell cycle and repair damaged DNA. As a consequence, patients are highly sensitive to ionizing radiation.

KEY POINTS: COMMON FEATURES OF ATAXIA-TELANGIECTASIA

1. Oculocutaneous telangiectasia
2. Cerebellar ataxia
3. Recurrent infection
4. Elevated alpha-fetoprotein level
5. High rate of malignancy

28. **What is the Nijmegen breakage syndrome (NBS)?**
A mutation in the ***NBS1*** **gene** is another disorder involved in **defective DNA repair** mechanisms. The *NBS1* gene, located on chromosome 8q21, encodes for a protein called nibrin, which acts as a substrate for ATM. The clinical features of this autosomal recessive disorder include micro-

cephaly, growth retardation, and recurrent sinopulmonary infections. A similar defect involving the *MRE11* gene has recently been reported. The *MRE11* gene encodes a protein associated with nibrin.

29. **What disease is characterized by an abnormal immune response to infection with Epstein-Barr virus (EBV)?**
    X-linked lymphoproliferative disease (XLP) or **Duncan's disease** is characterized by a selective susceptibility to EBV. Patients are initially immunologically intact, but 80% develop a fatal or severe mononucleosis or hepatic necrosis with exposure to EBV. Surviving patients develop an acquired agammaglobulinemia, bone marrow aplasia, or lymphoma. Laboratory values show T-cell impairment, inverted CD4/CD8 ratio, decreased proliferative mitogen response, and depressed NK-cell activity. Some patients were initially misdiagnosed with common variable immunodeficiency (CVID).

30. **Describe the molecular defect in XLP.**
    The *XLP* gene is encoded on Xq25. A mutation at this locus results in a **defect in SAP (SLAM-associated adapter protein)** or SH2D1A and allows the SLAM protein to mediate uncontrolled signal transduction and T-cell and NK-cell proliferation. Without SAP, there is no T-cell control of EBV infections. Bone marrow transplantation has been curative in some patients if performed at an early age, but there is no other effective treatment for XLP.

31. **What is chronic mucocutaneous candidiasis (CMC)?**
    CMC is a T-cell mediated immunodeficiency with susceptibility to *Candida* infections of the nails, skin, and mucous membranes. Despite extensive disfigurement by superficial involvement of *Candida*, disseminated infections are rare. Most patients have anergy to *Candida* in vivo. The genetic cause of CMC is unknown, but variants have a mutation in the AIRE (autoimmune regulator) gene.

32. **List the other acronyms associated with CMC.**
    CMC is also known as **autoimmune polyglandular syndrome type 1 (APS-1)** or **autoimmune polyendocrinopathy-candidiasis-ectodermal dystrophy (APECED)** due to the frequent association of autoimmune endocrine abnormalities such as hypothyroidism, hypoparathyroidism, hypoadrenalism, hypogonadism, pernicious anemia, vitiligo, alopecia, chronic active hepatitis, and keratoconjunctivitis.

33. **Name the immunodeficiency associated with CD8 lymphopenia.**
    CD8 lymphopenia is attributed to **zeta chain-associated protein-70 (ZAP-70) deficiency.** This autosomal recessive disease is due to a defective ZAP-70 tyrosine kinase encoded on chromosome 2q12 that is crucial for T-cell receptor transduction. No CD8+ cells are detected because ZAP-70 is responsible for positive and negative selection in the thymus, especially CD8+ cells. CD4+ cells, B cells, and NK cells are present with poorly functioning CD4+ cells and B cells. Another disorder with CD8 lymphopenia, called bare lymphocyte syndrome I, is discussed in question 35.

34. **How do patients with ZAP-70 immunodeficiency differ from patients with SCID?**
    Despite the similarities of severe, recurrent infections and failure to thrive, patients with ZAP-70 deficiency present at a later age and survive longer. The lymphoid tissue is present with normal thymus architecture. Flow cytometry demonstrates only an absence of CD8+ cells. The majority of cases of ZAP-70 deficiency have been reported in Mennonites.

35. **What is the bare lymphocyte syndrome (BLS)?**
    BLS is an autosomal recessive disorder associated with an MHC-I defect encoded on chromosome 6p21.3. **A mutation in the TAP1 or TAP2** (transporter associated with antigen presentation

protein) results in a **lack of MHC-I antigen expression** on lymphocytes, and CD8 lymphopenia ensues. Recurrent sinopulmonary infections, deep ulcers, and chronic pulmonary disease characterize this disease. BLS type I presents as a mild form of SCID and is less severe compared to BLS type II.

36. **Describe the defect in bare lymphocyte syndrome type II.**
    BLS type II is an autosomal recessive disorder related to a **defect** in the genes that regulate **MHC-II gene transcription:** RFX5, RFXAP, RFXANK, and CIITA. As a result, MHC-II antigen expression is undetectable. Laboratory studies demostrate low CD4+ cells and moderate lymphopenia. Clinical presentation resembles a milder version of SCID with hypoplastic lymphoid organs and infections with bacterial, viral, and opportunistic organisms. There is no susceptibility to GVHD with irradiated blood products or to BCG upon vaccination (as in patients with SCID).

37. **What is the molecular defect in Chediak-Higashi syndrome?**
    Chediak-Higashi syndrome is a rare autosomal recessive **phagocytic disorder.** The defect has been isolated to the **LYST protein** on chromosome 1q42 and is crucial for protein transport and phagolysosome formation. This disorder results in **giant granules** seen in all lysosomal-containing cells, **impaired chemotaxis,** and abnormal NK-cell activity.

38. **List the clinical features of Chediak-Higashi syndrome.**
    1. Recurrent bacterial infections
    2. Partial oculocutaneous albinism
    3. Neurologic abnormalities (mental retardation, seizures, nystagmus, neuropathy)
    4. Late-onset lymphoreticular malignancy
        Shiflett SL, Kaplan J, Ward DM: Chediak-Higashi syndrome: A rare disorder of lysosomes and lysosome related organelles. Pigment Cell Res 15: 251–257, 2002.

KEY POINTS: COMMON FEATURES OF CHEDIAK-HIGASHI SYNDROME

1. Oculocutaneous albinism

2. Neurologic abnormalities

3. Recurrent infections

4. Giant granules

---

39. **List some of the cellular deficiencies associated with the interferon (IFN)-γ/IL-12 axis.**
    1. IFNγ α chain receptor (IFNγR1)
    2. IFNγ β chain receptor (IFNγR2)
    3. IL-12 p40 subunit (IL-12β)
    4. IL-12 β1 chain receptor (IL-12Rβ1)
    5. STAT-1
    All of these mutations result in a susceptibility to intracellular organisms such as *Salmonella* or nontuberculous mycobacteria because of a defect in the IFNγ/IL-12 axis. IL-12 induces the pro-

duction of IFN-γ by Th1 T cells and NK cells. Without IFN-γ, mononuclear cells and phagocytes cannot initiate cytotoxic mechanisms.

40. **Name the five most common organisms that affect patients with chronic granulomatous disease (CGD).**
    - *Staphylococcus aureus*
    - *Serratia marcescens*
    - *Burkholderia cepacia*
    - *Nocardia* spp.
    - *Aspergillus* spp.

41. **Explain why patients with CGD are susceptible to infections with catalase-positive organisms.**
    CGD is a phagocytic disorder involving a **defect in the NADPH oxidase system** required for microbial intracellular killing through the production of hydrogen peroxide and hypochlorite. Because catalase-positive organisms are able to avoid the respiratory burst by breaking down their own hydrogen peroxide, patients with CGD are vulnerable to catalase-positive bacterial and fungal infections. Staphylococcal liver abscesses are pathognomonic for CGD. Infections with the above organisms result in lung, liver, skin, bone, and lymph node disease and obstructive granulomas in the gastrointestinal and genitourinary tracts.
    Holland SM: Update on phagocytic defects. Pediatr Infect Dis J 22:87–88, 2003.

42. **How is CGD diagnosed?**
    Diagnosis is made by demonstrating the inability of phagocytes to kill ingested organisms via a lack of dye reduction with nitro blue tetrazolium testing. Newer methods include measuring the reduced generation of superoxide ions by flow cytometry with dihydrorhodamine dye. Molecular analysis of the NADPH oxidase system confirms the diagnosis. Seventy percent of CGD cases are X-linked due to a defect in **gp 91^{phox}** subunit. The mutations in the other three subunits of the NADPH oxidase system result in an autosomal recessive form of CGD, with the **gp 47^{phox}** subunit being the second common mutation. Female carriers of the CGD gene can be detected by lyonization.

43. **What are the clinical features of hyperimmunoglobulinemia E (hyper-IgE) syndrome or Job's syndrome?**
    This syndrome is characterized by recurrent staphylococcal infections of the skin, lungs, and viscera that result in abscesses, pneumatoceles, and bronchiectasis. Severe eczema, coarse facial features, markedly elevated IgE, and structural abnormalities such as retained primary teeth, osteoporosis, and skeletal fractures are clinical features. Hyperimmunoglobulinemia E sydrome is a rare autosomal disorder with both dominant and recessive forms. The genetic defect is unknown but may be related to IL-4 overexpression or a mutation in T-cell regulation. Some kindred studies show a linkage to the proximal chromosome 4q region.

KEY POINTS: COMMON FEATURES OF HYPER-IGE SYNDROME

1. Elevated serum IgE

2. Coarse facial features

3. Staphylococcal abscesses of skin and viscera

4. Bone and dental abnormalities

44. **Characterize the clinical features of leukocyte adhesion deficiency (LAD).**
    - Delayed separation of the umbilical cord or omphalitis
    - Recurrent skin, upper and lower respiratory tract, and perirectal infections
    - Necrotizing enterocolitis
    - Gingivitis or periodontitis
    - Leukocytosis
    - Impaired wound healing
    - No evidence of suppuration
    - No leukocytes seen on rebuck skin window test

45. **Name the defect associated with LAD-1.**
    LAD type 1 is a mutation in the **gene encoding CD18** or the **common B-chain for B$_2$ integrin** molecules. CD18 complexes with CD11a, CD11b, and CD11c to form the heterodimers: leukocyte function-associated molecules LFA-1 and complement receptors CR3 and CR4. Without LFA-1, leukocyte cells are unable to bind to ICAM-1 and to mediate adhesion to endothelial cells for the subsequent diapedesis to infection sites.

46. **Name the defect associated with LAD-2.**
    LAD type 2 is a defect in the GDP-fucose transporter that results in the **absence of sialyl-Lewis-X binding** to the adhesion molecule, E-selectin. Leukocytes attach to the endothelium to initiate tethering and rolling with the binding of sialyl-Lewis-X to E-selectin. Mental retardation and short stature are seen in patients with LAD-2 in addition to the clinical scenario seen in patients with LAD-1.

47. **What are the clinical features of X-linked agammaglobulinemia (XLA)?**
    Eighty-five percent of **early-onset hypogammaglobulinemia** is secondary to XLA. XLA is an antibody deficiency that affects only males and usually presents when passive transfer of maternal antibodies decline by 6 months of age. Circulating B cells account for less than 2% of the lymphocytes. The absence of immunoglobulins results in **recurrent bacterial infections. No tonsil or lymphoid tissue is present.** T-cell numbers are unaffected and, therefore, respond well to viral infections with the exception of chronic enteroviral infections, vaccine-associated poliomyelitis, and *Ureaplasma* or *Mycoplasma* arthritis.

48. **Explain the genetic defect in XLA.**
    Bruton's tyrosine kinase (BTK) is a tyrosine kinase seen in the B-cell lineage that is important for B-cell differentiation and signal transduction of the B-cell receptor. A **mutation in BTK** is encoded in Xq22 and halts early B-cell development. Flow cytometry can be used to detect a lack of BTK expression. Female carriers of the BTK mutation may be identified by non-random X inactivation of their B-cells.

49. **List the genetic defects in agammaglobulinemia.**
    - BTK
    - IgM heavy-chain mutation
    - Surrogate light-chain λ5/14.1 mutation (CD179B)
    - Igα chain of the B-cell receptor mutation (CD79A)
    - BLNK (signal transducer B-cell linker protein)

    All of these molecular defects result in an absence of circulating B cells since B-cell development is arrested at any early stage. With the exception of the BTK mutation in X-linked agammaglobulinemia, the remaining four genetic defects are autosomal recessive.

50. **What is the cause of X-linked hyper-IgM (X-HIM) immunodeficiency?**
    X-HIM is encoded on Xq26 with a presentation of hypogammaglobulinemia similar to XLA with the exception of **normal or elevated serum IgM.** Patients with X-HIM deficiency cannot produce **CD40 ligand (CD154** or tumor necrosis factor superfamily member 5). CD40 ligand is

KEY POINTS: COMMON FEATURES OF X-LINKED AGAMMAGLOBULINEMIA

1. Absence or low levels of circulating B cells

2. No lymphoid tissue

3. Normal T cells

4. Recurrent sinopulmonary infections

5. Chronic enteroviral meningoencephalitis

6. Vaccine-associated paralytic poliomyelitis

expressed on activated T-cells and is required for immunoglobulin class switching by interacting with CD40 on B-cells. A CD40 defect on B cells has an identical phenotype to CD40 ligand deficiency but is inherited as an autosomal recessive trait.

51. What are the clinical features of X-HIM deficiency?
Because the mutation in X-HIM is a **T-cell defect,** patients have susceptibility to *Pneumocystis carinii, Histoplasma* spp., or cryptosporidia. The hypogammaglobulinemia leads to frequently recurring bacterial infections. Neutropenia and parvovirus-induced aplastic anemia are not uncommon. Malignancy and hepatobiliary disease, including sclerosing cholangitis, occur with increased incidence.

52. Summarize the genetic causes of XHIM immunodeficiency.
- X-linked CD40 ligand deficiency (Xq26)
- X-linked NEMO or IKKγ deficiency (Xq28)
- Autosomal recessive CD40 deficiency (chromosome 20)
- Autosomal recessive AID deficiency (chromosome 12p13)

53. What are the clinical features of X-HIM deficiency type 2 (X-HIM2)?
X-HIM2 is another autosomal recessive hyper-IgM deficiency due to a defect in an RNA-editing enzyme called activation-induced cytidine deaminase, which is required for class switching and somatic hypermutation of immunoglobulin genes. Unlike X-HIM, *Pneumocystis carinii* pneumo-

KEY POINTS: COMMON FEATURES OF X-LINKED HYPER-IGM IMMUNODEFICIENCY

1. CD40 ligand deficiency

2. Elevated serum IgM with low IgA, IgG, and IgE

3. Neutropenia

4. *Pneumocystis carinii* pneumonia

5. Recurrent pyogenic infections

nia, autoimmune hematologic disorders, and neutropenia are less common. Patients with X-HIM2 also have characteristic massive lymphadenopathy and intestinal lymphoid hyperplasia.

54. **How are the clinical features of X-HIM3 attributed to a NEMO mutation?**

X-HIM3 is encoded on Xq28 as a IKBKG gene mutation that affects nuclear factor Kβ essential modulator (NEMO). NEMO is critical for activation of transcription factor NF-Kβ. X-HIM3 presents with **dysgammaglobulinemia** and **anhidrotic ectodermal dysplasia** of the hair, teeth, and sweat glands. Variants of the IKBKG mutation are associated with osteopetrosis and lymphedema. An X-linked dominant germline loss of function is lethal in males and presents as incontinentia pigmenti in females.

Jain A, Ma CA, Liu S, et al: Specific missense mutations in NEMO result in hyper-IgM syndrome with hypohydrotic ectodermal dysplasia. Nat Immunol 2:223–228, 2001.

55. **Name the most common clinically significant primary immunodeficiency that presents in adulthood.**

Common variable immunodeficiency (CVID) or acquired hypogammaglobulinemia occurs at an incidence of 1/25,000 to 1/66,000. CVID is an antibody-mediated immunodeficiency disorder with variable inheritance. The cause of this heterogenous disease is unknown, but more than one gene is probably responsible for CVID. All cases are characterized by hypogammaglobulinemia greater than 2 standard deviations from the mean age-appropiate immunoglobulin level and impaired specific antibody response. Peripheral B-cell numbers are normal with variable T-cell function and mitogen response.

56. **Describe the clinical manifestations of CVID.**

- Recurrent sinopulmonary bacterial infections
- Noncaseating granulomas of the skin and viscera
- Bimodal age of onset at 5–15 years old and 25–45 years old
- Autoimmune disease and autoimmune cytopenias
- Increased incidence of gastrointestinal tract or lymphoid malignancy
- 10% incidence of atopy
- Chronic diarrhea and malabsorption
- Chronic enteroviral infections or meningoencephalitis
- Intestinal lymphoid hyperplasia and splenomegaly

Cunningham-Rundles C: Common variable immunodeficiency. Curr Allergy Asthma Rep 1:421–429, 2001.

57. **List the differential diagnosis for a patient with hypogammaglobulinemia.**

- X-linked agammaglobulinemia
- Common variable immunodeficiency disease
- X-linked lymphoproliferative disease
- Autosomal recessive agammaglobulinemia
- Hyper-IgM syndrome
- Transient hypogammaglobulinemia of infancy
- ICOS deficiency

58. **What is ICOS deficiency?**

ICOS deficiency is an autosomal recessive disorder that presents with panhypogammaglobulinemia. However, the lymphoproliferation and autoimmunity characteristically seen in CVID is absent. B-cell numbers are low (1–4%). ICOS is a CD28 costimulatory analog expressed on activated T-cells that stimulates the production of IL-10 needed for memory B-cells and plasma cells.

Grimbacher B, Hutloff A, Schlesier M, et al: Homozygous loss of ICOS is associated with adult-onset common variable immunodeficiency. Nat Immunol 4:261–268, 2003.

59. **How is CVID treated?**
Lifelong intravenous immunoglobulin (IVIG) infusions are given at a dose range of 300–600 mg/kg every 3–4 weeks and can be adjusted to achieve an IgG trough level greater than 500 mg/dL. Antibiotics may be needed in addition to IVIG. Prophylactic Bactrim is sometimes required for severely diminished T-cell function. Unlike T-cell immunodeficiencies, bone marrow transplant or gene therapy has not been a therapeutic treatment.

KEY POINTS: COMMON VARIABLE IMMUNODEFICIENCY

1. CVID is the most common clinically significant primary immunodeficiency that presents in adulthood.

2. CVID is an antibody-mediated immunodeficiency disorder with variable inheritance.

3. Diagnosis is based on findings of hypogammaglobulinemia and impaired antibody response.

4. CVID is treated with lifelong IVIG.

60. **What is the most common primary immunodeficiency?**
Selective IgA deficiency is the most common primary immunodeficiency with an incidence as high as 1/300–1/700 people. Most cases are **clinically asymptomatic.** There is, however, a frequent association of sinopulmonary infection, chronic lung disease, genitourinary infection, gastric cancer, lymphoma, atopy, and autoimmune disease in these patients. Infections are limited to the mucous membranes. A shared MHC haplotype may explain the high incidence of IgA deficiency and CVID among family members.

61. **List secondary causes of IgA immunodeficiency.**
A secondary IgA deficiency may occur with the use of drugs such as phenytoin, sulfasalazine, plaquenil, and D-penicillamine. The IgA decrease may or may not resolve with discontinuation of the drug.

62. **Name the four criteria that define selective IgA deficiency.**
1. Serum IgA < 7.0 mg/dL
2. Normal serum IgG and IgM levels
3. Normal cell-mediated immunity
5. Normal antibody production
   Cunningham-Rundles C: Physiology of IgA and IgA deficiency. J Clin Immunol 21:303–309, 2001.

63. **What other immunodeficiency disorders are commonly associated with IgA deficiency (IGAD)?**
IgA deficiency is commonly seen in CVID and ataxia-telangiectasia. Fifteen to 20% of IgA-deficient patients have an immunoglobulin subclass deficiency, especially to IGG2 and IGG4 subclasses.

64. **Can IVIG be used to treat symptomatic patients with selective IgA deficiency?**
No. Selective IgA deficiency results from a lack of secretory IgA. IVIG does not contain significant amounts of IgA for replacement. Anaphylactic reactions can occur if IVIG is given due to the

formation of anti-IgA antibodies. These antibodies are present in blood products, and transfusion reactions can ensue if packed red blood cells are not washed. Antibiotics are given to symptomatic people. IgA deficiency with an associated subclass deficiency may merit for a trial of IVIG treatment in selected cases.

KEY POINTS: SELECTIVE IGA DEFICIENCY

1. It is the **most common primary immunodeficiency** with an incidence as high as 1/300–1/700 people.

2. Most cases are clinically asymptomatic.

3. Symptoms may include sinopulmonary infection, chronic lung disease, genitourinary infection, gastric cancer, lymphoma, atopy, and autoimmune disease.

4. The four defining criteria are: (1) serum IgA < 7.0 mg/dL, (2) normal serum IgG and IgM levels, (3) normal cell-mediated immunity, and (4) normal antibody production.

65. **Explain transient hypogammaglobulinemia of infancy (THI).**
   This self-limited disorder generally presents with a prolonged and exaggerated hypogammaglobulinemia at 6 months of age and resolves by age 4 years. Clinically patients present with recurrent sinopulmonary infections typical of hypogammaglobulinemia but have normal specific antibody responses. Diagnosis is made retrospectively once immunoglobulin concentration returns to normal. This defect is likely due to a delay in maturation of T-cell assistance required for antibody production.

66. **Describe patients with specific antibody deficiency with normal immunoglobulins (SADNI) or functional antibody deficiency.**
   SADNI is seen in patients with impaired antibody response to infections or vaccinations but normal B-cell numbers, immunoglobulins, and subclass levels. T-cell number and function are also normal. Most patients present between age 3 and 6 with a poor response to polysaccharide antigens. This disorder may represent a delay in humoral maturation.

67. **What is the clinical significance of IgG subclass deficiency (IGGSD)?**
   Whether IgG subclass deficiency represents a true immunodeficiency is an ongoing debate. Healthy people without recurrent infections also have low serum IgG subclass levels. Most are clinically asymptomatic, but an increased incidence of viral and upper and lower respiratory infections has been reported. IgG subclasses deficiency is defined by any immunoglobulin subclass greater than 2 standard deviations below the age-appropriate mean.

68. **Name the most common subclass deficiencies in adults and children.**
   IGG3 and IGG2 are the most common subclass deficiencies in adults and children, respectively. The IGG2 subclass is an important response to polysaccharide antigens, such as pneumococci or *Haemophilus influenzae*. A protein antigen and conjugate vaccine response is usually demonstrated by the IGG3 and IGG1 subclass response.

69. **Which primary immunodeficiencies require treatment with IVIG?**
   IVIG is pooled plasma from 3000 to 10,000 healthy blood donors that contains mostly IgG antibodies and traces of IgA and IgM. IVIG is used for the treatment of antibody-mediated disorders

such as XLA, CVID, and HIM. IVIG is indicated for the antibody deficient component of combined immunodeficiencies such as SCID, WAS, AT, DiGeorge syndrome, and XLP. IVIG is considered in difficult or severe cases of IGAD, IGGSD with poor antibody response, THI, and SADNI after antibiotic prophylaxis fails.

Schwartz SA: Intravenous immunoglobulin treatment of immunodeficiency disorders. Pediatr Clin North Am 47:1355–1369, 2000.

70. **What are the most common organisms seen in complement defects?**
Complement deficiency can present with susceptibility to infections, angioedema, or rheumatologic disorders. Patients with deficiencies in the **early components (C1, C4, C2)** commonly present with **recurrent pyogenic bacterial infections** and **autoimmune disorders. Invasive neisserial infections** are usually seen in patients with defects in the **terminal lytic components (C5–C9)** and **properdin deficiency.** A deficiency of the pivotal factor C3 results in severe encapsulated bacterial infection, neisserial infections, and autoimmune disease.

71. **Name the most common complement deficiency.**
C2 deficiency is the most common inherited complement deficiency. It occurs in 1 in 10,000 people.

WEBSITES

1. Clinical Immunology Society: www.clinimmsoc.org

2. European Society for Immune Deficiencies (ESID): www.esid.org

3. Immune Deficiency Foundation: www.primaryimmune.org

4. Immunodeficiency Resource: www.uta.fi/imt/bioinfo/idr

5. Immunology Link: www.immunologylink.com

6. Jeffrey Modell Foundation: www.jmfworld.com

7. Online Mendelian Inheritance in Man (OMIM): www.ncbi.nlm.nih.gov/omim

BIBLIOGRAPHY

1. Ballow M: Primary immunodeficiency disorders: Antibody deficiency. J Allergy Clin Immunol 109:581–591, 2002.

2. Bonilla FA, Geha RS: Primary immunodeficiency diseases. J Allergy Clin Immunol 111:S571–S581, 2003.

3. Bonilla FA: Antibody deficiency. In Leung D, Sampson HA, Geha RS, Szefler SJ (eds): Pediatric Allergy: Principles and Practice. St. Louis, Mosby, 2003, pp 88–98.

4. Bonilla FA, Geha RS: CD154 deficiency and related syndromes. Immunol Allergy Clin North Am 21:65–89, 2001.

5. Buckley RH: Primary cellular immunodeficiencies. J Allergy Clin Immunol 109:747–757, 2002.

6. Buckley RH: Primary immunodeficiency diseases due to defects in lymphocytes. N Engl J Med 343:1313–1324, 2000.

7. Cunningham-Rundles C: Physiology of IgA and IgA deficiency. J Clin Immunol 21:303–309, 2001.

8. Cunningham-Rundles C: Common variable immunodeficiency. Curr Allergy Asthma Rep 1:421–429, 2001.

9. Cunningham-Rundles C: Primary immunodeficiency diseases. In Adelman DC, Casale TB, Corren J (eds): Manual of Allergy and Immunology, 4th ed. Philadelphia, Lippincott, 2002, pp 397–417.

10. Fischer TJ, Gruchalla RS, Alam R, et al (eds): Immunodeficiencies. In Allergy and Immunology Medical Knowledge Self-Assessment Program, 3rd ed. Milwaukee, AAAI-ACP, 2003, pp 289–346.

11. Geha RS: Approach to the child with recurrent infections. In Leung D, Sampson HA, Geha RS, Szefler SJ (eds): Pediatric Allergy: Principles and Practice. St. Louis, Mosby, 2003, pp 81–87.

12. Grimbacher B, Hutloff A, Schlesier M, et al: Homozygous loss of ICOS is associated with adult-onset common variable immunodeficiency. Nat Immunol 4:261–268, 2003.

13. Holland SM: Update on phagocytic defects. Pediatr Infect Dis J 22:87–88, 2003.

14. Jain A, Ma CA, Liu S, et al: Specific missense mutations in NEMO result in hyper-IgM syndrome with hypohy-drotic ectodermal dysplasia. Nat Immunol 2:223–228, 2001.

15. Javier FC, Moore CM, Sorenson RU: Distribution of primary immunodeficiency diseases diagnosed in a pediatric tertiary hospital. Ann Allergy 84:25–30, 2002.

16. Lekstrom-Himes JA, Gallin JI: Immunodeficiency diseases caused by defects in phagocytes. N Engl J Med 343:1703–1714, 2000.

17. Ming JE, Stiehm ER, Graham JM: Genetic syndromes associated with immunodeficiency. Immunol Allergy Clin North Am 22, 2002.

18. Notarangelo LD: T-cell immunodeficiencies. In Leung D, Sampson HA, Geha RS, Szefler SJ (eds): Pediatric Allergy: Principles and Practice. St. Louis, Mosby, 2003, pp 99–109.

19. Schwartz SA: Intravenous immunoglobulin treatment of immunodeficiency disorders. Pediatr Clin North Am 47:1355–1369, 2000.

20. Shiflett SL, Kaplan J, Ward DM: Chediak-Higashi syndrome: A rare disorder of lysosomes and lysosome related organelles. Pigment Cell Res 15: 251–257, 2002.

CHAPTER 18

IMMUNOTHERAPY

Cristina Porch-Curren, M.D.

1. **What is immunotherapy?**

   Immunotherapy is a treatment modality for IgE-mediated allergic disease. Incrementally increasing doses of specific allergen are injected into an allergic patient over time. In the build-up phase, injections are typically given 1–2 times/week, and in the maintenance phase patients receive a stable monthly injection. Maintenance can usually be achieved in 4–6 months.

2. **Describe maintenance dose.**

   The maintenance dose is the typical amount of allergen tolerated to achieve a sustained clinical response. This dose has been estimated to range from 5 to 20 μg for most allergens. The doses have been based on studies with dust mites, cats, grass, and ragweed. Maintenance for hymenoptera venom tends to be higher at 100 μg. These doses are often tailored to individual symptoms or reactions. When a patient reaches the maintenance dose the interval between injections can be increased to 4–6 weeks.

3. **How does immunotherapy affect the immune system?**

   There are still questions as to which specific immunologic change is the most important for a good clinical response (Table 18-1). The changes that seem to be the basis for symptom improvement include:

   - Antibody changes
   - Cytokine changes
   - Cellular changes

TABLE 18-1. IMMUNE CHANGES NOTED WITH IMMUNOTHERAPY	
Immune Parameter	**Change**
Allergen specific IgG	Increases
Allergen specific IgE-initially	Increases
Allergen specific IgE-over time	Decreases
Seasonal increase in allergen specific IgE	Decreases
TH2:TH1 (ratio)	Decreases
Basophil sensitivity	Decreases
Mast cell number	Decreases in target organ
Eosinophil number	Decreases in target organ
CD8 suppressor T cells	Increases in peripheral blood
CD4 T cells	Decreases in peripheral blood
Low affinity IgE receptor on B lymphocyte	Decreases

4. **Describe the antibody changes.**
   It has been proposed that the allergen-specific IgG may function as a "blocking antibody" to prevent the allergic cascade. However, data also suggest that such is not the case because the increase in IgG occurs after clinical benefit has been noted. Specifically, it appears that increases in IgG1 are followed by a rise in IgG4. Changes in IgE are also noted. Increases and decreases in IgE occur, depending on when immunotherapy is initiated.

5. **Describe the cytokine changes.**
   There remains some debate as to whether the shift from Th2 to Th1 is due to upregulation of Th1 or downregulation of Th2. Ultimately, the balance shift toward Th1 appears consistent. This shift reflects a relative decrease in the Th2 cytokines (interleukin [IL]-4, IL-5, and IL-13) and an increase in the Th1 cytokines (IL-2, interferon [IFN]-γ, and IL-12). In venom immunotherapy, IL-10 has been shown to be critical in developing a response to the treatment.

6. **What are the cellular changes?**
   Specific cellular changes have also been noted with immunotherapy. Changes in basophils, mast cells, eosinophills, and lymphocytes have been documented.

KEY POINTS: IMMUNE CHANGES WITH IMMUNOTHERAPY

1. Increase in allergen-specific IgG

2. Diminished typical seasonal increase in allergy-specific IgE

3. Shift from Th2 to Th1 cytokines

4. Decrease in allergy-mediating cells

7. **What clinical and lab evaluations are used to decide whether a patient will benefit from immunotherapy?**
   Candidates for immunotherapy are patients with IgE-mediated allergic disease, such as allergic rhinitis, allergic asthma, or hymenoptera venom allergy. Allergy should be well documented as the cause of symptoms by history, physical exam, and testing, including skin test, RAST, or both. Data also suggest that immunotherapy may work for atopic dermatitis.

8. **What other issues must be considered in evaluating a patient for immunotherapy?**
   It must be determined whether the patient can medically tolerate immunotherapy and a potential systemic reaction. For example, a patient with severe cardiovascular disease or pulmonary compromise with multiple medical comorbidities is not the ideal candidate. In evaluating pulmonary status, the FEV_1 should be > 70%. Other treatment modalities must also be considered, such as amount of medication used, degree of symptom control with medication, and ability to avoid the offending allergen. One may consider commencing immunotherapy after an informed discussion with the patient about adherence, risks, and benefits.

9. **Describe the risks of immunotherapy.**
   The greatest risk of immunotherapy is an anaphylactic reaction. Systemic reactions can vary in severity and range from mild pruritus to life-threatening anaphylaxis involving broncho-

constriction and cardiovascular collapse. A study evaluating fatalities secondary to allergy skin testing and immunotherapy from 1945 to 1987 documented 46 deaths. Forty occurred after immunotherapy injections and 6 after skin testing. The rate of systemic reactions has varied from 0.5–7% in different studies.

Lockey R, Benedict L, Turkeltaub P, et al: Fatalities from immunotherapy and skin testing. J Allergy and Clin Immunol 79:660–677, 1987.

10. **What are the contraindications of immunotherapy?**
   - Immunotherapy should not be started during pregnancy because of increased risk of anaphylaxis during the build-up phase and risk of fetal hypoxia with a systemic reaction. However, continuation of immunotherapy at maintenance doses has been accepted.
   - Malignancy, autoimmune disease, and immunodeficiency, are also contraindications. The effect on the immune system is not well understood.
   - Uncontrolled asthma poses an increased risk of fatal systemic reactions.
   - Beta-blocker use inhibits response to treatment of a reaction.
   - There are also concerns regarding response to treatment in patients taking an angiotensin-converting enzyme (ACE) inhibitor.

KEY POINTS: RISKS OF IMMUNOTHERAPY

1. The greatest risk of immunotherapy is an anaphylactic reaction.

2. Systemic reactions can vary in severity and range from mild pruritus to life-threatening anaphylaxis involving bronchoconstriction and cardiovascular collapse.

3. A study evaluating fatalities secondary to allergy skin testing and immunotherapy from 1945 to 1987 documented 46 deaths.

11. **What are skin testing and RAST?**
   Skin tests and radioallergosorbent testing (RAST) are used to help make a diagnosis of IgE-mediated allergic disease. RAST is an assay for allergen-specific IgE. It is highly specific but not as sensitive as skin testing. Allergists use the results of both tests for writing "recipes" for patient-specific immunotherapy.

12. **How are skin tests performed?**
   Skin tests can be done by either the percutaneous or the intradermal method. In the percutaneous, or prick, method, allergen extract is placed on the skin, and a device is used to prick through the extract. A positive control, typically histamine, is placed to evaluate for appropriate reactivity, and a negative control is used to evaluate for dermatographism. Intradermal testing involves injecting a small amount of allergen, usually for evaluation of hymenoptera allergy and drug allergy. It is used much less frequently for environmental allergens because of the increased sensitivity and decreased specificity.

13. **Can immunotherapy be used for any type of allergy?**
   Immunotherapy has been shown to decrease symptoms of allergic rhinitis, asthma, and ocular allergy. One study reports a decrease in allergic rhintis symptoms of 50–75%, and evidence indicates that immunotherapy may prevent the development of asthma in children with allergic rhinitis. Immunotherapy is also used for certain venom reactions. Allergen immunotherapy has

not been well documented for the treatment of food allergy, latex allergy, urticaria, or atopic dermatitis.

14. **Describe the time commitment for immunotherapy.**
Immunotherapy consists of a build-up and a maintenance phase. The patient comes to the office once or twice a week for injections during the build-up phase. Maintenance is typically reached in 4–6 months, and the shot frequency is decreased to a monthly interval. The benefit from immunotherapy increases and remains for a longer period if injections are continued for several allergy seasons. The World Health Organization states that immunotherapy should be continued until symptoms have markedly improved or resolved. The treatment typically lasts a total of 3–5 years.

15. **Why do patients have to wait in the office after receiving allergy shots?**
Most systemic reactions begin within 15–20 minutes of allergen injection, but they can occur later. An early reaction tends to be more severe. The allergen immunotherapy practice parameters recommend that the patient should remain in the office for at least 20 minutes, but many physicians request a 30-minute wait. A review of systemic reactions concluded that 70% occur within 30 minutes of injection.

16. **Is immunotherapy always an injection?**
Other modalities of immunotherapy have been investigated:
- Sublingual-swallow
- Sublingual-spit
- Oral
- Inhalation
- Nasal

Currently, the preferred route in the United States is subcutaneous injection, but there is much interest in the sublingual route.

17. **Describe sublingual-swallow immunotherapy.**
In Europe, the sublingual-swallow method is approved for certain circumstances. From 50 to 100 times the dose used in subcutaneous immunotherapy has been studied, and evidence indicates that it is more effective than placebo. A recent 9-year observational study in Europe concluded that sublingual therapy was clinically effective in respect to symptoms and decreased use of medication and that the method was safe and easy with good adherence. The study also noted a decreased trend toward asthma development in treated patients as opposed to those who remained on medications only. However, there are concerns about efficacy, dosing, treatment length to reach clinical efficacy, and effect on immune function.
Frew AJ, Smith HE: Sublingual immunotherapy. J Allergy Clin Immunol 107:441–444, 2001.

18. **What is the current status of sublingual-spit immunotherapy?**
This technique requires further evaluation.

19. **Is oral, inhalational, or nasal immunotherapy effective?**
Oral and inhalational immunotherapy have not been associated with clinical efficacy. Very high doses of allergen are used for oral immunotherapy, 20–200 times the dose used for subcutaneous injection. Adverse effects have been well documented, including oral and gastrointestinal side effects. Nasal immunotherapy has also been found to be effective for rhinitis, but when treatment is discontinued, the effect is not sustained.

20. **How and where should the injection be given?**
- Use a 26- or 27-gauge syringe with a three-eighths or one-half inch nonremovable needle.
- Expel any air in the hub of the syringe.

- Injection is usually given in the posterior portion in the middle third of the upper arm near the junction of the deltoid and triceps muscles. This area has more subcutaneous tissue. Subcutaneous injection allows slower absorption of vaccine.
- Wipe the area with an alcohol swab.
- Lift skin at injection site to avoid intravenous or intramuscular injection.
- Prior to injection, aspirate to check for blood return. If blood is present, withdraw the syringe. A fresh dose and syringe should be used to give injection in another location.
- Depress plunger at a rate slow enough to avoid a wheal or pain. Remove needle and apply mild pressure for 1 minute to avoid vaccine leakage.

21. **List risk factors for a systemic reaction.**
    - Asthma
    - High allergen sensitivity as determined by skin test or RAST
    - Dosing errors
    - Rush immunotherapy
    - Treatment with beta blocker
    - Build-up phase of immunotherapy
    - New vial for immunotherapy
    - Injection during symptom exacerbation

    Malling HJ: Minimising the risks of allergen-specific injection immunotherapy. Drug Safety 23:323–332, 2000.

    Nettis E, Giordano D, Ferrannini A, et al: Systemic reactions to allergen immunotherapy: A review of the literature. Immunopharmacol Immunotoxicol 25:1–11, 2003.

22. **What do we know about fatal systemic reactions?**
    Studies have looked at the cause of death in people who have sustained a systemic reaction. Uncontrolled asthma appears to be a major risk of poor outcome. An asthmatic with $FEV_1 < 70\%$ should not receive immunotherapy and peak expiratory flow rate (PEFR) should be checked before injection. In regard to beta-blocker therapy, it is not the medication itself that increases severity of a reaction but rather the medication's blockage of treatment; epinephrine is unable to bind the beta receptor, which leads to a more severe anaphylactic reaction.

    Lockey R, Benedict L, Turkeltaub P, et al: Fatalities from immunotherapy and skin testing. J Allergy and Clin Immunol 79:660–677, 1987.

23. **What is the most crucial treatment for a systemic reaction?**
    A systemic reaction or anaphylaxis can vary in presentation. The most crucial treatment is epinephrine, 1:1000 dilution 0.3–0.5 mL intramuscularly every 5 minutes as necessary (0.01 mL/kg in children; maximum = 0.3 mL). A randomized, blinded, placebo-controlled, 6-way crossover study comparing intramuscular and subcutaneous administration concluded that intramuscular injection into the anterolateral thigh results in quicker and higher plasma levels of epinephrine. Treatment is very easy with use of the EpiPen or EpiPen junior. These pens are preloaded with either 0.3 mL or 0.15 mL of 1:1000 epinephrine, and the medication can easily be injected through clothing.

    Simons FE, Simons KJ: Epinephrine absorption in adults: Intramuscular versus subcutaneous injection. J Allergy Clin Immunol 108:871–873, 2001.

24. **What secondary medications can be used to treat a systemic reaction?**
    Secondary medications are based on the clinical scenario. Examples include antihistamines, H_2 blocker, albuterol, and corticosteroids.

25. **Explain rush and cluster immunotherapy.**
    Both rush and cluster refer to an accelerated immunotherapy schedule. The build-up phase is much quicker so that maintenance can be achieved rapidly. Cluster schedules involve 1 or 2

visits/week with multiple escalating injections at each visit. Rush schedules are designed to achieve maintenance even more quickly than cluster schedules. Maintenance doses can be achieved in a matter of hours or days. Quicker schedules are more commonly used for venom immunotherapy in high-risk people.

Birnbaum J, Ramadour M, Magnan A, et al: Hymenoptera ultra-rush venom immunotherapy (210 min): A safety study and risk factors. Clin Exp Allergy 33:58–64, 2003.

26. Discuss the disadvantages of rush and cluster immunotherapy.
Quicker schedules have an increased risk of systemic reactions and should be reserved for exceptional situations. Reports of systemic reactions from the rush venom protocols range from 0% to 67%. In addition, systemic reactions occur at a longer time interval after the last injection. Therefore, patients should be monitored for longer than the standard 20–30 minutes recommended for standard schedules.

Portnoy J, King K, Horner S: Incidence of systemic reactions during rush immunotherapy. Ann Allergy 68:493–498, 1992.

Westall G, Thien F, Czarny D, et al: Adverse events associated with rush immunotherapy. MJA 174:227–230, 2001.

27. What results can be expected from immunotherapy?
Immunotherapy is efficacious in decreasing the symptoms of allergic rhinitis, the bronchial sensitivity of allergic asthma, and sensitivity to stinging insects. Benefits have been documented by symptom scores, reduction in medication use, and decreased bronchial hyperreposiveness. However, it is difficult to predict which patients will benefit most, and the degree of benefit varies. The best outcome is complete symptom resolution, but a reasonable goal is a decrease in symptom severity and medication use.

28. Explain the units used to label allergen extracts.
Not all allergen extracts are labeled with the same units, and this inconsistency tends to cause confusion. Standardized allergen vaccines have an allergen content compared with a national reference. In the United States, standardization is done with intradermal skin testing, known as ID50 EAL (intradermal dilution for 50-mm sum of erythema determines the bioequivalent allergy unit). The dilution is chosen when 50 mm of erythema is observed to the tested extract. This testing is performed in people with known allergy to the tested allergen. Once the testing is completed, extracts are labeled with the same unit, the bioequivalent allergy unit (BAU). In the past, they were labeled in potency units (PU). Despite being standardized, dust mites are still labeled as PU rather than BAU. Nonstandardized extracts are labeled as weight to volume (wt/vol), or protein nitrogen units (PNU). These extracts vary in biologic activity.

29. Are all allergen extracts standardized?
No. In the United States, cat dander, grasses, *Dermatophagoides pteronyssinus*, *Dermatophagoides farinae*, ragweed, and hymenoptera venom are available as standardized extracts. Ragweed is labeled as wt/vol, but because the dose necessary to achieve symptomatic improvement is well documented, it is considered a standardized extract.

30. What factors must be considered in mixing an allergen vaccine?
- Allergen cross-reactivity
- Optimal dosing of each extract
- Protease activity

31. Discuss the problems of allergen cross-reactivity and optimal dosing.
Many tree and grass pollens used in allergen vaccines cross-react. If the cross-reactivity is substantial, one representative may be used in the vaccine. In regard to dosing, the maintenance vial must contain a therapeutic dose of each constituent. Therefore, if too many allergens are in one

vial, the individual allergen may be diluted and ineffective. When this situation occurs, two separate vial mixtures may be necessary.

32. **How does protease activity affect mixing of allergen vaccines?**
Extracts with higher proteolytic enzyme activity may break down the allergens with lower proteolytic activity. For example molds, dust mite, and cockroach have higher proteolytic activity than the pollens and should be separated from them.

33. **Does immunotherapy prevent the development of asthma?**
Allergic rhinitis and allergic asthma are both IgE-mediated diseases. According to the Copenhagen allergy study, they appear to be manifestations of one disease entity. The PAT study looked at the issue of asthma development during immunotherapy. This study included 205 children for 3 years; ages ranged from 6 to 14 years. The children had allergic rhinitis and were assigned to immunotherapy or observation. Significantly fewer children in the immunotherapy group developed asthma, and the authors concluded that 3 years of immunotherapy in children with allergic rhinoconjunctivitis decreases the risk of developing asthma.
 Linneberg A, Henrik N, Frolund L, et al: Copenhagen Allergy Study. Allergy 57:1048–1052, 2002.
 Moller C, Dreborg S, Ferdousi HA, et al: Pollen immunotherapy reduces the development of asthma in children with seasonal rhinoconjunctivitis (the PAT study). J Allergy Clin Immunol 109:251–256, 2002.

34. **How efficacious is immunotherapy for Hymenoptera venom?**
It has been reported to be extremely effective in about 80–90% of patients. The risk of a systemic reaction from a sting after immunotherapy drops from 30–70% to less than 2%. Treatment of certain groups, including children under the age of 16 who only had a cutaneous systemic reaction, remains controversial. It is important to distinguish a cutaneous systemic reaction from a large local reaction, which is contiguous with the sting site. A cutaneous systemic reaction can be manifested by diffuse hives or angioedema in a location distant from the sting. It has been reported that children with cutaneous systemic reactions have a low likelihood of repeat systemic reactions. If they do, it is usually limited to the skin. These situations and the decision to treat with immunotherapy should be evaluated on a case-by-case basis.

35. **What is the difference between alum-precipitated allergen extract and aqueous allergen extract?**
Alum-precipitated extracts are modified allergen extracts used for immunotherapy. The allergens are absorbed on an alum hydroxide carrier. The purpose of this type of extract is to decrease the rate of allergen absorption, thus decreasing systemic reactions. Fewer injections are necessary to reach maintenance. Potency of the extract appears to be more stable than aqueous extracts. Treatment with alum-precipitated ragweed and grass allergen has revealed clinical and immunologic laboratory changes equivalent to aqueous extract.
 Nelson H: Long-term immunotherapy with aqueous and aluminum-precipitated grass extracts. Ann Allergy 45:333–337, 1980.

36. **Discuss the concerns related to alum-precipitated allergen extract.**
Concerns for using the alum-precipitated extracts include large local reactions and aluminum toxicity. Large subcutaneous nodules have been well reported in the literature as a result of the injections. The nodules are typically transient and resolve within 6 months of discontinuing the immunotherapy. Histology of the nodules is consistent with a foreign body reaction to the aluminum. Decreasing the dosage and frequency of injections may alleviate the problem. The amount of aluminum absorbed by the injections is reported to be minimal. A study evaluating serum and urine aluminum levels in patients treated with alum-precipitated extracts reported an increase in aluminum load but did not reveal any evidence of aluminum toxicity compared with controls.

Frost L, Johansen R, Pedersen S, et al: Persistent subcutaneous nodules in children hyposensitized with aluminum containing allergen extracts. Allergy 40:368–372, 1985.

Gilnert R, Burnatowska-Hledin M: Serum and urinary aluminum levels in patients receiving alum precipitated allergenic extracts. Ann Allergy 61:433–435, 1988.

37. **What other types of modified extracts are available?**
Other types of modified extracts have been evaluated but are not available in the United States. Examples include alum-precipitated pyridine-modified allergens, formalin-treated allergens, allergoids, and glutaraldehyde polymerization.

38. **Discuss the future role of DNA-based vaccines.**
Studies of DNA-based vaccines are promising. These vaccines use cytosine-phosphate-guanosine (CpG) oligodeoxynucleotides (ODN), which mimic bacterial DNA. This technique has been studied alone and coupled to an allergen.

The goal is to increase vaccine immunogenicity while decreasing the allergenicity seen with traditional immunotherapy. In vitro human studies looking at the coupled CpG ODN motifs have shown a decrease in Th2 response and shift to Th1 response.

Marshall J, Abtahi S, Eiden J, et al: Immunostimulatory sequence DNA linked to the Amb a1 allergen promotes Th1 cytokine expression while down regulating Th2 cytokine expression in PBMCs from human patients with ragweed allergy. J Allergy Clin Immunol 108:191–197, 2001.

KEY POINTS: RECENT AND FUTURE DEVELOPMENTS IN IMMUNOTHERAPY

1. Alum-precipitated allergen extract

2. Formalin-treated allergens, allergoids, and glutaraldehyde polymerization

3. DNA-based vaccines

4. Peptide fragments

5. Recombinant technology

6. Omalizumab

39. **What role may peptide fragments play in the future of immunotherapy?**
IgE recognizes three-dimensional allergen epitopes. This pathway ultimately leads to the clinical allergic reaction, while T cells recognize peptide antigen fragments and do not follow the allergic cascade. An in vivo study has looked at treatment of patients with bee sting allergy using peptide fragments. The patients were treated with a fragment resembling phospholipase A2, a major hymenoptera allergen. The results showed similar clinical and immunologic changes as with traditional allergen vaccines.

Muller U, Akdis C, Fricker M, et al: Successful immunotherapy with T-cell epitope peptides of bee venom phospholipase A2 induces specific T-cell anergy in patients allergic to bee venom. J Allergy Clin Immunol 101:747–754, 1998.

40. **What other approach to immunotherapy is under study?**
Recombinant technology is also affecting treatment of allergic disease. The development of recombinant allergens is being studied.

41. What is omalizumab (Xolair)?

Omalizumab is a recombinant humanized monoclonal anti-IgE antibody. It binds IgE at the Fc region of the antibody and forms an immune complex. This process ultimately leads to a decrease in free or unbound IgE, which is no longer available to bind to mast cells and basophils. There is also a reduction in the number of IgE receptors. Omalizumab has been approved by the Food and Drug Admnistration for the use in treatment of severe allergic asthma. This medication is recommended for people who have inadequately controlled symptoms with maximal medical therapy, side effects or complications secondary to their current regimen, recurrent asthma exacerbations requiring medical attention, issues with medication adherence, or continued interference with activities of daily living. The medication is given via subcutaneous injection every 2–4 weeks. The dose is based on weight on serum IgE level.

Busse W, Corren J, Lanier B, et al: Omalizumab, anti-IgE recombinant humanized monoclonal antibody, for the treatment of severe allergic asthma. J Allergy Clin Immunol 108:184–190, 2001.

WEBSITE

American College of Allergy, Asthma and Immunology: www.acaai.org

BIBLIOGRAPHY

1. Akdis CA, Blesken T, Wymann D, et al: Differential regulation of human T cell cytokine patterns and IgE and IgG4 responses by conformational antigen variants. Eur J Immunol 28:914–925, 1998.
2. Bielory L, Mongia A: Current opinion of immunotherapy for ocular allergy. Curr Opin Allergy Clin Immunol 2:447–452, 2002.
3. Birnbaum J, Ramadour M, Magnan A, et al: Hymenoptera ultra-rush venom immunotherapy (210 min): A safety study and risk factors. Clin Exp Allergy 33:58–64, 2003.
4. Bush R: The use of anti-IgE in the treatment of allergic asthma. Med Clin North Am 86:1113–1129, 2002.
5. Busse W, Corren J, Lanier B, et al: Omalizumab, anti-IgE recombinant humanized monoclonal antibody, for the treatment of severe allergic asthma. J Allergy Clin Immunol 108:184–190, 2001.
6. Durham SR, Walker SM, Varga EM, et al: Long-term clinical efficacy of grass pollen immunotherapy. N Engl J Med 341:468–475, 1999.
7. Fischer TJ, Gruchalla RS (eds): Allergy and Immunology: Medical Knowledge Self-Assessment Program, 3rd ed. Milwaukee, American Academy of Allergy, Asthma, and Immunology, 2003, pp 251–264.
8. Frew AJ: Immunotherapy of allergic disease. J Allergy Clin Immunol 111:s712–s719, 2003.
9. Frew AJ, Smith HE: Sublingual immunotherapy. J Allergy Clin Immunol 107:441–444, 2001.
10. Frost L, Johansen R, Pedersen S, et al: Persistent subcutaneous nodules in children hyposensitized with aluminum containing allergen extracts. Allergy 40:368–372, 1985.
11. Gilnert R, Burnatowska-Hledin M: Serum and urinary aluminum levels in patients receiving alum precipitated allergenic extracts. Ann Allergy 61:433–435, 1988.
12. Golden D, Kagey-Sobotka A, Lichtenstein L: Survey of patients after discontinuing immunotherapy. J Allergy Clin Immunol 105:385–390, 2000.
13. Greenberger P: Immunotherapy update: Mechanisms of action. Allergy Asthma Proc 23:373–376, 2002.
14. Li JT. Allergy testing. Am Fam Physician 66:621–624, 2002.
15. Li JT, Lockey R, Bernstein IL, et al (eds): Allergen Immunotherapy: A Practice Parameter. Ann Allergy Asthma Immunol 90(Suppl 1):1–40, 2003.
16. Lieberman P: Use of epinephrine in the treatment of anaphylaxis. Curr Opin Allergy Clin Immunol 3:313–318, 2003.

17. Linneberg A, Henrik N, Frolund L, et al: Copenhagen Allergy Study. Allergy 57:1048–1052, 2002.

18. Lockey R, Benedict L, Turkeltaub P, et al: Fatalities from immunotherapy and skin testing. J Allergy Clin Immunol 79:660–677, 1987.

19. Malling HJ: Minimising the risks of allergen-specific injection immunotherapy. Drug Safety 23:323–332, 2000.

20. Malling HJ, Abreu-Nogueira J, Alvarez-Cuesta E, et al: Local immunotherapy. Allergy 53:933–944, 1998.

21. Marogna M, Massolo A: Sublingual immunotherapy in the context of a clinical practice improvement program in the allergological setting: Results of a long term observational study. Allergy Immunol (Paris) 35:133–140, 2003.

22. Marshall J, Abtahi S, Eiden J, et al: Immunostimulatory sequence DNA linked to the Amb a1 allergen promotes Th1 cytokine expression while down regulating Th2 cytokine expression in PBMCs from human patients with ragweed allergy. J Allergy Clin Immunol 108:191–197, 2001.

23. Moller C, Dreborg S, Ferdousi HA, et al: Pollen immunotherapy reduces the development of asthma in children with seasonal rhinoconjunctivitis (the PAT study). J Allergy Clin Immunol 109:251–256, 2002.

24. Muller U, Akdis C, Fricker M, et al: Successful immunotherapy with T-cell epitope peptides of bee venom phospholipase A2 induces specific T-cell anergy in patients allergic to bee venom. J Allergy Clin Immunol 101: 747–754, 1998.

25. Muller U, Helbling A, Berchtold E: Immunotherapy with honeybee venom and yellow jacket venom is different regarding efficacy and safety. J Allergy Clin Immunol 89:529–535, 1992.

26. Nelson H: Immunotherapy for inhalant allergens. In Adkinson NF, Yuninger JW, Busse WW, et al (eds): Middleton's Allergy: Principles and Practice, 6th ed. St. Louis, Mosby, 2003, pp 1455–1473.

27. Nelson H: Long-term immunotherapy with aqueous and aluminum-precipitated grass extracts. Ann Allergy 45:333–337, 1980.

28. Nettis E, Giordano D, Ferrannini A, et al: Systemic reactions to allergen immunotherapy: A review of the literature. Immunopharmacol Immunotoxicol 25:1–11, 2003.

29. Norman P, Winkenwerder W, Lichtenstein L.:Trials of alum-precipitated pollen extracts in the treatment of hay fever. J Allergy Clin Immunol. 50:31–44, 1972.

30. Portnoy J, King K, Horner S: Incidence of systemic reactions during rush immunotherapy. Ann Allergy 68: 493–498, 1992.

31. Simons FE, Simons KJ: Epinephrine absorption in adults: Intramuscular versus subcutaneous injection. J Allergy Clin Immunol 108:871–873, 2001.

32. Stewart GE, Lockey RF. Systemic reactions from allergen immunotherapy, J Allergy Clin Immunol 90:567–578, 1992.

33. Sturm G, Kranke B, Rudolph C, et al: Rush hymenoptera venom immunotherapy: A safe and practical protocol for high-risk patients. J Allergy Clin Immunol 110:928–933, 2002.

34. Tighe H, Takabayashi K, Scwartz D, et al: Conjugation of immunostimulatory DNA to the short ragweed allergen Amb a1 enhances its immunogenicity and reduces its allergenicity. J Allergy Clin Immunol 106:124–134, 2000.

35. Westall G, Thien F, Czarny D, et al: Adverse events associated with rush immunotherapy. MJA 174:227–230, 2001.

COMPLEMENTARY AND ALTERNATIVE MEDICINE

Andrea T. Borchers, Ph.D.

CHAPTER 19

1. **Define complementary and alternative medicine (CAM).**

   The National Center for Complementary and Alternative Medicine (NCCAM) defines CAM as "a group of diverse medical and health care systems, practices, and products that are not presently considered to be part of conventional medicine." Once scientific evidence shows that certain CAM practices are safe and effective, they will eventually cease to be considered "complementary or alternative" and will become integrated into a comprehensive approach to treating patients. To date, well-designed scientific studies are still needed to establish the safety and efficacy of most CAM thereapies.

2. **What are the different types of CAM therapies?**

   See Table 19-1.

3. **Who uses CAM?**

   Several different surveys have attempted to assess the usage of CAM in the United States. The most recent and comprehensive survey (based on the National Health Interview Survey conducted by the National Center for Health Statistics) indicated that an estimated 29% of adults in the United States had used at least one of 12 types of CAM therapy in the preceding year. The estimates in other analyses ranged from 8% to 42%. Studies suggest that the prevalence of CAM usage, particularly of botanical preparations, is higher among patients with chronic conditions, including cancer, autoimmune diseases, asthma, and AIDS.

   Surveys indicate that women frequently report higher CAM usage than men; usage rises with increasing income and increasing education. The most frequently used type of CAM therapy varies among surveys and countries.

   Ni H, Simile C, Hardy AM: Utilization of complementary and alternative medicine by United States adults: Results from the 1999 national health interview survey. Med Care 40:353–358, 2002.

4. **Why do people use CAM?**

   The reasons for the increasing popularity of CAM therapies have not been investigated extensively. However, some surveys report that both the ineffectiveness of Western medicine in the treatment of chronic diseases and the side effects often associated with conventional Western pharmaceutical regimens emerge as primary reasons for patients to explore CAM. Other surveys of the general population, however, contradict such conclusions. The finding that people consider the combination of conventional medicine and CAM to be superior to either approach alone indicates that they perceive something to be missing from both.

   One of the main therapeutic purposes for which people use CAM therapies is pain, particularly chronic headaches and lower back pain as well as pain associated with inflammatory disease (e.g., rheumatoid arthritis), and also for anxiety and depression. Many others perceive CAM approaches as a way to maintain or improve health and well-being.

   Astin JA: Why patients use alternative medicine: Results of a national study. JAMA 279:1548–1553, 1998.

   Eisenberg D M, Kessler RC, Van Rompay MI, et al: Perceptions about complementary therapies relative to conventional therapies among adults who use both: Results from a national survey. Ann Intern Med 135:344–351, 2001.

TABLE 19–1. TYPES OF CAM THERAPIES

Type of CAM	Description	Examples
Alternative medical systems	Philosophies of medicine that integrate theory and practice; many of them evolved earlier than what is now called conventional medicine and are based on very different concepts of health, disease, diagnosis, and therapy.	Traditional Chinese medicine Ayurveda Homeopathy Naturopathy
Mind-body interventions	A variety of techniques designed to enhance the mind's capacity to affect bodily function and symptoms Note that some techniques have become mainstream (e.g., patient support groups and cognitive-behavioral therapy)	Meditation Prayer Mental healing Therapies using creative outlets (art, music, dance)
Biologically based therapies	Involves substances found in nature, such as herbs, foods, and vitamins. Examples include dietary supplements, herbal products, and other so-called natural but as yet scientifically unproven therapies (e.g., shark cartilage to treat cancer).	Dietary supplements*
Manipulative and body-based methods†	Methods based on manipulation and/or movement of one or more parts of the body.	Chiropractic manipulation Massage

Energy therapies

Biofield — Intended to affect energy fields that purportedly surround and penetrate the human body. Some forms of energy therapy manipulate biofields by applying pressure and/or manipulating the body by placing the hands in, or through, these fields.

Qi gong
Reiki
Therapeutic touch

Bioelectromagnetic — Involve the unconventional use of electromagnetic fields, such as pulsed fields, magnetic fields, or alternating current or direct current fields

*NCCAM adds: "Some uses of dietary supplements have been incorporated into conventional medicine. For example, scientists have found that folic acid prevents certain birth defects, and a regimen of vitamins and zinc can slow the progression of an eye disease called age-related macular degeneration (AMD)."

†NCCAM also lists osteopathic manipulation as an example of a manipulative and body-based methods. This listing may be correct for countries where practitioners of osteopathy, called osteopaths, are trained only in manipulative therapies. In the United States, however, the terms "osteopathic medicine" and "doctors of osteopathic medicine" (DOs) are used instead of "osteopathy" and "osteopath" to reflect the fact that DOs are physicians who receive the same 4-year medical school training as medical doctors, except that their training places special emphasis on the osteopathic philosophies As such, doctors of osteopathic medicine are conventional physicians, not CAM practitioners.

Modified from the NCCAM website (http://nccam.nih.gov).

Hilsden RJ, Scott CM, Verhoef MJ: Complementary medicine use by patients with inflammatory bowel disease. Am J Gastroenterol 93:697–701, 1998.

Sutherland LR, Verhoef MJ: Why do patients seek a second opinion or alternative medicine? J Clin Gastroenterol 19:194–197, 1994.

5. **Do patients tell their doctors about their CAM usage?**

Most patients do not tell their physician about CAM usage, although many do if specifically asked. Reasons given for lack of disclosure are that it does not concern the physicians, that the physician would not understand, and/or that the physician would discourage the use of CAM therapies. Many patients would like to be treated by a physician who is knowledgeable not only about conventional medicine but also about various forms of CAM. Knowledge of CAM use is particularly important with patients taking botanical supplements because of potential adverse reactions (allergies, toxicities) and drug-herb or herb-herb interactions. During the preoperative evaluation, patients should be asked to bring in all dietary supplements that they currently take.

Ang-Lee MK, Moss J, Yuan CS: Herbal medicines and perioperative care. JAMA 286: 208–216, 2001.

Eisenberg DM, Davis RB, Ettner SL, et al: Trends in alternative medicine use in the United States, 1990-1997: Results of a follow-up national survey. JAMA 280:1569–1575, 1998.

Eisenberg DM, Kessler RC, Van Rompay MI, et al: Perceptions about complementary therapies relative to conventional therapies among adults who use both: Results from a national survey. Ann Intern Med 135:344–351, 2001.

6. **What is a dietary supplement?**

The 1994 Dietary Supplement Health and Education Act broadened the definition of a dietary supplement from products made of one or more of the essential nutrients (such as vitamins, minerals, protein) to essentially any product—other than tobacco—intended for ingestion as a supplement to the diet. This definition includes vitamins, minerals, amino acids, herbs or other botanicals, "or a concentrate, metabolite, constituent, extract, or combination of any of the previously mentioned ingredients."

U.S. Food and Drug Administration: An FDA guide to dietary supplements. FDA Consumer. Sept-Oct, 1998.

7. **What is the label of a dietary supplement supposed to tell you?**

Among the information the label of a dietary supplement is required to provide are the name(s) of the ingredient(s), their concentration, and, in the case of botanicals, the plant part used. The FDA allows common names, as listed in a standard reference for the identification of plants; the Latin binomial name need not be included. Compliance with this regulation is still far from complete.

8. **Why is a label containing all of the required information not always helpful to consumers?**

Consumers may know certain botanicals only by their "generic" name and be unaware that this name can refer to several different species, which can differ substantially in their chemical constituents and biologic activities. For example, "ginseng" refers to a variety of plant species belonging to the genus *Panax*. These species are often subdivided into American ginseng (*P. quinquefolius)* and "Asian" ginseng, which includes *P. ginseng*, *P. notoginseng*, *P. japonicus*, and *P. vietnamensis*. The name "ginseng," however, can also designate a member of an entirely different genus, *Eleutherococcus senticosus* or Siberian ginseng.

9. **How reliable is the information provided on labels?**

Several research laboratories have analyzed and compared commercially available plant extracts. A key finding was a more than 100-fold difference in marker compounds among extracts or powders of the same plant species, with standardized (see below) extracts containing between 0% and > 300% of the concentration stated on the label.

Harkey MR, Henderson GL, Gershwin ME, et al: Variability in commercial ginseng products: An analysis of 25 preparations. Am J Clin Nutr 73:1101–1106, 2001.
http://www.consumerlab.com

10. **What factors may account for the variability in the chemical composition of plant extracts?**

Some of the variability is attributable to differences in plant maturity, plant part used, and the growing, harvesting, storing, and processing conditions, all of which are known to influence the types and amounts of chemical constituents and the proportions in which they are present in a particular plant. In addition, the chemical composition of a plant extract depends on the type of extraction procedure (e.g., water- or alcohol-based) used in its preparation.

11. **What is the purpose of standardization of botanical products?**

It is already common practice in many European countries to standardize botanical extracts, and American manufacturers are following suit. Standardization is intended to ensure that the same percentage of a certain ingredient or group of ingredients is present in every dose of a botanical preparation. It would be preferable, of course, if these ingredients were (among) the active ones.

12. **Discuss the problems involved in standardization of botanical products.**

In many cases, detailed information about the chemical constituents of botanicals is missing, and the active ingredients have not yet been identified. A further complication is that botanicals may have several different biologic activities, not all which are attributable to the same chemical compound or group of compounds.

There is also concern that manipulating the extraction procedure to obtain a standardized percentage of one ingredient may alter the amount or proportion of other compounds that modulate the activity of the "active" ingredient. They may do so by enhancing or inhibiting the absorption or metabolism of the active constituent or by forming complexes that modify its activity.

13. **Is standardization the solution to the problem?**

Although standardization is intended as quality assurance, it is by no means an assurance of biologic activity. Moreover, the finding that even supposedly standardized extracts contain concentrations of the marker compound(s) that differ strikingly from those stated on the label makes even the goal of quality assurance questionable.

14. **Are botanical supplements safe?**

Many consumers perceive botanical remedies as "natural" and therefore safe. Several recent papers, however, have highlighted that various herbal preparations can cause allergies and serious toxicities, including hepatotoxicity, nephrotoxicity, and death. In some cases, such effects may be attributable to the ingestion of higher-than-recommended doses due to considerably greater potency than indicated on the label. Toxicities, however, can also result from intentional or unintentional substitution of herbs, contamination, or admixture of pharmaceuticals. Some Ayurvedic and traditional Chinese remedies have been found to contain high levels of heavy metals, such as lead, mercury, and arsenic. In Chinese herbal remedies, a large variety of pharmaceuticals, including paracetamol, indomethacin, prednisolone, dexamethasone, diazepam, and many more, have been detected. A further cause of concern is the molds and fungi that are almost always associated with raw plant material. They can produce toxic substances and become a health hazard unless the raw material is properly stored and processed.

Ernst E: Harmless herbs? A review of the recent literature. Am J Med 104:170–178, 1998.
Halt M: Moulds and mycotoxins in herb tea and medicinal plants. Eur J Epidemiol 14: 269–274, 1998.
Tomlinson B, Chan TYK, Chan JCN, et al: Toxicity of complementary therapies: An eastern perspective. J Clin Pharmacol 40:451–456, 2000.

15. **Discuss the risk of herb-drug interactions.**

    Botanicals, even if safe when taken by themselves, can cause adverse events when combined with other herbs or pharmaceuticals. The constituents of such combinations can exert additive or synergistic effects or can inhibit each other by competing for absorption and/or metabolism. A majority of publicized herb-drug interaction cases involve St. John's wort (*Hypericum perforatum*), a botanical shown in clinical trials to be an effective antidepressant. St. John's wort increases the clearance of a large variety of pharmaceuticals, including cyclosporine, indinavir, digoxin, phenprocoumon, and several antidepressants. Numerous other botanicals, including *Panax ginseng*, Siberian ginseng (*Eleutherococcus senticosus*), *Ginkgo biloba*, garlic, chili pepper (source of capsaicin), valerian (*Valeriana officinalis*), licorice (*Glycyrrhiza glabra*) and others have also been implicated in herb-drug interactions.

    Fugh-Berman A, Ernst E: Herb-drug interactions: Review and assessment of report reliability. Br J Clin Pharmacol 52:587–595, 2001.

16. **How common is the concurrent use of botanicals and pharmaceuticals?**

    One survey of CAM usage found that almost 20% of people taking prescription medication reported the concurrent use of one or more botanical products and/or a high-dose vitamin supplement.

    Eisenberg DM, Davis RB, Ettner SL, et al: Trends in alternative medicine use in the United States, 1990-1997: Results of a follow-up national survey. JAMA 280:1569–1575, 1998.

17. **Discuss the risk of herb-herb interactions.**

    Even less is known about herb-herb interactions. This lack of knowledge is particularly worrisome in view of the fact that manufacturers offer combination products–and sometimes only the fine print on a label reveals the presence of other botanicals. With increasing frequency manufacturers incorporate combinations of botanicals in multi-vitamin and mineral supplements.

18. **Can dietary supplementation with essential nutrients affect immune responses?**

    It is well established that certain nutrient deficiencies are associated with imbalanced and suboptimal immune responses, which can be corrected and restored via supplementation with the appropriate essential nutrient(s). In addition, supplementation with pharmacologic amounts of certain essential nutrients may influence inflammatory processes.

19. **How do PUFAs affect the inflammatory process?**

    Essential long-chain polyunsaturated fatty acids (PUFAs) have the potential to affect inflammatory processes. Their mechanism of action involves their incorporation as phospholipids into the membranes of cells, where they can become precursors for the synthesis of eicosanoids via the cyclooxygenase and lipoxygenase enzymatic pathways. The eicosanoids (i.e., prostaglandins and leukotrienes) produced by these enzymes can be pro- or anti-inflammatory, depending on the fatty acid precursor. The ratio of these products is determined by competition of the various PUFAs for these two enzymes. Eicosanoids, in turn, play an important role in regulating the production of cytokines, particularly those that promote inflammation.

20. **What is gamma-linolenic acid (GLA)?**

    GLA is an n-6 PUFA present in a variety of plant oils, including evening primrose, black currant, borage, and fungal oils. The products of its metabolism by cyclooxygenase and lipoxygenase have been found to exhibit anti-inflammatory activities in a variety of experimental systems.

21. **Is GLA an effective therapy in inflammatory diseases?**

    Supplementation with GLA has been investigated in patients with a variety of inflammatory diseases, such as atopic dermatitis, ulcerative colitis, and asthma, but the results have been contradictory. More encouraging effects have been observed in patients with rheumatoid arthritis (RA).

KEY POINTS: COMPLEMENTARY AND ALTERNATIVE MEDICINE

1. Allergists should ask patients about their use of CAM therapy.

2. The efficacy of CAM therapy in allergy/asthma is minimal, if it exists at all.

3. Allergists should be aware of the appropriate websites for CAM therapy.

4. Interactions of dietary supplements and conventional drugs may produce toxicity.

22. **What evidence supports the efficacy of GLA in RA?**
A Cochrane review of herbal therapies for RA included seven randomized, double-blind, placebo-controlled studies comparing GLA with various oils intended as placebo (two studies used olive oil, which appears to have some effects of its own). Although reporting of the data was considered inadequate in some of the studies, the overall results indicated that GLA was associated with improvement in pain, joint tenderness score, and joint tenderness count. The effects on joint swelling were inconsistent, with two studies reporting a decrease, but one reporting an increase in both the active treatment and the placebo groups.

Little C, Parsons T: Herbal therapy for treating rheumatoid arthritis. Cochrane Database Syst Rev 3 2003 [last substantive amendment August 2003].

23. **Does GLA have adverse effects?**
To date, only minor adverse effects from consumption of supplemental GLA have been reported, mostly associated with abdominal discomfort.

24. **Discuss the optimal dosage and duration of treatment for GLA.**
Although optimal dosage and duration of treatment have not yet been established, availble data suggest that a dose of 1.4 gm/day of GLA or greater may be necessary to achieve clinically relevant improvements and that a period of supplementation of at least 6–12 months may be necessary for GLA to become fully effective in reducing signs and symptoms of synovitis.

25. **Can plant extracts affect immune responses?**
Various botanicals are offered as dietary supplements with the claim of enhancing or stimulating the immune system. Examples include several species of *Echinacea*, Siberian ginseng *(Eleutherococcus senticosus),* ginger root *(Zingiber officinale),* licorice root *(Glycyrrhiza glabra),* cat's claw *(Uncaria tomentosa),* goldenseal *(Hydrastis canadensis),* pau d'arco *(Tabebuia impetiginosa),* atractylodes *(A. macrocephala, A. lancea),* astragalus *(A. membranaceus),* and various mushrooms or mushroom constituents, among others. For most of these botanicals, data from in vitro experiments and, in most cases, animal studies suggest that they can modulate some immune responses. Data from randomized, controlled clinical trials, however, are rare or lacking entirely.

26. **Discuss the evidence from in vitro and animal studies supporting the usefulness of echinacea as an immunostimulant.**
Echinacea (common name: coneflower) is not only one of the most widely sold supplements but also one of the most extensively studied, both in vitro and in vivo. Data from in vitro experiments and animal studies suggest that various preparations can enhance nonadaptive immune responses, particularly stimulation of the motility and phagocytic activity of polymorphonuclear leukocytes as well as macrophage cytokine production and natural killer activity.

27. **Discuss the effects of echinacea on phagocytosis in humans.**
The results of human studies investigating the effects of echinacea on phagocytosis have been conflicting. Methodologic factors may have contributed to the discrepancies. Specifically, the

time points after the last ingested dose at which blood is drawn and immune cells are isolated are likely to play a major role. Only a few studies have addressed the question of whether echinacea preparations can modulate adaptive immune responses. One of them recently reported that *E. angustifolia* root extract administered to rats in drinking water significantly enhanced antigen-specific production of immunoglobulin G.

Rehman J, Dillow JM, Carter SM, et al: Increased production of antigen-specific immunoglobulins G and M following in vivo treatment with the medicinal plants *Echinacea angustifolia* and *Hydrastis canadensis*. Immunol Lett 68:391–395, 1999.

28. **Give examples of the contradictory findings in clinical trials evaluating the efficacy of echinacea preparations for preventing and treating upper respiratory infections.**

A Cochrane systematic review identified 16 randomized clinical trials published up to 1998 addressing the efficacy of echinacea (as monopreparation or as the major ingredient in combination with other plant extracts and, in some cases, vitamin C) in preventing or treating the common cold. Interestingly, all but two of the studies had been conducted in Germany. None was published in a Medline-listed journal, according to the authors (although two of them now are in Pubmed). The authors concluded that some echinacea preparations appeared to be superior to placebo. The data were insufficient, however, to recommend a specific product or preparation.

A prevention trial by Turner et al. tested an echinacea preparation in induced rhinovirus colds and failed to find a significant effect of the echinacea preparation in reducing the incidence of upper respiratory infections.

Melchart D, Linde K, Fischer P, Kaesmayr J: Echinacea for preventing and treating the common cold. Cochrane Database Syst Rev 3 2003 [last substantive amendment October 1998].

Turner RB, Riker DK, Gangemi JD: Ineffectiveness of echinacea for prevention of experimental rhinovirus colds. Antimicrob Agents Chemother 44:1708–1709, 2000.

29. **As a whole, what does the current evidence suggest about the efficacy of echinacea?**

Taken together, the currently available evidence suggests that certain echinacea preparations may be able to prevent upper respiratory infections and, if taken shortly after their onset, shorten the duration of symptoms. The overall effect size appears to be small, however, with a reduction in the relative risk of 10–20% and shortening of the duration of symptoms by 0.25 days, although others found a reduction of up to 3 days.

Barrett BP, Brown RL, Locken K, et al: Treatment of the common cold with unrefined echinacea: A randomized, double-blind, placebo-controlled trial. Ann Intern Med 137:939–946 2002.

Schulten B, Bulitta M, Ballering-Bruhl B, et al: Efficacy of *Echinacea purpurea* in patients with a common cold:A placebo-controlled, randomised, double-blind clinical trial. Arzneimittelforschung 51:563–568, 2001.

30. **What makes the evidence on echinacea preparations so inconclusive?**

Although the quality of several of the recent trials with echinacea is somewhat higher than many of those included in the Cochrane Review, these studies still do not allow definitive conclusions about the efficacy or inefficacy of echinacea for the same reasons given by the authors of the systematic review. Comparison of study results is made very difficult by the administration of a different echinacea preparation in almost every study due to the use of:

- Three different echinacea species *(E. purpurea, E. pallida,* and *E. angustifolia)*
- Different parts of the plant (roots, herbs, whole plant)
- Different methods of extraction (e.g., alcohol extracts, water extracts, or no extraction [i.e., encapsulated powder of whole dried herbs])
- Additional plant extracts or homeopathic components in some preparations

In addition, no validated instruments are available for the assessment of the common cold, which adds to the difficulties in determining the efficacy of any therapy in ameliorating and/or shortening symptoms. Furthermore, a serious shortcoming in existing knowledge about *Echinacea* species is the almost complete lack of dose-response data from clinical studies.

31. **How can such confounding issues be addressed in future studies?**

The use of many different echinacea preparations of undefined or poorly defined chemical composition in various studies not only makes comparisons of the results impossible but also severely limits reproducibility. Having worked extensively with various *Echinacea* species, Wagner and colleagues have urged that investigators should provide detailed information about the exact chemical composition of the extract used in the study. In addition to enhancing reproducibility, this strategy would eventually make it possible to correlate specific chemical constituents with observed biologic activities. It is not very helpful, however, to provide a detailed chemical analysis of the extract under investigation without mentioning the extraction procedure or the species and plant parts used, as was done in a recent investigation.

Turner RB, Riker DK, Gangemi JD: Ineffectiveness of echinacea for prevention of experimental rhinovirus colds. Antimicrob Agents Chemother 44:1708–1709, 2000.

32. **Define acupuncture.**

In traditional Chinese medicine, acupuncture is used to correct disturbances in the flow of *qi*, the life force or energy that is channeled through 12 primary and 8 "extraordinary" meridians. Approximately 360 acupuncture points are located along these meridians. Chinese acupuncturists use a variety of diagnostic techniques to determine the nature of the imbalance and to choose the appropriate points at which acupuncture needs to be applied. The traditional method consists of inserting a long, thin needle into the skin at these points and then manipulating it manually. Other mechanisms of manipulation include heat, pressure, friction, suction, or electric stimulation.

33. **What are the difficulties in designing a controlled trial of acupuncture?**

One of the most basic decisions in planning a trial of acupuncture concerns the question of whether to follow the Western practice of using a formula approach (the same acupuncture points are stimulated in all patients) or the traditional Chinese medicine approach (the acupuncture points are individually tailored to each patient). The formula approach will always be open to the criticism that a lack of response is the inevitable result of the fact that therapy was not individualized. In addition, the study design needs to take into account and control for a large number of parameters, including siting of needles, number of acupuncture points, needle insertion depth, type and duration of needle manipulation (manual, electrical, moxibustion), duration of insertion, and achievement of *dachi (de qui)*, a tingling or irradiating sensation after needling that is thought to indicate effectiveness. Furthermore, the acupuncturist knows whether she or he is giving real or sham acupuncture. As a consequence, blinding can be only partial in any randomized, controlled trial of acupuncture, and the effects of the suggestion potentially resulting from this knowledge cannot be controlled for.

34. **Can acupuncture modulate the immune response?**

In a recent randomized trial by Joos et al. of acupuncture in patients with asthma, a significant decrease in peripheral blood eosinophils and an increase in $CD3^+$ and $CD4^+$ T cells were reported in the group receiving acupuncture according to the principles of traditional Chinese medicine but not in those in whom points not specific for asthma were treated. In addition, true acupuncture was associated with increased lymphocyte proliferation and changes in the production of a variety of cytokines. Medici et al also reported a decrease in blood and sputum eosinophil concentrations in asthmatic patients after acupuncture, but in that study, the groups receiving real and sham acupuncture both exhibited greater changes than the group receiving no treatment. Similarly, Karst et al. found that the neutrophil respiratory burst was increased by both real and sham acupuncture compared with baseline. In addition, there are reports of acupuncture resulting in increased serum cortisol levels, which in turn are likely to affect inflammatory processes. Taken together, these results suggest that acupuncture can modulate a variety of immune responses.

Joos S, Schott C, Zou H, et al: Immunomodulatory effects of acupuncture in the treatment of allergic asthma: A randomized controlled study. J Altern Complement Med 6:519–525, 2000.

Medici TC, Grebski E, Wu J, et al: Acupuncture and bronchial asthma: A long-term randomized study of the effects of real versus sham acupuncture compared to controls in patients with bronchial asthma. J Altern Complement Med 8:737–750; discussion, 751–754, 2002.

Karst M., Scheinichen D, Rueckert T, et al: Effect of acupuncture on the neutrophil respiratory burst: A placebo-controlled single-blinded study. Complement Ther Med 11:4–10, 2003.

35. **Summarize the Cochrane review of evidence related to the efficacy of acupuncture in asthma.**
A Cochrane systematic review identified seven small randomized, controlled trials (involving a total of 174 patients) that studied the use of acupuncture in chronic asthma and met the inclusion criteria. Subjective symptoms were significantly improved in two trials. The differences in lung function parameters between real and "dummy" acupuncture, however, were neither statistically significant nor clinically relevant. In some of the studies, the control groups received acupuncture at true acupuncture points that were thought not to affect asthma but may have resulted in therapeutic benefit (see above), thereby masking the effect of acupuncture treatment specific for asthma.

Linde K, Jobst K, Panton J: Acupuncture for chronic asthma. Cochrane Database Syst Rev 3 2003 [last substantive amendment October 1998].

36. **What other evidence is relevant to the efficacy of acupuncture in patients with asthma?**
Not included in the Cochrane review was a recent trial of acupuncture in patients with mild-to-moderate persistent asthma that included not only a real and a sham acupuncture group but also a group of patients that did not receive any treatment besides standard asthma medications. This study included only patients with asthma of the *Shi* (excess) type in order to use a formula approach while still adhering to the concepts of traditional Chinese medicine. For two treatment periods of 4 weeks each, separated by a 2-month period without treatment, patients received acupuncture twice weekly. They were then followed for 10 months. Both real and sham acupuncture significantly reduced the variability in peak expiratory flow (PEF) compared with no treatment, although to varying degrees of significance at different time points. They did not, however, affect other lung function parameters. The authors themselves questioned the clinical relevance of this finding since PEF variability in their group of patients was low even at the beginning of the study.

Medici TC, Grebski E, Wu J, et al: Acupuncture and bronchial asthma: A long-term randomized study of the effects of real versus sham acupuncture compared to controls in patients with bronchial asthma. J Altern Complement Med 8:737–750; discussion, 751–754, 2002.

37. **Where can you find information on CAM and individual CAM therapies?**
For information about a particular botanical or therapy, it is advisable to use literature reviews as starting points only but not to rely on them exclusively. The best source of information is original literature, but it needs to be read critically. Table 19-2 lists various criteria that may help in determining whether a study can be considered of adequate quality or whether the reporting of the results is so inadequate that the methodological soundness of the study is questionable.

Since a vast majority of studies of botanicals are published in Europe, EMBASE is likely to yield more citations than Medline; and Biosis can be helpful especially for studies addressing chemical composition and mechanistic questions.

Table 19-3 lists websites related to CAM and dietary supplements, particularly botanicals. The NCCAM Website (http://nccam.nih.gov) is particularly useful.

TABLE 19–2. CRITERIA FOR EVALUATING STUDIES

Criterion	Questions	Comment
Randomization	Is it adequate and adequately described?	Alternation or assignment based on odd/even birthdays is considered quasi-randomization at best
	Was it successful? Were the groups similar, or did they differ significantly at baseline?	Major differences at baseline may leave little room for improvement in one of the groups, thereby skewing the results in favor of the other group
Blinding	Was blinding adequate?	Botanical products and some of their constituents tend to have very characteristic smells and tastes that are difficult to mask and almost impossible to duplicate in a placebo.
		Note that the practitioner providing both the real and the sham acupuncture can never be blinded to the treatment of the patient; only the person evaluating the effects of treatment can be blinded.
		Blinding may be presented in such a way as to appear adequate, but the actual question of whether patients were able to tell which treatment they received may allow a better assessment of the success of blinding.
	Did the authors try to assess whether the patients were able to tell which treatment they received?	
Controls	Are they adequate?	Ask yourself whether a significant change observed in a placebo group can be attributed to normal fluctuations in disease activity or is likely to have arisen from a therapeutic effect of what was assumed to be an ineffective treatment.
Primary outcome measures	Is a primary outcome measure clearly stated?	The lack of a clearly defined outcome measure is a flaw particularly of older studies. This makes it difficult to determine whether the study was designed to assess the outcomes that are reported or only reported a particular outcome from a post-hoc analysis because other parameters failed to exhibit significant differences.

(continued)

TABLE 19–2.   CRITERIA FOR EVALUATING STUDIES (continued)

Criterion	Questions	Comment
Intention to treat analysis	Is the statistical analysis based on the intention to treat, or are only those subjects analyzed that completed the study?	Lack of efficacy may be a major reason for withdrawal from the study in both the active treatment and placebo groups; hence, exclusion of drop-outs from the final analysis is likely to skew the results.
Drop-outs	Are the reasons why people dropped out of the study clearly stated for all drop-outs?	A comparison of the number of subjects dropping out of the active treatment and the placebo group and the reasons for dropping out may provide important insights into whether patients perceived the treatment as acceptable and effective. It may also give some indications about the adverse effects and toxicities associated with the treatment.
Results	Are the results only statistically significant or also clinically relevant? Is the clinical relevancy discussed by the authors?	
Treatment period	Was it long enough?	The optimal duration of treatment has not been established for many alternative therapies. It can be assumed, however, that many of them—not being as potent as pharmaceuticals—require prolonged periods of treatment before taking effect (see section on GLA in RA). Continuous improvement in the treatment group that did not reach statistical significance compared to placebo by the end of the study but also showed no signs of reaching a plateau may indicate that the treatment effect would have increased over time
Test compound	Is it well characterized?	The authors of numerous clinical trials with botanicals provide little information (e.g., plant species and part[s] used, extraction procedure, chemical composition) on the extracts they used. Detailed information about these characteristics is a prerequisite for comparability and reproducibility of results.

TABLE 19–3.   VALUABLE RESOURCES FOR FURTHER INFORMATION

Organization	Web Address	Type of Information Contained in the Website
NCCAM, NIH	http://nccam.nih.gov	Definition of CAM and CAM categories, information about ongoing trials, but also advisories and warnings on various individual products or product categories, their potential toxicities and their interactions with pharmaceuticals
Center for Food Safety and Applied Nutrition, FDA	http://vm.cfsan.fda.gov/~dms/supplmnt.html	Definition of dietary supplements, labeling requirements, and other regulatory and industry information. *Adverse events associated with dietary supplements should be reported to the FDA using the instructions provided on this site.*
Agricultural Research Service, United States Department of Agriculture	http://www.ars-grin.gov/duke	Information about the chemical composition of botanicals.
HerbMed	http://www.herbmed.org	Information about > 160 botanical compounds, including available evidence, although no clear distinction is made between in vitro, animal, and human studies. When available, studies of pharmacodynamics, adverse effects/toxicities, and drug interactions are also listed.
Consumer Lab	http://www.consumerlab.com	Reports on independent laboratory testing of dietary supplements, including comparisons of potency; also information on recalls and warnings about individual products or product categories.

WEBSITES

See Table 19-3.

BIBLIOGRAPHY

1. Ang-Lee MK, Moss J, Yuan CS: Herbal medicines and perioperative care. JAMA 286:208–216, 2001.

2. Astin JA: Why patients use alternative medicine: Results of a national study. JAMA 279:1548–1553, 1998.

3. Barrett BP, Brown RL, Locken K, et al: Treatment of the common cold with unrefined echinacea: A randomized, double-blind, placebo-controlled trial. Ann Intern Med 137:939–946 2002.

4. Brinkeborn RM, Shah DV, Degenring FH: Echinaforce and other Echinacea fresh plant preparations in the treatment of the common cold. A randomized, placebo controlled, double-blind clinical trial. Phytomedicine 6:1–6, 1999.

5. Eisenberg DM, Davis RB, Ettner SL, et al: Trends in alternative medicine use in the United States, 1990–1997: Results of a follow-up national survey. JAMA 280:1569–1575, 1998.

6. Eisenberg DM, Kessler RC, Van Rompay MI, et al: Perceptions about complementary therapies relative to conventional therapies among adults who use both: Results from a national survey. Ann Intern Med 135:344–351, 2001.

7. Ernst E: Harmless herbs? A review of the recent literature. Am J Med 104:170–178, 1998.

8. Fugh-Berman A, Ernst E: Herb-drug interactions: Review and assessment of report reliability. Br J Clin Pharmacol 52:587–595, 2001.

9. Grimm W, Müller HH: A randomized controlled trial of the effect of fluid extract of *Echinacea purpurea* on the incidence and severity of colds and respiratory infections. Am J Med 106:138–143, 1999.

10. Halt M: Moulds and mycotoxins in herb tea and medicinal plants. Eur J Epidemiol 14:269–274, 1998.

11. Harkey MR, Henderson GL, Gershwin ME, et al: Variability in commercial ginseng products: An analysis of 25 preparations. Am J Clin Nutr 73:1101–1106, 2001.

12. Henneicke-von Zepelin H., Hentschel C, Schnitker J, et al: Efficacy and safety of a fixed combination phytomedicine in the treatment of the common cold (acute viral respiratory tract infection): Results of a randomised, double blind, placebo controlled, multicentre study. Curr Med Res Opin 15:214–227, 1999.

13. Hilsden RJ, Scott CM, Verhoef MJ: Complementary medicine use by patients with inflammatory bowel disease. Am J Gastroenterol 93:697–701, 1998.

14. Joos S, Schott C, Zou H, et al: Immunomodulatory effects of acupuncture in the treatment of allergic asthma: A randomized controlled study. J Altern Complement Med 6:519–525, 2000.

15. Karst M., Scheinichen D, Rueckert T, et al: Effect of acupuncture on the neutrophil respiratory burst: A placebo-controlled single-blinded study. Complement Ther Med 11:4–10, 2003.

16. Linde K, Jobst K, Panton J: Acupuncture for chronic asthma. Cochrane Database Syst Rev 3 2003 [last substantive amendment October 1998].

17. Lindenmuth GF, Lindenmuth EB: The efficacy of echinacea compound herbal tea preparation on the severity and duration of upper respiratory and flu symptoms: A randomized, double-blind placebo-controlled study. J Altern Complement Med 6:327–334, 2000.

18. Little C, Parsons T: Herbal therapy for treating rheumatoid arthritis. Cochrane Database Syst Rev 3 2003 [last substantive amendment August 2000.]

19. Medici TC, Grebski E, Wu J, et al: Acupuncture and bronchial asthma: A long-term randomized study of the effects of real versus sham acupuncture compared to controls in patients with bronchial asthma. J Altern Complement Med 8:737–750; discussion, 751–754, 2002.

20. Melchart D, Linde K, Fischer P, Kaesmayr J: Echinacea for preventing and treating the common cold. Cochrane Database Syst Rev 3 2003 [last substantive amendment October 1998].

21. Ni H, Simile C, Hardy AM: Utilization of complementary and alternative medicine by United States adults: Results from the 1999 national health interview survey. Med Care 40:353–358, 2002.

22. Rehman J, Dillow JM, Carter SM, et al: Increased production of antigen-specific immunoglobulins G and M following in vivo treatment with the medicinal plants *Echinacea angustifolia* and *Hydrastis canadensis*. Immunol Lett 68:391–395, 1999.

23. Schulten B, Bulitta M, Ballering-Bruhl B, et al: Efficacy of *Echinacea purpurea* in patients with a common cold: A placebo-controlled, randomised, double-blind clinical trial. Arzneimittelforschung 51:563–568, 2001.

24. Sutherland LR, Verhoef MJ: Why do patients seek a second opinion or alternative medicine? J Clin Gastroenterol 19:194–197, 1994.

25. Tomlinson B, Chan TYK, Chan JCN, et al: Toxicity of complementary therapies: An eastern perspective. J Clin Pharmacol 40:451–456, 2000.

26. Turner RB, Riker DK, Gangemi JD: Ineffectiveness of echinacea for prevention of experimental rhinovirus colds. Antimicrob Agents Chemother 44:1708–1709, 2000.

27. U.S. Food and Drug Administration: An FDA guide to dietary supplements. FDA Consumer. Sept–Oct, 1998.

CHAPTER 20

SYSTEMIC MAST-CELL DISEASES

Christopher Chang, M.D., Ph.D.

1. **What are mast cells?**

   Mast cells are mononuclear cells that are rarely seen in peripheral blood but are present in tissue. Mast cells are particularly abundant in the connective tissue that surrounds areas of the body that interface with the environment, such as the respiratory tract, gastrointestinal tract, and skin.

2. **When were mast cells discovered?**

   Mast cells were discovered in rabbit mesentery in 1877 by Paul Ehrlich at Freiburg University. Ehrlich derived the name from the Greek *mastos* (= feeding), because he thought that the cytoplasmic granules that he observed were a result of phagocytosis.

3. **Summarize the function of mast cells.**

   The function of mast cells remained unknown for many years. Mast cells are now known to be an integral part of inflammation and play an important role in allergic diseases. They are also involved in infectious diseases, particularly parasitic infestations, and neoplastic conditions. Mast cells are present in all mammalian species. Initially, they were thought to be the tissue equivalents of basophils in the peripheral circulation. Recently, they have been well characterized in humans and mice and have been found to be distinct from basophils.

   Church MK, Lei-Schaffer F: The human mast cell. J Allergy Clin Immunol 99:155–160, 1997.

KEY POINTS: CHARACTERISTICS OF MAST CELLS

1. Mast cells originate from a pluripotent CD34+ stem cell derived from the bone marrow.

2. Mast cells are mononuclear cells that are present in various tissues.

3. Mast cells are usually round but can be spindly or elongated in shape.

4. Mast cells release both preformed and newly generated mediators.

5. The primary cell-surface receptor of the mast cell is the high-affinity FcεRI receptor.

4. **How are mast cells identified?**

   Mast cells can be seen on examination of nasal mucosal cells, skin, intestinal mucosa, respiratory tract tissue, and conjunctival scrapings. Under light microscopy, mast cells have a rounded shape, and the cytoplasm contains numerous intracellular granules, which stain characteristically with toluidine or Alcian dye to the color of violet to reddish purple. The color is a result of a reaction between highly acidic heparin in mast cells and the basic aniline blue dyes. In contrast, basophils are smaller, and possess a multilobular nucleus. Basophils are similarly stained with toluidine and Alcian dye. Mast cells do not stain with hematoxylin-eosin. Mast cells can also be identified (1) under electron microscopy, (2) by virtue of specific proteases in their cytoplasmic granules, and (3) by characterization of cell-surface markers specific for mast cells.

5. **Describe the structure of a mast cell.**
   Mast cells are usually round but can be spindly or elongated in shape, typically between 9 and 12 microns in diameter. The nuclei of mast cells are ovoid in shape. The cytoplasm of the mast cell contains many granules. These secretory granules have a unique bilaminar phospholipid membrane containing lysosomes, which carry oxidative enzymes and acid hydrolases.

6. **Summarize the ontogeny of the mast cell.**
   Mast cells originate from a pluripotent CD34+ stem cell derived from the bone marrow. When cultured in the presence of stem cell factor, these stem cells are triggered to produce inordinately high numbers of mast cells. Cytokines that enhance the development of mast cells include interleukin (IL)-3, IL-5, and IL-6. Contrary to earlier belief, mast cells and basophils do not share a common lineage. Basophils share a common lineage with eosinophils. Mast cells complete their final maturation and differentiation in the tissues and can survive for several months.

   McNeil HP, Austen KF: Biology of the mast cell. In Frank MM, Austen KR, Claman HN, Unanue ER (eds): Samter's Immunological Diseases, 5th ed. Boston, Little, Brown, 1995, pp 185–204.

7. **Explain the heterogeneity in the structure and formation of mast cells in different tissues.**
   Heterogeneity in the structure and function of mast cells in different tissues is based on microenvironmental stimuli during the differentiation and maturation phase. Mast cell growth factors include the c-kit ligand or stem cell factor (stem cell factor is the high affinity ligand of a c-kit proto-oncogene), which is secreted by fibroblasts. Mast cell precursors cultured with fibroblasts give rise to more mature cell lines than those cultured only with IL-3. When both fibroblasts and IL-3 are present in the cultures, mast cell differentiation increases due to the synergistic activity of stem cell factor and other growth factors, such as granulocyte-macrophage colony-stimulating factor (GM-CSF), IL-3, and IL-6.

   Galli SJ: New concepts about the mast cell. N Engl J Med 328:257–65, 1993.

8. **What is "kit"?**
   Kit or c-kit is the cellular homolog of the oncogene of the v-kit gene found in feline sarcoma virus. The c-kit gene, located on chromosome at 4q11-12, is a member of the type 3 tyrosine kinase family.

9. **What is the relationship between stem cell factor and kit?**
   Signaling through c-kit is important for differentiation and maturation and survival of mast cells. The c-kit gene also serves as a receptor for platelet differentiation and growth factor (PDGF), macrophage colony-stimulating factor (M-CSF), and stem cell factor (also called kit-ligand)

10. **How does one distinguish a mast cell from a basophil?**
    See Table 20-1.

11. **Define the two kinds of mast cells in humans.**
    Humans have two kinds of mast cells: those that secrete the neutral protease tryptase (designated MC_T) and those that also secrete other enzymes, primarily carboxypeptidase, cathepsin G, and chymase (designated MC_{TC}). Both forms of human mast cells contain similar amounts of histamine. The different forms of mast cells are preferentially found in different tissues of the body.

12. **Where are MC_T cells found? Describe their function.**
    MC_T cells are predominantly found in gastrointestinal submucosa, skin, and vascular structures. They appear to be more closely linked with inflammatory disorders or allergic diseases and are referred to as immune system-associated mast cells. They also play a role in host defense and

TABLE 20-1.	HOW TO DISTINGUISH A MAST CELL FROM A BASOPHIL
Mast Cells	**Basophils**
Larger (9–12 μm)	Smaller (5–7 μm)
Round nucleus	Multilobular nucleus
Contain prostaglandin D_2	No prostaglandin D_2
High level of tryptase	Low level of tryptase
Chymase in MC_{TC} mast cells	No chymase

are decreased in immunodeficiency syndromes. Mast cells have been linked to defense against parasitic diseases of the gut as well as involvement in innate immunity against bacterial invasion. They are increased around areas of Th2-cell activation.

13. **Where are MC_{TC} cells found?**
MC_{TC} cells are more commonly found in the connective tissue of the lung, upper respiratory tract, and small intestine. They are sometimes referred to as the nonimmune-system associated mast cell.

14. **Discuss the cell surface receptors of the mast cell.**
The primary cell-surface receptor of the mast cell is the high-affinity FcεRI receptor. The FcεRI receptor consists of an α chain, a β chain, and two γ chains. Signal transduction across the cell membrane is regulated by alterations in the carboxyterminal cytoplasmic tail of the β or γ chains. Other cell-surface receptors include CD43, CD44, CD45, CD68, kit, and IL4R. Mast cells also possess receptors for IgG and the anaphylatoxins, complements C3a and C5a.

KEY POINTS: RECEPTORS ON THE SURFACE OF THE MAST CELL

1. IgE
2. CD43
3. CD44
4. CD45
5. CD68
6. Kit
7. IL4R
8. IgG

15. **What types of mediators are released by mast cells?**
Mast cells release both preformed and newly generated mediators. The clinical effects of mastocytosis syndromes are directly related to the effects of release of both categories of mast cell mediators.

Church MK, Holgate ST, Shute JK, et al: Mast cell-derived mediators. In Middleton E Jr, Ellis EF, Yuninger JW, et al (eds). Allergy: Principles and Practice, 5th ed. St. Louis, Mosby, 1998, pp 146–167.

16. **What are the best known preformed mediators released by mast cells?**
The best known of the preformed mast cell mediators is **histamine**. Histamine is derived from the amino acid histidine and is spontaneously secreted from mast cells at low levels. The

amount of histamine contained in a human mast cell is on the order of 3–8 pg. The biogenic amine **serotonin** is another of the preformed mediators. **Heparin** is also present in large amounts in mast cells. Effects of heparin include endothelial cell stimulation and kinin pathway activation.

17. **What other preformed mediators do mast cells contain?**
Mast cells also have a high concentration of neutral proteases (about 60 pg per cell). The neutral protease, tryptase, is present in both human and rodent mast cells. Tryptase is a serine protease present in tetrameric form, with a total molecular weight of 200 to 560 kD. There are two pairs of subunits, designated α and β, with variable molecular weights (due to varying degrees of glycosylation) between 31 and 38 kD.

Mast cells also contain proteoglycans; chemotactic factors, such as eosinophil chemotactic factor (ECF) and neutrophil chemotactic factor (NCF); oxidative enzymes; other biogenic amines; and acid hydrolases, such as β-hexosaminidase, β-glucuronidase, β-D-galactosidase, and aryl-sulfatase.

Church MK, Holgate ST, Shute JK, et al: Mast cell-derived mediators. In Middleton E Jr, Ellis EF, Yunginger JW, et al (eds). Allergy: Principles and Practice, 5th ed. St. Louis, Mosby, 1998, pp 146–167.

18. **Summarize the primary mechanism by which mast cells are activated.**
Mast cells are primarily activated as a result of antigen-triggered IgE binding to the high-affinity FcϵRI receptor on the surface of the mast cell, followed by cross-linking. Mast cells also possess the low-affinity IgG receptors FcγRII and FcγRIII. Antigen-IgE interaction leads to cross-linking of FcϵRI molecules on the surface of the mast cell.

19. **What are the next steps in the activation of mast cells?**
Cross-linking of FcϵRI molecules on the surface of the mast cell leads to activation of tyrosine kinase, which catalyzes phosphorylation of a number of substrates, including phospholipase Cg1 and the β and γ chains of the FcϵRI receptor. In turn, this phosphorylation leads to activation of protein kinase and mobilization of intracellular calcium ions, which then leads to phospholipase A2 activation. Activation of phospholipase results in the cleavage of arachidonic acid from the membrane phospholipids. The resulting lysophospholipids are active in fusion of plasma membrane with the secretory granule membrane and lead to extrusion of bioactive mediators such as histamine from the cell (degranulation).

20. **How else may histamine release be induced?**
Histamine release from mast cells can also be induced by autoantibodies to the IgE FcϵRI receptor in patients with chronic idiophathic urticaria (CIU). Non-immune-related factors, such as exercise, pressure, trauma, or cold, may also lead to activation of the FcϵRI receptor.

21. **Describe the characteristics of the FcϵRI receptor.**
The FcϵRI receptor is the high-affinity IgE receptor. It is a tetrameric protein consisting of an α chain, a β chain, and two γ chains. The α chain extends outside the cell and contains the IgE receptor. The β subunit is responsible for amplification of the signal. The FcϵRI receptor correlates with serum IgE levels.

22. **How many FcϵRI receptors are on the surface of a mast cell?**
There are 10,000 to 1,000,000 FcϵRI receptors on the surface of a mast cell. Aggregation of anywhere from 1% to 15% of these receptors leads to degranulation.

23. **What are the biologic effects of histamine?**
Histamine is a hormone that exerts its effects on other cells by binding to cell-surface receptors of both inflammatory and noninflammatory cells. There are two common types of histamine

receptors, designated H$_1$ and H$_2$. A third type of histamine receptor, H$_3$, is found on presynaptic nerve endings in both the peripheral and central nervous systems. There does not appear to be a significant role for the H$_3$-receptor in allergic or inflammatory conditions.

24. **What are the physiologic effects of histamine?**
    - Gastrointestinal and bronchial smooth muscle contraction
    - Gastric acid secretion
    - Endothelial cell retraction
    - Increased vascular permeability
    - Vasodilation
    - Increased permeability of plasma membranes
    - Stimulation of chemotaxis
    - Infiltration of neutrophils and eosinophils
    - Stimulation of the release of other neuropeptide mediators

25. **List the clinical effects of histamine on skin.**
    - Pruritus
    - Wheal and flare response
    - Hives

26. **What are the clinical effects of histamine on the respiratory system?**
    - Wheezing
    - Bronchial hyperresponsiveness
    - Pulmonary edema
    - Mucus production

27. **How does histamine affect the vascular system?**
    Histamine may lead to circulatory instability and circulatory collapse.

28. **List the clinical effects of histamine on the gastrointestinal system.**
    - Cramping
    - Gastritis
    - Peptic ulcers

KEY POINTS: CLINICAL FEATURES OF SYSTEMIC MASTOCYTOSIS

1. Urticaria pigmentosa
2. Solitary mastocytomas
3. Peripheral blood abnormalities
4. Lytic bone lesions
5. Mast cell leukemia
6. Peptic ulcer disease
7. Malabsorption
8. Hepatic or splenic involvement
9. Peripheral lymphadenopathy

---

29. **How serious are the clinical effects of histamine?**
    Severe manifestations of the above symptoms can result in death.

30. **What is the role of tryptase in acute inflammation and mastocytosis?**
Tryptase can comprise up to 20% of the total cellular protein of a mast cell. Because tryptase is not released by basophils, measurement of tryptase levels can be a more specific indicator of mast cell activation and degranulation than histamine. In patients with asthma, anaphylaxis, or systemic mastocytosis, tryptase can be found in bronchoalveolar lavage fluid after an exacerbation. Tryptase has been found to have complement activation activity and can cleave fibrinogen.

31. **What are the newly generated mediators of mast cells?**
In contrast to preformed mediators, mast cells also generate mediators upon activation by antigen binding to the FcεRI receptor or other stimuli. These mediators include the arachidonic acid metabolites prostaglandin D2 (PGD2), leukotriene C4 (LTC4), and platelet-activating factor (PAF), which are synthesized through the action of lipoxygenase and cyclooxygenase, both of which are present in mast cells. Mast cell degranulation is also an important cytokine-releasing event. Mast cells generate and release proinflammatory and immunomodulatory cytokines, including tumor necrosis factor-alpha (TNF-α), interleukins (IL-1, IL-2, IL-3, IL-4, IL-5, II-6, IL-8, IL-16), lymphotoxin, transforming growth factor-β (TGF-β), and endothelin. Some of the interleukins have both proinflammatory and mitogenic activity.

Church MK, Holgate ST, Shute JK, et al: Mast cell-derived mediators. In Middleton E Jr, Ellis EF, Yunginger JW, et al (eds). Allergy: Principles and Practice, 5th ed. St. Louis, Mosby, 1998, pp 146–167.

32. **What are the triggers of mast cell degranulation?**
Many different types of stimuli can trigger mast cell degranulation:
- Antigen-induced cross-linking of the FcεRI receptor on the surface of the mast cell
- IgG-autoantibodies to IgE or the FcεRI receptor
- Physical events (e.g., cold, heat, pressure, water, ultraviolet light, vibration, exercise)
- Cellular mediators (e.g., major basic protein, interleukins such as IL-3, stem cell factor)
- Chemicals (e.g., dextran, compound 40/80, phorbol myristate acetate, ionophore A23187, protamine sulfate)
- Medications and drugs
- Naturally occurring substances (e.g., anaphylatoxins C3a and C5a, neuropeptides such as substance P, venoms)

33. **Which drugs can trigger mast cell degranulation?**
- Radiocontrast
- Adrenocorticotropic hormone (ACTH)
- Doxorubicin
- Daunorubicin
- Codeine
- Morphine
- Vancomycin
- Vitamin A
- Polymyxin B

34. **Define systemic mastocytosis.**
Systemic mastocytosis is a heterogeneous collection of disorders with clinical symptoms resulting from an increase in mast cells in the tissues. Organ systems involved may include skin, gastrointestinal tract, lung, brain, bone, bone marrow, liver, spleen, and lymph nodes.

35. **How is mastocytosis classified?**
Based on the World Health Organization Classification of Tumors of Hematopoietic and Lymphoid Tissues and the Mastocytosis Concensus Classification established in Vienna in 2000, mastocytosis can be classified into the following categories:

1. Cutaneous mastocytosis
2. Systemic indolent mastocytosis without an associated hematologic disorder
   - Smoldering systemic mastocytosis
   - Isolated bone marrow mastocytosis
3. Systemic mastocytosis with an associated nonhematologic mast cell disorder
   - Myelodysplastic syndrome
   - Myeloproliferative disease
   - Acute myeloblastic leukemia
   - Non-Hodgkin's lymphoma
4. Systemic aggressive mastocytosis
5. Mast cell sarcoma
6. Mast cell leukemia
7. Extracutaneous mastocytoma

36. **At what age does mastocytosis present?**
Mastocytosis can occur at any age, but about 60% of cases develop before the age of 2 years, 75% occur before the age of 15 years, and most other cases occur before age 40 years.

37. **What are the consequences of a codon 816 c-kit mutation in mastocytosis?**
The mutation in the c-kit gene at codon 816 can cause activation of mast cells in systemic mastocytosis in the absence of stem cell factor. This fact is important because it means that ligand-independent activation of mast cells can be a primary defect leading to the overproduction of mast cells and causing mastocytosis.

38. **How is the diagnosis of systemic mastocytosis made?**
Accurate diagnosis of mastocytosis requires (1) the major criterion of characteristic multifocal, dense infiltrates of mast cells in the bone marrow and one minor criterion or (2) three minor criteria. The four minor criteria are listed below:
1. Serum tryptase level greater than 20
2. Detection of a codon 816 c-kit mutation
3. Spindle-shaped morphology of mast cells
4. Flow cytometric coexpression of CD117, CD25, and CD2 by the bone marrow mast cell population

39. **Discuss the frequency with which the various organ systems are involved in mastocytosis.**
The skin is the most commonly affected organ system in systemic mastocytosis, followed by the gastrointestinal tract, bone marrow, liver, spleen, and lymph nodes. The specific frequency with which organ systems are involved in systemic mastocytosis varies from study to study. With that in mind, some often-quoted frequency rates are shown in Table 20-2.

TABLE 20-2. FREQUENCY OF ORGAN SYSTEM INVOLVEMENT IN MASTOCYTOSIS		
Organ System	**Percentage**	**Conditions Most Frequently Seen**
Skin	90–100	Urticaria pigmentosa, solitary mastocytomas
Hematologic	28–70	To various degrees, including peripheral blood abnormalities, lytic bone lesions, mast cell leukemia
Gastrointestinal	70	Peptic ulcer disease, malabsorption, hepatic or splenic involvement
Lymphatic	26	Peripheral lymphadenopathy

40. **What is urticaria pigmentosa?**

One of the most common skin presentations of systemic mastocytosis is urticaria pigmentosa. Its appearance can vary, but it is typically described as tan to red-brown macules that first appear on the trunk and then spread outward. Urticaria pigmentosa tends to spare the palms and the soles. In general, the lesions are highly pruritic. The pruritus can be exacerbated by environmental changes, including heat or friction. Biopsy specimens of urticaria pigmentosa show large numbers of mast cells, spanning all of the dermal layers.

Venzor J, Baer SC, Huston DP: Urticaria pigmentosa. Immunol Allergy Clin North Am 15:775–784, 1995.

41. **Who first described urticaria pigmentosa?**

The skin condition was first described by Nettleship in the mid-19th century. Snagster first used the term "urticaria pigmentosa" in 1878. Initially, all cases were described in patients only a few days to a few months of age, with spontaneous resolution followed by hyperpigmentation. Urticaria pigmentosa, however, can occur in any age group.

42. **In addition to urticaria pigmentosa, what are the other two skin manifestations of systemic mast cell disease?**

The other cutaneous presentations of systemic mast cell disease are a solitary mastocytoma and telangiectasia macularis eruptiva perstans.

43. **Describe a solitary mastocytoma.**

The mastocytoma is a single nodule; it may be present at birth. It is usually hyperpigmented and located on a distal extremity. There may be associated local pruritus. Solitary mastocytoma is the most common presentation of mastocytosis in children less than 2 years of age.

44. **Describe telangiectasia macularis eruptiva perstans.**

Approximately 1% of patients with systemic mast cell disease may present with telangiectasia macularis eruptiva perstans. This condition usually occurs in adults, and the appearance is one of numerous telangiectatic macules, primarily on the trunk. Pruritus may vary. Lesions are 3–6 mm in diameter and worsen with trauma.

45. **Which of the three skin conditions may appear in a bullous form?**

Any of the above forms of mastocytosis, including urticaria pigmentosa, can appear in a bullous form. Bullous urticaria pigmentosa usually occurs in children less than 3 years of age. Hemorrhagic blister formation and ulceration are characteristic of the lesions. Other organ system involvement is common.

Kettelhut BV, Metcalfe DD. Pediatric mastocytosis. Ann Allergy 73:197–202, 1994.

46. **What is diffuse cutaneous mast cell disease?**

Diffuse cutaneous mast cell disease is another rare presentation of mastocytosis in young children. A yellowish brown or red color, thickening, and lichenification characterize the affected skin.

47. **Describe Darier's sign.**

In patients with urticaria pigmentosa, scratching of the macular lesions leads to a wheal-and-flare reaction around the original lesion. This reaction is known as Darier's sign (Fig. 20-1).

48. **Summarize the skin biopsy findings in urticaria pigmentosa and diffuse cutaneous mastocytosis.**

In urticaria pigmentosa, biopsy shows an increase in the number of dermal mast cells. Most of the mast cells identified in the skin of the patients are of the MC_{TC} variety. Mast cells primarily infiltrate the upper third of the dermis, but increased numbers can be seen throughout. In

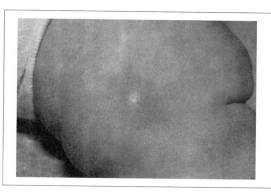

Figure 20-1. Darier's sign (wheal and flare of a brown papule after scratching). (From Morelli JG: Pediatric dermatology. In Fitzpatrick JE, Aeling JL: Dermatology Secrets, 2nd ed. Philadelphia, Hanley & Belfus, 2001, Fig. 7, p 399.)

patients with systemic involvement, the mast cells may have an atypical morphology. Mast cells may also aggregate perivascularly. The skin biopsy findings in diffuse cutaneous mastocytosis are similar to those of urticaria pigmentosa.

49. **List the most common sites of bone marrow lesions in systemic mastocytosis.**
In order of decreasing frequency: the long bones, pelvis, ribs, and skull.

50. **Is there a genetic component to systemic mastocytosis?**
Systemic mastocytosis is generally sporadic but has also been found to have an autosomal dominant familial pattern. Systemic mastocytosis of pediatric onset is more commonly seen in Caucasians. There appears to be a slight male predominance.

51. **What is the differential diagnosis of urticaria pigmentosa?**
Because the skin is the most commonly affected organ system in systemic mastocytosis, the differential diagnosis is often dictated by the appearance of the skin lesions. One must consider idiopathic urticaria and angioedema. Other possibilities may include recurrent anaphylaxis and scleroderma. Pheochromocytoma and carcinoid tumor may also present with the same signs of vascular instability that are commonly seen in systemic mastocytosis. These conditions may be ruled in or out by the measurement of urinary catecholamines.

52. **What is the differential diagnosis of systemic mastocytosis?**
In the absence of skin changes, the presence of unexplained flushing, peripheral blood changes, or visceral organ enlargement may support the diagnosis of mastocytosis. Other confounding diagnoses include other forms of shock (cardiogenic, endotoxic, and hemorrhagic); reactions to medications or physical factors; hereditary angioedema; nonorganic diseases such as vocal cord dysfunction; and panic or hysteric attacks. If the diagnosis is suspected, it is particularly important to obtain a bone marrow biopsy for confirmation and to categorize the disease because category plays a role in prognosis.

53. **Describe the gastrointestinal manifestations of systemic mastocytosis.**
Patients with systemic mastocytosis generally complain of abdominal pain, diarrhea, nausea, and vomiting. Some patients may present with gastric ulcers. Malabsorption can be seen. Liver and spleen involvement can also occur in systemic mastocytosis, although less frequently. Fibrosis of the liver has been observed, and vitamin B_{12} deficiency has been reported.

54. **Define xanthelasmoidea.**
Xanthelasmoidea is the term used by Fox in 1875 to describe the hyperpigmented skin of patients with urticaria pigmentosa. The pigmented skin was described as smooth, prominent, and firm.

55. What are normal plasma histamine levels?

The half-life of histamine in blood is only about 20 seconds, and measurement of histamine levels as a marker of mast cell activation is not practical. Histamine release is not solely a function of mast cell activation because histamine is also largely released by basophils. Histamine levels in asthmatics have been found to be higher than levels from nonatopic people and atopic nonasthmatic people. Histamine levels in the latter group range from 1 to 5 nmol/L, while those in asthmatics range from 3 to 14 nmol/L. Histamine levels are increased in asthmatics during acute asthma symptoms.

56. How are histamine and tryptase levels measured?

Both histamine and tryptase levels can be measured by immunoassay. Tryptase is measured with the B12 and G5 antibody-based immunoassay. G5 is a mouse monoclonal antibody that recognizes a linear epitope on denatured and inactive tryptase. The active tetramer is not detected by the G5 antibody immunoassay. The sensitivity of the current G5-tryptase assay is 1 ng/ml. The G5-capture monoclonal antibody immunoassay preferentially recognizes the β subunit. In contrast, the B12-capture monoclonal antibody immunoassay detects both the β and α subunits. Of patients with systemic mastocytosis, 50% have baseline levels of tryptase significantly greater than 1 ng/ml.

57. What is the significance of plasma histamine levels?

Unfortunately, because of the short plasma half-life of histamine, measurement of histamine levels in patients with mastocytosis or anaphylaxis has limited utility. In addition, because histamine is released from basophils during blood sampling, histamine levels are not entirely reflective of mast cell activation. However, a rise in plasma histamine levels has been observed in patients with severe cold urticaria, with peak levels reached at about 8 minutes after cold stimuli. This finding corresponds to histamine release observed in skin biopsy specimens.

58. What is the significance of plasma tryptase levels?

Tryptase has been used in the diagnosis of systemic anaphylaxis because its half-life is somewhat longer (1.5 to 2.5 hours). The mean normal serum or plasma levels for α-tryptase is 4.5 ng/ml. Beta tryptase is normally undetectable. Measurement of serum or plasma tryptase levels can be helpful in determining response to therapy that is directed toward decreasing the degree of mast cell activation.

Schwartz LB: Laboratory assessment of immediate hypersensitivity and anaphylaxis. Use of tryptase as a marker of mast cell-dependent events. Immunol Allergy Clin North Am 14: 339–50, 1994.

59. Discuss the role of the mast cell in anaphylaxis.

Anaphylaxis is not a typical syndrome associated with systemic mastocytosis, but it occurs as a result of degranulation of mast cells with release of mediators into the circulation. The clinical symptoms of anaphylaxis result directly from the release of histamine, tryptase, and other vasoactive mediators. β-Tryptase is involved in mast cell-dependent systemic anaphylaxis, while α-tryptase is found to be elevated in systemic mastocytosis. Substance P, vasoactive intestinal peptide, and calcitonin gene-related peptide are released during an anaphylactic reaction. Mast cells also release kininogenase. Other mast cell mediators released in anaphylaxis include heparin, prostaglandin D2 and F2a; leukotrienes B4, C4 and D4; platelet-activating factor; lymphokines such as IL-3, IL-5, and TNF; eosinophilic chemotactic factor and neutrophilic chemotactic factor; neutral proteases; major basic protein; and arachidonic acid-stimulating factors.

60. **Discuss the role of the mast cell in anaphylactoid reaction.**
Anaphylactoid reactions are clinicaly indistinguishable from anaphylactic events but are not mediated by IgE or mast cells. Degranulation of mast cells in anaphylactoid reactions may be triggered by the activation of the FcεRI receptor by non-immune-related stimuli.

61. **What is the significance of mast cells in urticaria?**
Urticaria occurs in about 10–20% of the population at some point during their lifetime. Signs of urticaria include pruritus, vasodilatation, and increased vascular permeability of the superficial dermis. The wheal-and-flare reaction is a hallmark of urticarial lesions. Histamine, prostaglandin D2, the cysteinyl leukotrienes, platelet-activating factor, and bradykinin mediate wheal-and-flare production. Flare production is indicative of increased vasodilatation. A 10-fold rise has been found in mast cell number in skin biopsies of active urticarial lesions.

62. **What are the effects of arachidonic acid metabolites in systemic mastocytosis?**
Arachidonic acid is a precursor of a number of newly generated mast cell mediators, including prostaglandin D2, leukotriene C4, and thromboxane A2. Leukotriene C4 is the predominant product of the lipoxygenase pathway. The effects of leukotriene C4 include vasodilation and increased increased vascular permeability. LTC4 is also an arteriolar constrictor. Mast cells also produce small amounts of LTB4, which plays a role in neutrophil chemotaxis. The effects of PGD2 include increased vasopermeability and vasodilation. PGD2 can also cause pulmonary vasoconstriction and augmentation of basophil histamine release. It is also a neutrophil chemoattractant that contributes to the skin and gastrointestinal effects seen in mastocytosis. Platelet-activating factor (PAF) can also be released during mast cell activation. In addition to increasing vascular permeability, PAF can also induce neutrophil and eosinophil chemotaxis and activation.

63. **Describe the biologic functions of the cytokines released by mast cells.**
Cytokines released by mast cells can have proinflammatory, immunomodulatory, and/or mitogenic biologic activity, as shown in Table 20-3.

64. **Outline the general approach to treatment of systemic mastocytosis.**
There is no known cure for systemic mastocytosis. Thus, the treatment of mast cell disorders is focused on control of symptoms related to the release of mast cell mediators. Avoidance of common physical and chemical triggers is of the utmost importance. The most common treatable effects of histamine include urticaria and pruritus, gastrointestinal cramps, increase in gastric acid production, and episodes of anaphylaxis. The patient should carry epinephrine at all times.

65. **How are histamine-related symptoms controlled?**
While most of the inflammatory effects of mast cells are mediated through H_1-receptor activation, gastrointestinal symptoms, in particular, may be related to H_2 receptors, which are present in high concentrations in the acid-secreting parietal cells in the gut. Consequently, both H_1 and H_2 antagonists may be needed. The availability of second-generation antihistamines, including cetirizine, loratadine, desloratadine, and fexofenadine, has provided advances in the control of the above symptoms because of the absence of sedative side effects and because of their long half-life. For this reason, these agents are preferable to over-the-counter medications such as diphenhydramine.

TABLE 20-3.	BIOLOGIC EFFECTS OF THE CYTOKINES RELEASED BY MAST CELLS
Cytokine	Effects
IL-1α, IL-1β	Augments histamine release; stimulates IL-10 secretion; increased expression of endothelial cell adhesion molecules, lymphocyte activating factor; stimulates synthesis of IL-2 and IL-2 receptor; stimulates inflammation in allergic disease
IL-2	Inhibits IL-4 activity
IL-3	Activation, degranulation and chemotaxis of eosinophils; degranulation of mast cells; activation of monocytes, prolongation of eosinophil survival; induces mast cell prolilferation
IL-4	Activates T cells; triggers isotype switching to IgE production; induces IL-6 production by endothelial cells; induces VCAM-1 production
IL-5	Chemotaxis and activation of eosinophils
IL-6	Augments histamine release; inhibits IL-1 and TNF production
IL-8	Chemotaxis of neutrophils; activates neutrophils; inhibits histamine release; induces production of leukotriene B4
IL-10	Inhibits eosinophil survival; inhibits IL-4 induced IgE synthesis, cytokine synthesis inhibitory factor, and mast cell proliferation
IL-13	Plays a role in allergic inflammation; closely related to IL-4 and may share a common receptor
IL-16	Role in inflammatory disorders such as asthma; modulates lymphocyte chemotactic response of CD4+ cells
TNF-α	Activates a variety of proinflammatory cells, including T lymphocytes, monocytes, eosinophils and neutrophils; Up-regulates endothelial cell adhesion molecule expression; stimulates ICAM-1 production
INF-γ	Inhibits IL-4 and IL-13 induced IgE isotope switching
GM-CSF	Prolongs survival of eosinophils; eosinophil, monocyte, and neutrophil activation; autostimulatory mast cell degranulation; eosinophil chemotaxis

Antihistamines such as hydroxyzine or the tricyclic antidepressant doxepin may be added for severe cases. Doxepin is known to have highly potent H_1 and H_2 antihistaminic activity. They should be used primarily at night because of their sedative side effects. Cyproheptadine, which has both antihistaminic and antiserotonin activity, has been shown to be of benefit in the treatment of mastocytosis. Examples of H_2-receptor antagonists include ranitidine and cimetidine.

66. **How are the clinical effects of other mast cell mediators controlled?**
Control of the clinical effects of the other mast cell mediators poses a more difficult problem because of the lack of specific blocking agents for the other mediators. As yet, no clinical data support the efficacy of leukotriene receptor antagonists in mast cell disorders. Mast cell-stabilizing

agents, such as oral disodium cromoglycate, may be particularly useful in control of gastrointestinal symptoms; however, it is costly. The daily regimen is 20–40 mg/kg/day in 4 divided doses. Ketotifen may also be used and may have some benefit in controlling skin symptomatology.

67. **Discuss the role of steroids in the treatment of mastocytosis.**
Steroids may be used to control the inflammation resulting from release of mast cell mediators. Methylprednisolone has been used in conjunction with cyclosporine to treat aggressive systemic mastocytosis. High-potency topical steroids such as betamethasone dipropionate may be used to treat skin manifestations. Some success has been reported with the use of psoralen with long-wave ultraviolet radiation over time. For isolated lesions, local injections of corticosteroids may be effective.

68. **How are the more aggressive forms of mastocytosis treated?**
Unfortunately, there is little effective treatment for the more aggressive forms of systemic mastocytosis or for mast cell leukemia. Interferon γ-2b at a dose of 0.5 million units per day has been found to be effective in decreasing lymphadenopathy in retroperitoneal and mesenteric locations. Some decrease in the number of mast cells in the bone marrow also was noted. Although the authors of the interferon study detected a decrease in urinary excretion of histamine metabolites, there was no effect on serum tryptase levels. Frequent side effects of interferon γ-2b include hypothyroidism, thrombocytopenia, and depression.

69. **Describe the approach to patients with severe liver involvement and ascites.**
In patients with severe liver involvement and ascites, steroids may be beneficial, and the use of a portacaval shunt for management of portal hypertension may occasionally be necessary.

70. **What newer modalities of therapy are under investigation?**
Newer modalities of therapy under investigation include interferon-α, which targets the mast cell precursor; 2-CDA (cladribine); imatinib, which targets tyrosine kinase; and bone marrow transplantation. Results from these therapeutic modalities have been mixed.

71. **Discuss the prognosis of systemic mastocytosis.**
The prognosis of systemic mastocytosis depends on the degree of severity of the disease. Mast cell leukemia is a serious disease with a median survival rate of only 6 months. Bone marrow biopsy can be useful for prognosis. Patients with indolent disease can be managed by pharmacologic intervention; the disease may even spontaneously regress. Prognosis of systemic mastocytosis is better in children when the onset is under 10 years of age. Overall, 50% of children with urticaria pigmentosa have spontaneous resolution of the disorder by the second decade of life.

Kettelhut BV, Metcalfe DD. Pediatric mastocytosis. Ann Allergy 73:197–202, 1994.

72. **Define mast cell leukemia.**
Patients with mast cell leukemia have a poor prognosis. The bone marrow of these patients is infiltrated with abnormal mast cells. Mast cells can be seen in the peripheral circulation, sometimes comprising up to 90% of the peripheral white blood cells. Mast cell leukemia occurs in less than 2% of all patients with systemic mastocytosis.

73. **Discuss the dosages and indications of commonly prescribed H_1 and H_2 antagonists.**
A large number of prescription and nonprescription antihistamines are available to the allergic patient. The only nonsedating antihistamine available over the counter is loratadine. Characteristics of antihistamines are shown in Table 20-4. With respect to use of antihistamines in lactating mothers, both sedating and nonsedating antihistamines are secreted in breast milk, but only the sedating ones produce side effects such as sedation or irritability in the breast-fed infant.

TABLE 20-4. ANTIHISTAMINE DOSAGES

Drug	Adult Dose	Pediatric Dose	Available In	Over-the-Counter	Pregnancy Category
H₁ antagonists					
First-generation antihistamines					
Diphenhydramine	25–50 mg q6h	1–2 mg/kg q4–6h	Liquid, tablet, and others	Yes	NA
Hydroxyzine	12.5–25 mg q6h	12.5 mg q6h (<6 yr) 12.5–25 mg q6h (>6 yr)	Liquid, tablet	No	NA
Cyproheptadine	4 mg qid	0.25 mg/kg/d (2–6 yr) 4 mg tid (7–14 yr)	Tablet	No	B
Clemastine fumarate	1 mg bid	0.25–1 mg/kg bid	Tablet	Yes	NA
Chlorpheniramine maleate	8–12 mg bid	0.2 mg/kg bid	Tablet and liquid in combination with other meds	Yes	NA
Second-generation antihistamines					
Fexofenadine	180 mg qd	30 mg bid (> 6 yr)	Tablet	No	C
Loratadine	10 mg qd	5 mg qd (> 2 yr)	Syrup, tablet, Reditab	Yes	B
Desloratadine	5 mg qd	5 mg qd (> 12 yr)	Tablet	No	C
Cetirizine	10 mg qd	2.5 mg (6–23 mon) 5 mg qd (> 2 yr)	Tablet, chewable tablet, syrup	No	B
H₂ antagonists					
Cimetidine	300 mg qid	20–40 mg/kg/d	Tablet, liquid, injection	Yes	B
Ranitidine	150 mg bid	6–10 mg/kg/d	Tablet	No	B
Famotidine	20 mg bid	1 mg/kg/d	Tablet, suspension	No	B
Nazitidine	150 mg bid	NA			

74. **What is the role of mast cell activation in sudden infant death syndrome?**
Postmortem signs of mast cell activation have been found in some cases of sudden infant death syndrome (SIDS). These findings include elevated tryptase levels in 50 infants with SIDS compared with 15 normal controls. The suggestion of mast cell activation leads to speculation that anaphylaxis may be a cause of SIDS.
    Platt MS, Yunginger JW, Sekula-Perlman A, et al: Involvement of mast cells in sudden infant death syndrome. J Allergy Clin Immunol 94:250–256, 1994.

WEBSITES

1. American College of Allergy, Asthma and Immunology: www.acaai.org
2. National Library of Medicine: www.nlm.nih.org

BIBLIOGRAPHY

1. Benjamini E, Leskowitz, S. Immunology: A Short Course, 2nd ed. New York, Wiley-Liss, 1991.
2. Bier OG, Dias Da Silva W, Gotze D, Mota I: Fundamentals of Immunology. New York, Springer-Verlag, 1981.
3. Bierman CW, Pearlman DS: Allergic Diseases from Infancy to Adulthood, 2nd ed. Philadelphia, W.B. Saunders, 1988
4. Church MK, Holgate ST, Shute JK, et al: Mast cell-derived mediators. In Middleton E Jr, Ellis EF, Yunginger JW, et al (eds). Allergy: Principles and Practice, 5th ed. St. Louis, Mosby, 1998, pp 146–167.
5. Church MK, Lei-Schaffer F: The human mast cell. J Allergy Clin Immunol 99:155–160, 1997.
6. Galli SJ: New concepts about the mast cell. N Engl J Med 328:257–265, 1993.
7. Hurwitz S: Unclassified disorders. In Clinical Pediatric Dermatology: A Textbook of Skin Disorders of Childhood and Adolescence. Philadelphia, W.B. Saunders, 1993, pp 663–694.
8. Kaposi M: Pathology and Treatment of Diseases of the Skin. New York, William Wood & Company, 1895.
9. Kennard CD. Evaluation and treatment of urticaria. Immunol Allergy Clin North Am 15:785–802, 1995
10. Kettelhut BV, Metcalfe DD. Pediatric mastocytosis. Ann Allergy 73:197–202, 1994.
11. McNeil HP, Austen KF: Biology of the mast cell. In Frank MM, Austen KR, Claman HN, Unanue ER (eds): Samter's Immunological Diseases, 5th ed. Boston, Little, Brown, 1995, pp 185–204.
12. Metcalf D: Mastocytosis syndromes. In Middleton E Jr, Ellis EF, Yunginger JW, et al (eds): Allergy: Principles and Practice, 5th ed. St. Louis, Mosby, 1998, pp 1093–1103.
13. Metcalfe DD, Austen KF: Mastocytosis. In Frank MM, Austen KR, Claman HN, Unanue ER (eds). Samter's Immunological Diseases, 5th ed. Boston, Little, Brown, 1995, pp 599–606.
14. Platt MS, Yunginger JW, Sekula-Perlman A, et al: Involvement of mast cells in sudden infant death syndrome. J Allergy Clin Immunol 94:250–256, 1994.
15. Schwartz LB: Laboratory assessment of immediate hypersensitivity and anaphylaxis. Use of tryptase as a marker of mast cell-dependent events. Immunol Allergy Clin North Am 14: 339–350, 1994.
16. Venzor J, Baer SC, Huston DP: Urticaria pigmentosa. Immunol Allergy Clin North Am 15:775–784, 1995.

INDEX

Page numbers in **boldface type** indicate complete chapters.